The Soul Dimension of Yoga
Heinz Grill

The Soul Dimension of Yoga

Heinz Grill

ISBN: (English Edition) 978-1-916732-32-2

English Edition Published By:

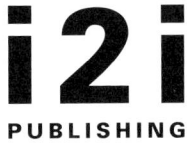

i2i Publishing. Manchester.
www.i2ipublishing.co.uk

Copyright 2024

All rights reserved. No part of this publication may be reproduced, stored in a retrieval system or transmitted in any form or by any means, electronic, mechanical, photocopy, recording or otherwise, without prior written consent of the copyright owner. Nor can it be circulated in any form of binding or cover other than that in which it is published and without similar condition including this condition being imposed on a subsequent purchaser.

The right of Heinz Grill to be identified as the author of this work has been asserted in accordance with the Copyright Designs and Patents Act 1988.

A copy of this book is deposited with the British Library.

Translated from the original German title: Die Seelendimension des Yoga – Praktische Grundlagen zu einem spirituellen Übungsweg by Heinz Grill: German Edition published by Stephan Wunderlich Verlag.

English Translation by:
Karen Patterson, Claudia Edwards and Emily Scott Bolton

Illustrations: Axel Berberich

Layout: Albert Wimmer

Contents

Foreword	8
How to use this book	13
The Soul Dimension of Yoga	17
The practice of yoga and its meaning	17
The three basic forces of the soul	19
Where is the home of the soul?	21
Breathing and the life of the soul	26
The meaning of inhalation and exhalation	26
The difference between free breathing and guided breath	27
Forming mental pictures has an effect on the breath	30
The different regions of the soul-life	32
Mūlādhāra-cakra and the earth element	37
Svādhiṣṭhāna-cakra and the water element	43
Maṇipūra-cakra and the air element	48
Anāhata-cakra and the warmth element	54
Viśuddha-cakra, and learning to differentiate between a consciousness free from the body and a consciousness bound to the body	58
Ājñā-cakra and the development of a freely creating power of thought	62
Sahasrāra-cakra and the experiencing of soul content	68
Attention, Concentration and Relationship	74
A practical example for attention	79
The beginning of a path of consciousness to develop the soul	81
The different energies in yoga, three different radiations of the aura	86
Different demands in the exercises	90
Rhythmically building up an exercise and developing yoga out of the social context	97
An exercise does not lead to escape from the world	97
Rhythmically building up an exercise in three phases	99

Inner calm and relaxation	105
The development of the soul-life takes place in three steps	111
Shaping life with content – *anāhata-cakra*	112
Exercises for experiencing the spine pictorially – *pārśva parivṛtta trikoṇāsana*	114
The tip-toe pose – *pādāṅguṣṭhāsana*	120
The tree – *tāḍāsana*	126
The St Andrew's cross – *saṁdhisthāna*	134
The shoulderstand – *sarvāṅgāsana*	136
The development of expansiveness – *maṇipūra-cakra*	142
A basic exercise for expansiveness: *vihāyas* – free space	144
The plough – *halāsana*	148
The head to knee pose – *paścimottānāsana*	156
The bow – *dhanurāsana*	166
The camel – *uṣṭrāsana*	170
The triangle – *trikoṇāsana*	176
The lying triangle – *anantāsana*	184
Openness through developing mental pictures, releasing the old and beginning anew – *viśuddha-cakra*	188
The wings – *pakṣati*	190
The yoga gesture – *yoga mudrā*	194
The fish – *matsyāsana*	198
The half moon – *āñjaneyāsana*	202
The head to knee pose in half lotus – *eka pāda padma paścimottānāsana*	208
Water and the movement of gathering – *svādhiṣṭhāna-cakra*	216
A soul exercise	218
The standing head to knee pose – *uttānāsana*	220
The locust – *śalabhāsana*	226
The wide stretch and forward-bending variations – *koṇāsana, eka pāda paścimottānāsana*	232

Developing a power of consciousness free from projection – *ājñā-cakra*	244
A basic exercise for developing the mid-point in the head	246
The sitting twist – *ardha matsyendrāsana*	248
The headstand – *śīrṣāsana*	254
The cobra – *bhujaṅgāsana*	260
Encouraging primordial strength and developing a freely available decisiveness – *mūlādhāra-cakra*	266
The earth – *bhūmi*	269
The leg pose – *utthita eka pāda hastāsana*	272
The inclined plane – *pūrvottānāsana*	280
The peacock pose – *māyūrāsana*	284
The development of complete freedom from the body – *sahasrāra-cakra*	292
The fire of lengthening – *dīrghāsana*	294
The lotus – *padmāsana*	296
The half diamond – *supta vajrāsana*	298
The scorpion – *vṛścikāsana*	302
The horse – *vātāyanāsana*	304
The crow – *kākāsana*	309
The scales – *tulādaṇḍāsana*	313
The dove – *kapotāsana*	320
A methodical sequence with which to construct a practice session	330
The sun prayer – *sūrya namaskāra*	334
A meditation on the three circles	342
Author's notes	350
Translator's notes from the text	351
General notes on the translation	352
Recommended literature	354
About Heinz Grill	355

Foreword

If you have just picked up this book for the first time, the front cover may already have conveyed to you something that sets it apart from the many and varied yoga books on the market today. It does not have a picture of a yogi in lotus pose, eyes closed immersed in ancient flavours of Eastern mysticism. Neither does it present a picture of glowing health and vitality, achieved through scientifically verified methods. The image on the front cover, and also the many photos you will see as you flick through the book, express first and foremost an artistic and aesthetic quality of gracefulness and beauty. They speak not just to the intellectual mind, nor to the nostalgic emotions, but to the sensitively feeling soul.

The soul, and its development, is the chief subject of this book. But how can we really understand this term "soul", above all in a time when people question whether we have a soul at all? Until recently, the soul was deemed as far more essential to our identity than the body, but now we live in an age where only what can be perceived with the physical senses is accepted as "real". However, many authors, including for example Rudolf Steiner (i), Bede Griffiths (ii), and also Heinz Grill himself, have described how this was not always the case, and how human consciousness has changed through the millennia.

Steiner for example, described how up until about 4000 years ago, people experienced themselves less as separate individuals, but rather as part of a much greater cosmos. They experienced not segmented spaces but vast distances, not hours and minutes but simultaneous time. Human thinking and feeling did not centre around individual concerns and emotions but were merged with a sense of a greater whole. People felt what was around them as shades of light and dark, connection or separation. One could say that they were more "soul beings", expanded into space, than physical beings contained within the confines of the skin. With this, human beings experienced themselves as being part of a natural order maintained by Gods. They had no individual will but were governed by a wisdom-filled lawfulness.

Bede Griffiths has written how the period around 600 BC marked a huge turning point in human consciousness. He described how prior to that time, ancient man had not thought in a logical, theoretical manner but more intuitively and pictorially. Teachings and truths about life had been conveyed using myths. But now the first Greek philosophers emerged, employing logic and reason to question, rather than simply accepting myths. With this emergence of logical, conceptual thinking, people began to experience themselves as individuals, separate from the whole, or from the cosmos. Whereas ancient man had lacked his own individual will, now, with the capacity to form abstract thoughts and concepts, a greater sense of self and individual autonomy began to develop. Yet with this, at the same time came a growing sense of isolation, of separation from a cosmic whole.

Today these two trends have clearly become extreme. Technology and automation have become highly advanced, and yet we have lost touch with the higher wisdom and order into which we are integrated. While comfort and material wealth have increased more than ever before, I meet people again and again who experience a sense of emptiness or meaninglessness in their lives; people who feel they are on a treadmill that is leading nowhere.

And so today we have countless paths of spirituality, meditation and yoga which seek to fill this void and find meaning. Some of them do so by emptying the mind in an attempt to take people back to an ancient consciousness of mystical oneness. Others use highly advanced scientific research methods to establish how many grams of protein we need to eat to build up our muscles, how many minutes we need to stand on our head to lower our blood pressure, and which yoga mat will give the ideal non-slip surface for our practice. The yoga industry is thriving on the consumerist attitude of our times.

But what is it that can really re-fill that void in people's souls? According to Heinz Grill, we cannot go back to that time of blissful oneness because humanity has evolved. We now have different capacities of thinking and feeling that we need to train and to use.

This book, like many yoga books on the market, is a practical handbook for yoga. It contains clear pictures and precise descriptions of almost forty different yoga poses, with step by step instructions for their practice. But it is also a handbook for training our capacity to think, to feel, and the way we use our will, or, as Heinz Grill puts is, our "soul forces".

And so how does Heinz Grill approach this enormous task of training the soul? Unlike the body, he explains, the soul cannot be trained by following purely technical instructions. Rather it needs a more artistic approach, involving pictures, metaphors and mental images which conjure up new subtle-feelings and experiences. Today we need not only practical methods, but thoughts and words, combined with physical perceptions, to ignite in us new and deeper experiences, "soul" experiences.

The soul experiences not the outer physical appearance of something, but its meaning, what it expresses. So, for example Bede Griffiths described how in ancient times people would look at the sky and would experience it not as a mass of air consisting of oxygen and nitrogen, but as an expression of infinity, eternity, vastness. Infinity, eternity and vastness could be said to be the inner meaning of what we see as "sky", and the act of perceiving that inner meaning is a perceptive activity of the soul.

For thousands of years, different forms of art have been used by those with deep wisdom and vision in order to help people rekindle a connection to the inner meanings of the world's phenomena. And so now, alongside its practical function as a handbook, The Soul Dimension of Yoga uses artistic words and pictures to present deep, inner meanings that lie hidden within the various yoga poses, so that new, inner experiences can gradually unfold in the souls of those who work with this book over a period of time.

Addressing readers of the 21st century, this book serves both to rekindle an intuitive sensitivity that has been lost, as well as to ignite a new capacity of consciousness that has never previously existed. It combines philosophy with movement, artistic expression with physical health, poetic words with practical instructions and brings a timeless wisdom into contemporary life. It is both a reservoir of spiritual wisdom and a practical handbook for life, taking its readers on a journey of soul development.

As a yoga teacher, The Soul Dimension of Yoga has become for me a life time's companion. Its depth seems inexhaustible, with new insights emerging with each revisit. It continues to form an essential foundation for my own path of spiritual development, and a reservoir of inspiration for my yoga teaching. In working with these thoughts in my yoga classes, I am repeatedly surprised by the way my students seem to open out of their mechanical way of thinking and are taken into a life-refreshing, expansive dimension of awareness; – the dimension of the soul.

Karen Patterson

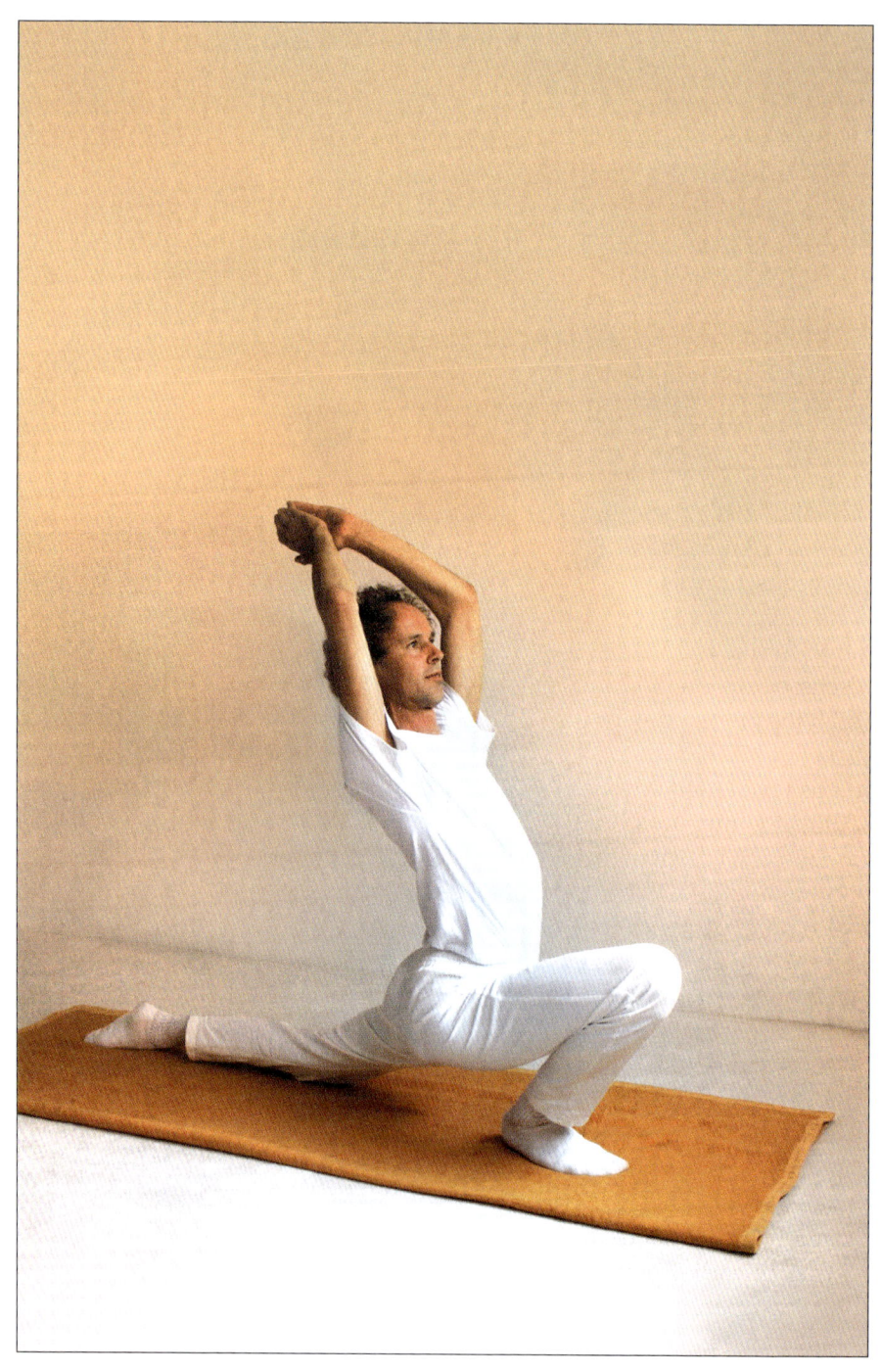

How to use this book

There are different ways in which a practical guide to an ancient spiritual discipline, like yoga from the far shores of India, can be written. One way, and this is the most common and best known way, is that Westerners follow the Eastern yoga traditions, and link these with the Western way of thinking and understanding in a form which is practical, achievable and useful. However, by passing on a reproduction and guide to the yoga exercises in this very general and materialistic way, a real connection between a former, Eastern yoga culture and our familiar, current, more scientifically oriented world does not yet come about. The more metaphysically inclined thinking patterns of the Indian-spirited yoga-culture, and particularly of ancient India, from where yoga originated, are so very different from the Western mentality that it seems highly questionable and inappropriate to place these in an unthinking and rapid utilitarian context. Yoga and its instruction today needs a precise conceptual interpretation and a concrete, nuanced use of its exercises, so that it can be viewed in a way that illuminates its original depth for the thinking and perception of today. When concepts have been discussed sufficiently, and contextual pictures have been acquired, yoga can reach the present day human consciousness in a way that is progressive.

In this text, attention is given, in a rhythmically repeating way, to the concept of the human soul, and in the chapters that follow, the soul dimension which can potentially be introduced into the practice of yoga should become illuminated through active mental picturing. In order now to explain more closely some of the terms addressed in the following text, it is necessary to explore their content with increasing care. This clarification of terms and content becomes extremely important, as most people embarking on a spiritual path – and yoga is ultimately a spiritual path – associate all sorts of different and imprecise ideas with the exercises, thus burdening their souls with feelings and emotions, which often do more harm than good to their development. For these reasons it even becomes necessary to characterise the term "content" prior to the exercise instructions.

Formerly the terms used in yoga had a more spiritual and intensive content, as in earlier periods of yoga human beings had a clear-sighted and thus vivid, intuitive perception of metaphysical phenomena and spiritual connections. At the time of origin of the Vedas, the Upanishads or the

Bhagavad Gītā, (these are the spiritual texts that shaped the yoga culture), human beings still experienced very clearly the unified connections between a cosmic life after death and mortal culture, and so they could transfer and apply their beheld wisdoms to a path of yoga exercises. Today, however, this clear-seeing consciousness has become lost due to a material hardening and an overemphasis of the intellect, and so the formerly clear-sighted perceptions have also been lost. For present day culture and our current time, the terms found in yoga are therefore at first empty, seemingly void of content, out of context, and so cannot be used as direct prescriptions.

So that yoga today can once again be understood and further developed within the context of social and human life, it seems absolutely necessary to repeat this almost banal sounding, but nonetheless interesting question: What is a content, a soul content, a spiritual content? If such a thing as a soul or spiritual content is to exist, it needs a concrete thought, which is led in the direction of an understandable, logical and also true relationship. This directional relationship taken with the thought brings about an appropriate feeling or sentiment, which eventually can be grasped and experienced consciously. As long as a term appears in isolation in a text, or is used in a way that is absolute, definitive, or bound to a specific tradition, its inner connection or inner and true relationship is missing. Then its real essence, its characteristic colour, or its proportions and form are missing and so it is actually only a superficiality, a kind of shell without a kernel. A content, on the other hand, shows characteristic traits and reveals its identity through its logical interconnectedness, its truth and also through the vision inherent in it.

The antithesis to this path of consciousness through content can be seen in the so widespread consumerist orientation, which particularly in recent decades has become a natural part of human will. The spiritual seeker of today will almost automatically also transfer this consumerist orientation to a practice like yoga. It is not the case that yoga can generate only misunderstanding for the western world because it originated from a distant land and from earlier civilisations, but much more that our contemporary mindset itself has elevated the principle of profit, or of material usefulness, to the highest maxim. This present mindset is now leading yoga, with its former high ideals and content, into a materialistic sphere, mixing and interpreting the terms and concepts in an unhealthy way and so leading human soul-development into a hidden and unrecognised bondage.

The examination of terms and descriptions that now follows leads specifically and intentionally to an articulation and differentiation of the consciousness, and ultimately to a more concrete relationship to the thoughts with their objects, and so to a deeper experience of their content. Consciously approaching and developing the content and the resulting relationships in this clear sequence must therefore be highlighted at the start, because through this sequence the will in yoga develops a dimension of soul, as will be clarified in the course of this book. The thinking, picturing, sensitive and deepening work of consciousness, and only then the practice with the body, leads to the development of the kind of experience that can be described as a soul experience. This is the kind of experience that should be discovered today in its true depth and in its potential and broader context, in order to actually overcome the materialism of the time from within.

Particularly at the beginning of this yoga practice, it can seem very difficult for the untrained reader to comprehend the thoughts and content correctly, and also to think them themselves, in a way that is authentic to their meaning. This independent thinking is actually a requirement in this way of practice. A consumerist kind of practice, which mainly takes from an exercise, and does not have to concern itself with the content in a careful and clear sense, would certainly be the easier way, but it would also be unsuitable for comprehending the depths of the soul and its dimensions in creation. For this reason, a closer understanding of the path described here needs some time and patience. The real meaning contained in a term, and its context, cannot be comprehended and conceived through rapid reading. Rather, it is only through repeated, sensitive and concentrated seeing, and independent, conscious imagining and picturing, that the central thought comes closer and can be experienced in its position here in this context. This discipline is as if the reader were listening to a faraway sound, which only reaches the inner ear through cultivating careful attention, and so becomes heard in its sensitivity, its start and its end. In the same way, the stated thought gradually comes closer with its context, its real content, its scope, its start, its centre and its end, and through the activity of thinking it can become personally integrated.

When reading these texts, it is a good idea to refrain from premature, emotional evaluations or intellectual, pedantic, rapid judgements. To work with the exercises and read the texts, one's human, creative power should instead be stimulated in the sense of a growing, authentic activity of picturing content. In order to achieve this it is helpful to study the thoughts found in the text, thinking them until they open up a greater, truer, subject-related capacity for judgement. There are critics who assert that people would become dependent if they did not immediately offer criticism and judgement of what they had read, and of the exercises. But dedication to these texts does not mean giving up a capacity for judgement, rather it means enhancing and perfecting the capacity for criticism and judgement by meaningfully activating the thinking of thought-contents and mental pictures. If we were to speak of dependency with this discipline, which is certainly relatively unfamiliar to most paths of yoga, we would waste the opportunity we have, through studying texts and through giving thoughtful attention to terms and exercises, of attuning the soul to a higher correlations and enriching it with content. For a spiritual discipline, we must not remain at the surface of the terms, rather we do ourselves a great favour when we look right into the depth of their meaning, and learn to think and ultimately feel them through experience in the different ways they interrelate, both authentically and also in a greater context. The picturing activity stimulated in this way, connected with the practice of exercises, brings that longed-for consciousness of the hidden life of the soul.

The Soul Dimension of Yoga

The practice of yoga and its meaning

The word "yoga" comes from the Sanskrit root *yuj*, which in general terms described the activity of connecting. A discussion of the traditions of yoga, its ancient culture, its various forms and meanings, would exceed the scope of this book and so this will not be included. Purely the inner meaning of the word "connection", which can be thought of as encompassing the broadest planes of human and spiritual existence, will be of specific interest for this practical guide. This word "connection" will receive a detailed description and analysis from the angle of deep, personal-human existence, as well as from the angle of its superordinate and spiritual sense. The longing for a connection to others, to the earth, to natural phenomena, but ultimately also to the higher worlds rests within the human being as a great desiring and driving force, and at the same time it is that dimension that can be described as "soul". The individual soul, known as *jīva* in Sanskrit, seeks, even if often secretly, its wise convergence and connection with the so-called cosmos, which constitutes for the human being a reality beyond the senses, or it seeks, so to speak, a vivid and experienceable relationship to a universal whole or to the higher worlds. From within, a desire is inherent in human beings and this desire strives towards a growing consciousness of conformity and unity with a greater spirit, and at the same time preserves a palpable uniqueness in human individuality. This deep motive belongs to every single soul.

The systems of yoga in the way they are given, for example with the classical path of *rāja-yoga*, the so-called royal path of meditation, and which cannot obtain an adequate mention here in this book, consist of various exercises which include the body, the breath, one's attitude in life, and an appropriate development of concentration and meditation. The path involving physical exercises, speaking more specifically, is generally known as *haṭha-yoga* or sometimes also as *kuṇḍalinī-yoga*. They are paths that have developed an encompassing methodology and which, starting with the body, aspire first and foremost to transcend life. However, for the discussions that follow they are not very important, as the descriptions of the soul dimension of yoga are based on new fields of reference and have been formulated with a new methodology. The further great and all-encompassing, chief paths of yoga are *bhakti-yoga*, which in its outer principles elects reverential devotion as its deepest motive, *jñāna-yoga*, the path of developing wisdom-filled knowledge, which likewise, considered from a more external standpoint, places the consciousness and the work with thoughts at the centre of its efforts, and finally karma-yoga, the path of active doing and active thinking. These three paths are described as the *trimārga*. If the trouble is taken to investigate this *trimārga* in its multifaceted and various qualities, it will be found not only in Indian culture but in all the religious and spiritual endeavours of other paths. In the following descriptions of the soul dimension of yoga, these chief paths are integrated in a practical synthesis, for the soul, through its nature, seeks from within a connection to others, as well as to active life and to the world, and it also naturally seeks this connection to the higher truths and wisdoms of the life beyond death. Through its own desiring urge, therefore, the soul seeks a form of three-fold activity, and it will not wish for and realise something one-sided, like for example to direct its desire only towards the world or to fix it only on the spirit, but rather it will further the urge for an integral realisation, which is directed both to the world, to the societal and human fabric as well as to the higher and spiritual world. The soul and its desiring urge brings about, from within, a path of *trimārga* and it will learn, with increasing development, to express this path in the different phases of life.

The paths which take the body as the starting point for practice have spread widely in recent decades in the West, surprisingly in a greater quantity that in their land of origin, India. Westerners have probably learnt to appreciate the physical exercises more on account of their value for health than because of their spiritual meaning. Nevertheless, as the great and more spiritually oriented, chief paths show, the term "yoga" encompasses far more than the methodical practice of physical exercises. Yoga itself is much more an inner, growing attitude of consciousness of the individual; in its precise sense it can even be seen more as the maturing-step of the consciousness, developed through lengthy experience, towards a progressive, spiritual and universal development of wisdom and love, which comes ever closer to the higher worlds and integrates these worlds into life. In this sense yoga is an extraordinary and challenging aim. Through a lengthy journey of experience with multifaceted steps of exploration, combined with the right work of concentration and consciousness, with endeavours for pure thinking, refined feeling and purposeful action, individuals acquire the power of guidance over life that can be described with the general term "yoga". The term "yoga" would therefore be very scant and flimsy if it were to limit itself to a methodical, physical practice, and it would also be very one-sided if it were to describe a practice that took place in isolation from life and from social circumstances. At the beginning of these discussions it will not yet be possible to define and describe the term "yoga" precisely, as it is so all-encompassing in its depth and in its scope that it can initially be taken more as an over-arching aim and considered in that way.

Tadā yogam avāpsyasi – "Then you will attain yoga" says the master to his student in the Bhagavad Gītā (II/53), as he reveals to him the high worlds of the spirit. The Bhagavad Gītā contains a spiritual description, which explains the chief paths of yoga and which presents an exceptionally high dialogue between Krishna and Arjuna or, to express it differently, between a divine person and a fully-prepared student of many years. The typical mental attitude of guidance and mastery, which is characteristic of yoga according to its classical image, is only attained after lengthy practice, perseverance and experience. Therefore, it is not favourable if people attend yoga classes and say they practise yoga, because they will merely be practising a few yoga exercises and will certainly not yet have arrived at the knowledge and consciousness of yoga. By refraining from integrating the word "yoga" into the usual terse and material custom of speech, but by first moving this word into the light of contemplation, and now gradually forming a consciousness that with this high aim an all-encompassing spirituality is addressed, interested students more easily experience a first true subtle-feeling of the soul. They experience this truer subtle-feeling because they make the effort to form an encompassing and concrete seeing of a term in its full potential. The effort for an articulated, more concrete and objective seeing brings closer that process of consciousness that corresponds to the life of the soul.

The three basic forces of the soul

The soul, as it is being described here, has three basic forces, which to name them explicitly are the thinking, the feeling and the willing. Through the thinking, the soul receives the external world and through the feeling the soul becomes established in itself, while with the will it works back on the external world making impressions on it. In this sense the soul is divided into three active limbs, each of which works specifically and yet together with the others in a precisely calculated way. The thinking process is in a sense like the rising sun, which emanates light into its surrounding sphere, illuminating the objects of the world. As the sun rises, the starry night-sky disappears. When at this point a thinking process is spoken of, this does not mean intellectualising, but rather a conscious, content-related, attentive contemplation with very clear, thoughtful evaluation. The feeling, however, is like the sun's manifestation within, and if it is taken in its purer, original meaning of real subtle-feeling, and is not confused with emotion or sentimentality, the feeling is the centre of the soul-life itself. It forms, as it were, the midst of the soul. Now the willing is like the starry night-sky, which in the sun's absence emanates with an exceptionally high impact onto the world and therefore leaves behind a change in the external dimension. Were the soul to be rooted only in feeling, and were the thinking and also the will to be excluded as basic forces, then people would have in the soul neither a receiving nor a giving reality. Because the soul-forces work together in a precisely calculated interplay, active development can occur.

The methodical practice of yoga, particularly of yoga with physical exercises, which originated predominately in the East, cannot be adopted by us in the West without knowledge of the three soul-forces and their interaction. The mentality of the yoga culture has established and preserved a deep tradition in a kind of emotional willing and often rejects in general the thinking aspect of being. However, development here in the West needs to take specific and attentive account of the activity of thinking, as only thinking is in a position to overcome the intellectualism and also the materialism of the time. It might at first seem contradictory to say that precisely the thinking activity can overcome materialism, as one would assume that intellectualism is caused through thinking itself and one ought now to discard thinking in favour of better feeling. This rash conclusion, however, is not right, as thinking can provide a luminous expansion for the consciousness and, if it is used in the right way it also builds and strengthens the feelings and will-impulses. In the thinking itself, when properly applied, there lives a sun-like content of thought, and it is this that enriches the life of the soul.

In this sense the soul possesses three wishes or needs. These constitute its healthy existence and its harmonising and ordered position in life. So right from within, the *jīva* or the individual soul wishes for progress in learning or, to express it still more clearly, a new horizon, an expansion of consciousness, to get to know a reality it does not yet understand or has not yet acknowledged. This new step happens through the thinking. Secondly, the soul wants to discover itself in itself through a deep feeling, and it wants to know that in this feeling it is connected both with a higher truth as well as with worldly criteria. It desires that authentic feeling of truth that gives it congruity with itself and with the reality of the external world or of other people. Finally, however, the soul's desire urges for a body of work in the world, and wants to convey to the world or to others a part of the inner truth and reality it has gained so far.

Where is the home of the soul?

What dimension encompasses the soul through its three basic forces of thinking, feeling and willing? Where is the home of the soul? Where does it live, how does it live and what force is inherent in it? The soul is feminine in nature, while the spirit is masculine. In the basic three-fold articulation into body, soul and spirit, the soul adopts the connecting mid-position between above and below. The body belongs to the earthly world, to the so-called sensory sphere or manifest world of matter. Now the spirit belongs to the upper world, but it is not the intellect, rather it is a dimension more of self-awareness, which becomes represented through thought. Because there is a sphere of thought, and because the human individuality or the human thinking activity, through its own over-seeing and experiencing consciousness, can become aware of this plane in which thought exists, the spirit can be recognised directly in its being-existent. The process of consciousness that takes place though this attention belongs to the soul and so consciousness can be equated with the essence of the soul. To experience the spirit, however, is a deep process of becoming aware, which cannot be attained through the existing intellect or emotions. Intellectuality and also emotional feelings are only the outermost imprint of a kind of inner binding that manifests within the soul-forces themselves and therefore they do not allow the building of a clear thought process or of an unequivocal, insightful knowledge.

In former cultures yoga, with its various contemplative exercises, would not have been achievable without careful asceticism and a certain retreat from life. In the West too, a realisation of deep, mystical Christian experiences was unthinkable without renouncing the world. The consciousness however, or in this context we could say the soul's constitution, has changed over the centuries, and if people were to retreat into a monastery, into an ashram or into solitude today, it would probably be difficult for them to grow and develop in a way that would fulfil the real desire in the soul. They would be more exposed to feelings of pain, desolation and loneliness and would be unable to experience that so valuable link to harmonious connections with society. A developing spiritual discipline that would make sense in the West should not be accompanied by great outer changes, by a retreat from life and hard, ascetic exercises, for this would contradict the basic needs of the life of the soul. Life can, for the most part, remain in the same position as before outwardly, and those who live in families or are married, should continue to remain in their communities. Life does not attain its transformative enrichment through great external changes, but rather from within. By attuning life more deeply from the soul, through thinking and through subsequently developing corresponding and suitable feelings, which are integrated into external life with well-proportioned forms, one's personal position and organisation into societal and social existence ultimately changes. The path describes a progressive self-development, which goes hand in hand with real, authentic and understandable processes of consciousness from the thinking to the feeling and finally to the will, and pervades life to an extent that is meaningful and reasonable.

The soul is the middle limb in our human existence. It is, so to speak, the link between the manifest body and the unmanifest spirit. The soul encompasses both the consciousness and the subconscious. If we equate the soul with the entire consciousness, then we can also equate it with the esoteric term "astral body". In a sense the soul is the microcosmic part in the interior of a personality, within a great macrocosmic whole. Belonging to this cosmos are the stars, as well as the sun and moon. The astral body, or the cosmos, holds in itself that substance that in an encompassing sense can be described as soul.

The soul receives the impulses from physical existence and it also receives influences and stimuli from the thought-life and thus from the spirit. The impulses that the soul receives from the body can serve merely as information, but they cannot expand the consciousness. In all exercises, particularly physical exercises but also in any concentration or meditation exercises, the soul should receive its attunement from a superordinate spirit. The sense-bound or involved bodily consciousness must not be allowed to motivate the yoga practice. The practice of yoga must be accompanied by very concrete thoughts which are formed out of a consciousness of spiritual truth. In simple terminology we can recognise a direction of action that can be pictured or imagined as an influence, or to be more precise, as a thought process, which streams from above down into the soul and which, starting from the spirit or from a transcendent reality, enriches the soul-fabric within. The path from above to below, or from thought to feeling, from the non-manifest to the experienceable and ultimately to the manifest is exceptionally important for a contemporary practice. In the way that the sun rises in the morning, so the thought-life awakens, and in the way it ascends up to the zenith, bringing all the stars, even the morning star, to fade, so the feelings and experiences manifest deep within the unconscious, and in the way the sun descends to the nadir and disappears, so with the rising night-sky of stars, these feelings and impulses work via the hidden inclinations of will, in the broadest of ways, back onto the external world.

Generally, the conditions of our time today are shaped by the principle of benefiting, using, consuming and seeking advantage. These principles of taking and expending are commonly and succinctly denoted by the term "materialistic". They come from an illusionary consciousness or from a soul constitution that has become sick, and they say something along the lines of: "If we can acquire more, we are richer." Although this utilitarian principle has a certain validity for life's physical circumstances, this one-sided and customary axiom must not be used for the inner world of the soul. On the contrary, in the world of the soul a reverse principle to materialism holds true. The principle that actually applies is: "Whatever in their being someone does for another, whatever someone gives or gives away for the sake of a whole, that is what they are in their soul itself." The seers and wise-men of old described this axiom with the sentence *tat tvam asi*, "That you are". This principle of the soul world does not just demonstrate a moral rule, but points to a law that exists deep within life and encompasses the true soul-existence of a human being. In the soul, human beings are by no means what they can acquire for themselves in earthly life, they are far more what they provide for life, what they do for the existence of society and what they truly give for others. The soul lives in the capacity for conception of the thought, and in a deepest truth of the feelings, and in an insatiable wish to pass these forces on to life again.

A path that goes from below to above, in other words starts from the corporeal worlds and also from the principles of the earthly world, from materialistic, consumerist thinking or from the emotions of the body, cannot really lead to the inner, true soul-basis of existence. In the practice described here, great emphasis is placed on this distinction, so that the discipline remains free from emotional and unrecognised dependencies and does not fall into a putative consciousness and follow the principles of the material world. Because most of the Western yoga schools today have excluded the former asceticism and strictness in their methods, and use in their practice the terms that at that time were still alive but today have become empty, they rid the practice of any real or potential spirituality. During the day the soul is enclosed in the body. With the soul, one could say, the whole cosmos is also enclosed. In the night during deep sleep, however, the soul is free from the body and it streams out into the universal space of the stars. Seen in this way, the soul is that closed-in aspect, which exists in an alternating play with the flowing-out aspect. However, this was not always the case, for when the Indian in the time of the former yoga-culture looked out into the universal space, he could confidently say that this universal space revealed an important truth. This universal space was for him the tat, the so-called "that", and even by looking he felt that the home of his true identity was in the universal space: *tat tvam asi*. This universal space is your own essence: "You yourself are that". A vast cosmology with an unmistakable physical freedom revealed itself for the yogin of old, for he experienced much more vividly the reality of the stars and macrocosmic soul-space, and he did not yet feel himself to be completely enclosed in the body with feelings and emotions. Asceticism was not connected with strain or force for him at that time, rather it was natural for him as he did not want to turn away too far from his cosmic soul-space and submerge himself in the body with feelings. Today, however, individuals only gradually become reacquainted with this vast cosmic dimension, and with the out-pouring of their soul into the cosmos during the night. Their practical path is not to draw the soul only onto themselves and their feelings, but to turn towards others and towards the world in an appropriate way and gradually to learn to recognise that this cosmos, with its effects, lives in their social surroundings. *tat tvam asi* – "You are not the person you can become through asceticism or through solitary practice, but you are as you affect others, you are the moral and noble relationships you establish, the beautiful and aesthetic forms you create and the way you ultimately carry these into the night sea of stars."

The soul dimension of yoga needs to be described and expanded in this conceptual way, because what human beings can initially achieve from the body, and can shape materially through exercises, merely serves the world and will return to the world. But by getting to know the soul as that dimension that is enclosed in the body during the day and streams out into the universal space of the stars during the deep-sleep of the night, and there is utterly free, aspirants become acquainted with the concept of yoga in its content and from a new perspective. The practice, the methods and the interpretation of this soul-inspired yoga are not derived from previously known paths, and yet they lead directly into the sensitive, sacred realm of *bhakti-, jñāna-* and *karma-yoga*. However, they lead into this realm in a new way and imbue these terms with the freedom that is achievable for the thinking and creating human being today. The content of this soul-yoga can be understood on a logical level, pictured through the consciousness, and implemented in an artistic form. This discipline of a thorough forming of yoga from the soul, because it develops the soul-forces, provides moral improvements for the whole of life, insights into interconnections, a more stable resilience in health and mental well-being, and opens up to individual practitioners a way to begin mastering and guiding their lives. A high, inner sense of honour is expressed in an exercise when it is shaped with active thoughts and authentic feelings. Individuals can discover the spiritual worlds and, in the face of the higher truths, their soul raises up the inner self-awareness and sense of honour. Once again, however, it should be emphasised that yoga is not something that can be performed or done like any other task. This activity is more a discipline of consciousness, which forms itself out of the spirit, out of true and noble thoughts and sentiments, and places a purposeful, ongoing and stabilising guidance into life. *Tadā yogam avāpsyasi* – "Only then will yoga be attained." The form of mastery of the consciousness is a school for life, and it begins with the study of thoughts and subtle-feelings which, from above to below, from the spiritual basis of existence, via the soul, ultimately are expressed in earthly life.

Breathing and the life of the soul

The meaning of inhalation and exhalation

Anatomically speaking, human breathing happens approximately in the middle of the body, in the regions of the trachea, the bronchi and the lungs. In rhythmic waves the motion of inhalation and exhalation stimulates the abdominal organs and metabolic processes down below, and keeps the consciousness present and alert up above. Breathing is always an activity that is both rhythmic and balancing, so that a healthy movement of breath can always strengthen the life forces of the body and at the same time maintain mental concentration. Beyond this, the rhythm that lives in the breathing is also connected with the cosmos, or with the higher principles of creation.

Upon breathing in, human beings take the air from their surroundings into themselves and upon breathing out they rid themselves of this air again. Physical, physiological analysis tells us that the oxygen which is breathed in maintains the life functions of the body, and therefore oxygen is given most attention, while the carbon dioxide that is breathed out, being toxic to the body if retained, and the waste product of a whole process, is not given any noteworthy physiological significance. Now beside their pure physiological function, it is also possible to investigate the individual basis of these substances right into a spiritual depth, and so create some clarity about the higher meaning contained in oxygen and carbon dioxide. Everything that is material carries within it a hidden dimension that is spiritual, and therefore oxygen is not just a carrier of life but also a substance that leads the consciousness into the earthly world and keeps it in this world with alertness. Carbon dioxide, however, which in the first instance must be rated as an unusable toxin for humans, can be assigned to the regions of death. Two far distant poles therefore live in the breathing, the pole of life and also the pole of death. But both these poles exist in the physical, physiological world, and because it is on this plane that their effect spreads, if we now want to discover the soul-life, different criteria must be considered. As stated previously, the soul weaves and lives not only on a physical plane, but in its own soul regions. For this reason the question arises as to how the movements of breath in their waves, in particular inhalation and exhalation, are to be understood with regard to the soul.

The two poles of inhalation and exhalation constitute a natural response of the will, which is controlled in an automated way according to the particular needs. With physical movement the need to inhale increases, while with calmness and relaxation it decreases. What is essential for exploring the soul dimension in the breathing is that the breathing is appropriate for the natural needs of the human will and therefore as a rule happens unconsciously. It is governed automatically by the autonomic nervous system. It is a basic requirement in life and is also an existential need.

As soon as people engage with a yoga exercise, they also notice the different qualities and rhythms of the breathing. Because a yoga exercise is practised with careful consciousness and calmness, the question arises as to how practitioners can approach the breathing. Do they leave the rhythm of the breath and the intensity of breathing in a natural flow, or do they begin to intervene consciously into this flow, thus changing the natural course of the autonomically governed functions of the will? Do they for example introduce a higher intensity into the in-breath, or impose a harmonising rhythm to obtain a particular, contemplative calmness? Practitioners will very quickly discover the different possibilities the breathing has, and then they will notice that the way in which they use or modulate the breath also changes the quality that is produced in the exercise. Long, calm breaths lead to more reverent moods, while faster, shorter breaths make physical exertion easier. An infinite number of possibilities for manipulation could be discovered in this domain of influencing the quality, rhythm and intensity of the breath.

The difference between free breathing and guided breath

The breath itself, however, is subject in normal life to the autonomically controlled will and because of this it is linked to the autonomic nervous system. The will itself manifests the deepest of the three soul-forces and in its full entirety it embraces the human individuality. Now through suitable manipulation of the breath, this individuality could be transformed in a very rapid and accessible manner. So in yoga there are the so-called *prāṇāyāma* methods, the control of the breath, which ultimately also leads to a control of *prāṇa* or energy in the human body. The use of *prāṇāyāma* always represents an intervention into the individual will fabric, and for this reason it is on the one hand an extremely powerful *yoga-vidhi*, a yoga method, but on the other hand also an extremely critical one. Just as we should not intervene into the will of other people, it would be favourable if practitioners were also careful themselves and left the fabric of their own autonomically controlled will-body in peace. The will is connected in its mysterious depths with extremely high spiritual mysteries, with hidden planes, which are anchored, for example, deep within the organs through autonomic control systems. As soon as human beings intervene[1] rashly or without wisdom into these planes and alter them via a physical component, then perhaps not at the outset but after some time they all too easily experience a strong reattachment to the body.

For this reason, the *prāṇāyāma* methods are not practised in the soul dimension of yoga. The rhythm-bringing and intensifying breath exercises of *prāṇāyāma* are replaced by the practice of the so-called free breath, which leaves both the natural rhythm and also the intensity of the breathing to take its most natural course. Practitioners therefore take care not to manipulate the autonomically controlled breath process and they also do not use the breath, for example to better their practice of an exercise. For example, in the so-called head to knee pose, *paścimottānāsana*, people could use the method of gathering power with the inhalation and moving farther outwards into the stretch forwards with the exhalation. Or in the plough, *halāsana*, with the help of the breath they could breathe away the pressures of constriction or the pains that arise in the limbs, and thus gain access to the position. These methods of exploiting and using the breath, although they seem to happen almost naturally, are firmly rejected in this yoga and there are also specific reasons for this.

As long as practitioners use the breath for themselves or for a benefit in the exercise, they cannot yet build their consciousness objectively and freely. Through the utilitarian connection with the breathing process, and interested students can discover this very quickly, they immediately immerse themselves in, or rather dive down into, their own subjective inner life. They become involved in their own hidden will and in this way they bind their thinking, and also their feeling-life, to the forces that are stored in the autonomic nervous system. However, this strong and one-sided, subjective reattachment should be avoided. In fact on closer inspection there are no longer any students today who could fulfil all the precepts that would be required to integrate *prāṇāyāma* in a way that makes sense.[2] Therefore for the development of the soul dimension of yoga, and particularly also for a socially applicable way of working with the exercises, it seems important to further a high and free quality in the breath, and a naturally appropriate quality and rhythm.

When practising an *āsana*, practitioners will make sure that on the one hand they don't forget the breathing as a result of the demands of the movement, and on the other hand they make a calm effort to leave the breath flowing naturally in and out. Strenuous exercises will naturally challenge them, bringing intensified breathing, and contemplative movements will calm the waves of their breath. Principally, however, when practising, practitioners can make sure that they come fluidly to a natural, permeating breath and enliven the different regions of the chest and abdomen in accordance with the exercises.

If the breathing remains free, then the consciousness can also move more freely into a progressive unfolding of thought. The importance and significance of free breathing will probably be underestimated by students at the beginning of their practice, as they only gradually become familiar with the laws of the soul and spiritual life. Although these laws are exceptionally complex and difficult, and are connected with the so-called *karma*[3], with a person's previous life, students can nevertheless acquire a first idea of how the breathing process interacts with the human soul-life.

For example, we could imagine entering into a wide open space and experiencing this space in its freedom. The breathing that individuals will feel in themselves will probably display a clear and pleasant relaxation. The opposite would be the case if someone entered into a confined space and allowed the constrictions they experienced to affect them. Their breathing would become more cramped and tightened. Constriction, oppression or openness and freedom express polar emotional responses and the human being takes these up via a perceivable awareness, and carries them forth into the breathing process. Now practitioners must not succumb to the error of saying that a constricted space also directly makes their breath tense up and an expanding space leads their breath to relax. In reality it is our own consciousness of the space, the perception through the nerves, which conveys the feeling of constriction on the one hand or expansiveness on the other, and only as a result of this awareness does the breath adopt the corresponding quality. The human being therefore acquires the rhythm and quality of the breath via the active, living consciousness, and in this way shapes the inner, subjective fabric of the will.

If individuals were now to intervene prematurely into the breath process and manipulate it, as generally happens in most of the systematic instructions used in yoga, they would not notice the subtle forms of consciousness, which seem to live like an over-arching, subtly dispersed sea of stars in the head, and they would prematurely alter a fundamental equilibrium in the autonomic nervous system. Although the yoga methods of *prāṇāyāma* deliver rapid and excellent success, the essential fact is almost always overlooked that the living consciousness, which exists above one's own subconscious will-regions, needs to attain an independent and autonomous development, and the breath process ought only be controlled on this basis. For the reason explained in this example, the breath process should find the most natural balance possible, but the consciousness should move increasingly in a direction of meaningful development.[4]

Forming mental pictures has an effect on the breath

To give an example, we could practise an exercise in which we picture a wide open space and observe how this activity of picturing in turn affects the breath process. Then we can also think the opposite and picture a confined space, and again observe the effect on the breath quality. With these simple mental pictures we create a first perception of the all important connection between our own activity of thinking and picturing, and the quality of the breathing.

The more, in human existence, the active work of consciousness strengthens in its objectivity and care, the more the quality of the breath becomes suffused and lifted, and this breath, in its function, then begins naturally to build up human life in the will and in the individuality. The route therefore is not from the breath to the awareness but from activation of the conscious processes naturally back onto the breath. The free breath can adopt many different qualities and depths. The greater the human soul-spiritual activity, the more the breath process will take form and become ordered as a result. Instead of manipulating and directing the breath directly, the possibility now begins for the growing consciousness to build a creating force, and from this a profound quality and natural rhythm develops in the breath.

To summarise, therefore, the breathing movement, with inhalation and exhalation, can be characterised in terms of the soul. With the inhalation, practitioners take in the air from their surroundings, and with the exhalation they release it. Besides taking in oxygen from the air and giving out carbon dioxide with the exhalation, with every inhalation the individual human awareness connects with the body or also with the will. We can say it connects with the body because the will is submerged in the body. The breathing is the connecting line between a higher and a lower process, between a state of awareness and a bodily will-disposition. With the poles of inhalation and exhalation, the breathing forms a rhythmic centre, which builds life and then gives this life back again to the higher worlds. But the significant thing with this breath movement is the process of developing the individuality and the will, because individuals who pursue this happening very precisely will reach the following conclusion: On the one hand, they will find that with every breath they participate in the life that surrounds them, exchanging with a universal whole in the rhythmic alternation of the breath. On the other hand, however, they will notice that they can only attain real expansiveness and freedom when their consciousness becomes open for the external world and its various manifest forms, and when they explore these forms.

The soul dimension of free breath begins with the work of consciousness, and this in turn begins with the exploration that takes place outside the circumstances of one's own subjective will.[5] For this reason the breath is left as free as possible. With the inhalation, practitioners take into themselves the forms of consciousness from their own thinking and picturing processes, and with the exhalation they then give out all those forms of movement, which lie within their capacity of consciousness, to the external world. When this fact is recognised as belonging to the soul, it becomes clear how important the edifying, aesthetic and increasingly moral path of human consciousness is becoming.

The different regions of the soul-life

The human soul is not limited to discrete feelings or isolated sensations. In its hidden and inwardly housed existence of light and being, it is infinitely multilayered and multiplexed, elemental, creating and connecting in a precisely measured way through the activities of thinking, feeling and willing, and finally it has no end of active desire in its longing to reach out, expand, participate and empathetically touch the phenomena of the worlds. Just as light aspires to sensitively touch the world outside, so the soul inside strives for the most subtle, sensitive feelings of identity in participating in the inner as well as the outer reality. The soul seeks, in its mysterious inner movement, the depth of phenomena, the profound nature of life, it seeks the true identity of a feeling, an impression or a matter. With this reaching out for a creating and connecting touch with the phenomena of the worlds, the consciousness equally reaches out and human life becomes richer, more fulfilled and ultimately wiser. The more human beings become conscious of the inherent needs and hidden drives of the soul, the more they avoid the superficial and biased emotions of life and no longer give themselves up in their self-being so easily. Access to the soul-life makes minds more stable and provides less vulnerability to manipulation from world propaganda. The soul-life gives a feeling of inner contentment and fulfilment and brings about a connection with others on a deeper level, so that truer and more stable feelings of belonging together, of growing relationship to unity and peace can arise.

Overall, the movements of the soul-life are outwardly characterised by sympathy and antipathy. Sympathy and antipathy depict the two great poles of feeling in life, or also, to use an esoteric term, the poles of the astral body. The astral body, which is represented in the macrocosm through the stars and exists as a microcosm in human beings through the nervous system, gives rise to the infinite variety of feelings, perceptions, impressions, experiences, needs, hardships, pain, suffering, longing, joys and subtle-feelings of life.

Behind all those feelings of life, behind the joys and sufferings, behind the highs and lows of success and failure, behind fears and hopes, which declare themselves through the body and the bodily existence, there rest deep subtle-feelings of truth, which are beyond the polar opposites of pleasant and unpleasant. These deeper subtle-feelings and true experiences of identity shall be developed in this new yoga, for the soul possesses, through its own desirous yearning for truth, the urge to know the undivided and authentic connection of beings.

If students were to meditate or work directly into a spiritual sphere without developing these deeper subtle-feelings in the soul, as is often the aim today in yoga and places of meditation, they would not yet be able to establish any deep synthesis between spirit and world. Only the developed soul-life, with its sensitive truth-impressions and empathies, provides home on earth and at the same time opens the consciousness for the highest, eternal spheres of being human. This soul-life, with its connecting and stabilising inner force, can be compared with the spinal cord itself. This spinal cord holds the spine upright in fluid elegance. In its absence, the spine too would immediately collapse. A developed feeling transforms itself further to a stabilising subtle-feeling and to a radiating life-force, and it works like a creative force itself, which lives within as a health promoting being-nature or "creation" of its own. In the technical language of the mystery schools, one speaks of an ordering, attuning and expanding of the astral body, so that the soul-forces of thinking, feeling and willing become strong enough and can take up the creative, unique and highest reality of the eternal existence. The conscious development of a soul-life prepares human beings for their true humanness and for integration of the truths of the highest worlds. Without the development of a soul-life and an expanding consciousness, no real, practical, life-integrating, pious, religious and wisdom-filled expressions of will proceed forth from human beings and edify social and interactive life.

Infinitely varied are the feelings of the astral body. From these diverse feelings of sympathy and antipathy there are a great and essential number of further basic subtle-feelings, which rest beyond opposites, and have an important role in stabilising life and leading it into a synthesis with the spirit and the world. These basic subtle-feelings rest deep and undeveloped in every single soul, and yet they form an axis of mature humanness. Just as water of the sea at depth is calm and clear and at the surface choppy, foamy and effervescent, so too the human astral body at the surface is more emotional, desirous and passionate; deep down, however, it is wise, calm and acts to guide life. The surface of the astral body is characterised more through bodily feelings and worldly impressions of life, while the deeper subtle-feelings wait, as if latently and innocently, behind all movements, for their discovery. In the soul human beings are therefore what they have actually achieved in the depth of their being by way of experiences and feelings of expansiveness, feelings of appreciation and connection; in this sense, as already mentioned, they are then connected with the cosmos. They are, however, least that which, by way of external successes, enthusiasms, emotions, vital forces and sympathies, moves them on the surface.

Only after the demise of the body, when death has occurred in earthly life, does the soul after some time enter these inner worlds of the cosmos, in which it discovers its true feelings of identity and the connections it has established. It then enters into the deep region of its own existence. In the mystery schools the learned speak of the soul passing over into heaven or into the cosmos and occupying its home in the real and true spheres of light, which are alive, sensitive and salutary. The soul itself lives on after death. This fact can be relied on whatever the circumstances. The soul cannot die like a body in the earthly world. And with the death of the body, upon leaving the earthly sphere, there begins the inevitable soul existence of every human being. The soul itself belongs to the astral reality of the universe, for it is the microcosmic astral body itself. After it has given up being embedded in a body, it witnesses itself in the light spheres of the cosmos and there it experiences itself from now on in a very precise integration and appropriate new positioning, from which it looks back to the past earthly existence in much more authentic and sensitive ways.

By practising the various physical exercises and soul exercises, aspirants of this yoga study the most varied, subtly-felt impressions, and they feel their way into a profound depth of soul-life. Not outer sympathies and outer feelings should be the gauge for practice, but a deep search for the truths and inner impressions of an actually existing reality. The exercises serve to build a discernment between the different planes in which life takes place, and at the same time they should encourage the attention in that direction of becoming acquainted with actual, inner subtle-feelings, which rest in the soul's deep source of being and silently accompany life. Through a suitable development of thinking and mental picturing, the latent feelings eventually develop into true creations. For those who think and practise the content in this way, the yoga practice is a path of training, which brings the soul and spiritual worlds closer and develops the experiences gained so that they can enter into life in a deeper way, makes these experiences tangible and gives a more radiant and creative sense of feeling for life. By more profoundly coming to know and shaping the soul-life, and at the same time developing clear forces of thinking, feeling and purposeful acting, practitioners of this yoga can more easily free themselves from outer compulsions, they can identify overwhelming, outwardly imposed moral ideas in their true sense and then, in their life, out of their own experience, they can begin an orientation to the spirit with greater responsibility. The developed soul-life out of profound depths makes human beings more independent, less able to be influenced from outside, and more creative in developing relationships to the various conditions of life.

The deep region of the soul, according to the mystery schools, can be divided into seven chief sections or domains. Terms like "domain" or "section" must not be seen by the reader from too worldly an understanding as purely spacial regions, for it is much more a case of deep light-soul-regions, which are like qualities in themselves, and from these qualities they possess their specific expression and longing for enhancement, for completion. The soul domains, as qualities of inner being, exist as animated, elemental organisms of the cosmos and rest right in the depth of every single human being. They wait for their discovery and for their consciously developed expansion and completion.

In a simplified, roughly accurate analogy, these different soul domains can be assigned to the so-called seven energy centres, the *cakrāḥ*, the gathering places for subtle energy. The term "energy centre" must be one of the most beguiling terms in the yoga scene, for energy is actually always unspecific and can take the most different movements and directions, thus simulating perceptions that erroneously become taken for subtle-feelings of the higher worlds. Better for this description would be to depict the general term "energy centre" with the wider, slightly more elegant picture of the so-called lotus flower, and to give this lotus flower, with its petals of soul qualities, a very characterising and concrete description. For it is not some kind of undefined energy that exists in the *cakrāḥ*, the wheels, but qualities of the soul of a specific kind, which when they are developed, enrich life from within. These seven centres are located from bottom to top, from the coccyx along the spine up to the head and crown. The individual exercises of yoga should promote the specific qualities of the *cakrāḥ* in conscious ways and increase their associated soul substance. The path to this development does not, in fact not ever, function with "energies" in a way that people understand them in the yoga scene today, but only through a very intensive exploration, in which practitioners learn to involve their consciousness, in thinking, perceiving and in a reserved and yet well-positioned wanting, in all stages of the exercises. Not out of the unconscious or out of passive participation in the exercises do practitioners build up the inner soul worlds, but through a focused, active forming of pictured content, and subsequent observing of the subtle-feelings arising, they come to know and also build up those regions that hide behind life's outer feelings of sympathy and antipathy.

Mūlādhāra-cakra and the earth element

The first region of this soul-life can be brought into connection with primordial strength, or direct strength of the nervous system. The *cakra* that encompasses these strengths is called *mūlādhāra-cakra* and can be translated as "root centre". It rests at the base of the spine and is generally equated with the earth element. Those people who have developed this centre well, display in their personality structure a very characteristic image. They usually possess a good mental and wilful ability to make decisions and to follow their decisions through. They can make decisions independently from the feelings signalised by their body, they can more easily override petty fears through their personal and clear form and therefore possess a great deal of strength to maintain their composure, even in difficult situations. Those people value forms and structures for life, as these are an expression for earthly life and the earth element. They do not easily become dependent on desirous urges, inclinations of the body, superficialities and despondencies. This region of the soul-life is also provided with the strength for uprightness, for a pure feeling of form in terms of moral attitude and thus for innermost human dignity. Uprightness in being human is the primordial substance of personality. If it is inherent, individuals possess, to a greater degree, that characterful capacity for confrontation, for truth, for opposition and because of the standpoint they have attained, they can make decisions and declare their decisions.

Now, however, the question arises as to how someone interested can grow towards this human ideal of a clear, upright "earthly attitude" with the help of exercises and a good exploration of spirituality. This capacity for decisions matures in a human life when, for example, the individual explores a fact noticeable in the soul worlds after death. Particularly through exploring what is communicated about the life after death, the human consciousness matures, and develops that morality which is solid and true and thus can be integrated into the human personality structure. It is that morality that does not necessarily correspond to the traditions, which point their moralising, lofty teaching finger, but exists as spiritual substance in world creation. Therefore, for the development of morality, a practical, plausible exploration of the worlds beyond is also important.

After the physical body departs, the soul goes over into its own body-free realm and now it can carry out a learning experience that it cannot normally accomplish in earthly life. So now a very compact and brief outline of the life of the soul after death will be depicted here, giving a description of this region of experience, so that readers can form a picture of the criteria and the forms of subtle-feeling concerned, and use these for their own self-knowledge and training of consciousness. The description of the experience in the soul world after death is given so that readers can form their own thoughts, and this in turn helps them to develop a new feeling, a feeling that already slumbers in the soul but, because the concepts have not been ascertained, has remained as yet undeveloped, unformed and thus unknown.

The soul, which enters into this realm beyond death, experiences the circumstances of its own desires and the relationships that have resulted from these. In the first realm into which it enters it is literally confronted with the classical substance of desire, the astral substance or, to use the Sanskrit name, *kāma*. This first region of the soul realm can also be described as a region in which the soul most clearly starts to explore the solid, earthy aspects of the world once again in a new way. It then experiences what is solid or worldly as a quality that is actually material and inherently free from any moral judgement. Thus, what is solid is solid and it is neither good nor bad. However, solidity or earthiness signalises death, severance, separation. The human body in its physical manifestation belongs to the realm of this solid matter, to the world of coarse matter, and it will also return to this world with its passing. It is born out of the elements of the earth and will become entirely earth once again. Desire comes therefore not directly from solid matter and thus not from the physical corporeality either. It originates out of its very astral kernel and in the earthly world it actually feels like a form of energy, and for this reason it represents one of the greatest temptations, particularly in the sense of yoga.

Here, however, in the life after death, in the realm of the soul-life, this *kāma* is now in no sense any longer an energy, rather it is a form in its own right, a *kāma-rūpa*, as expressed in the Bhagavad Gītā, the working of a being in its nature, a being which either isolates itself or connects, which either becomes detached or is organised to become a being of a higher rank. The *kāma-rūpa* in its being-nature, in its form and working, is now experienced by the soul in this plane into which it enters, and therefore the soul can recognise which beings are indeed subject to death and to the transient cycle, and must therefore be relinquished.

Now when our desires are directed towards the world and towards the physicality, our mind does not let this world and our own body rest, it does not leave other people in peace, and with an infinite array of expectations, demands, compulsions, manipulations, suggestions and criticisms, it begins, with the substance of desire, *kāma*, to coat and ultimately even corrode this matter or these various physical forms. This can happen in a forceful or also in a pedantic way. Desire directed towards the world and towards matter is therefore an error which saddles the soul in the realm beyond death. This desire neither builds up ideals nor brings solid matter into a synthesis with these ideals, but rather we can picture this desire, which is directed so very much towards the world and towards other people, as if it produces obscuring, shadowing clouds which clothe matter and, when it is directed towards other people with secret greed or inappropriate expectation, even produces actual holes in their subtle astral body. The act of directing desire towards the world with unwarranted and, therefore, always to some degree violent demands, is now experienced by the soul, in its true sphere beyond, like a perforation of matter. It is indeed as if someone is boring holes into solid substance. If the desiring is directed too deeply and expectantly towards the world or towards the body, the primordial substance is weakened and the soul can soon no longer demonstrate its upright and clear attitude with a free decisiveness. The soul experiences this connection in the realm beyond, as it directly senses the actions of the beings and the orientations their relationships take.

A healthy decisiveness, which when achieved strengthens the first centre in the subtle body, can attain definitive development when students explore this plane of *kāmaloka*, the plane of desires that exists beyond death, with the distinguishing criteria presented here. Desire itself is a necessary property of the soul, a life-essential and substantial kind of material of its own, and if we were to deny it on principle, it would be as if we were removing the spinal cord from people and yet still then wanting to declare them as existent. However, at the same time it is also inappropriate to offer the desirous urges of one's disposition a completely free run and thus to lead life not to yoga, to self-control, but rather to *bhoga*, to maximum indulgence.

This behaviour would be like settling into an instinctive and animal-like sphere, or like a conceited growth of all egoism. Since desire represents a divine and great driving force in human beings, through the course of a lifetime it must be integrated into an order in its right place. Solid matter, physical existence, must not be desired by individuals on their path, at least not beyond the natural and existential needs, but rather they must learn to form this solid matter, to mould it and ultimately even to build it, so that the physical or earthy and solid element finds its way to the natural order, beauty and purity that is appropriate for it. When individuals apply this differentiation in the right sense, they will notice how they find a more concrete and upright way of dealing with other people and with societal life, and they will also enjoy a growing capacity for decision. The earth element becomes matter that draws back to itself, action becomes action in the edifying sense, and decision becomes an independent, spiritual force of personal existence.

In the exercises concerning this region, personal decisiveness should move to the forefront and practitioners should not make themselves too dependent on the whims of the body. Most particularly however, practitioners can notice the nature and behaviour of the feelings and learn to discern their different orientations and qualities. The feelings should not be attached to the body, and the consciousness must not slip dreamily or suggestively into the internal world of the organs as it so often does in yoga practice. The movements carried out in the exercises attain their beautiful and free expression when they are performed by means of the concrete will, accompanied by a clear subtle-feeling. Practitioners lead the body with concrete and clear mental pictures, but at the same time they leave it free from feelings and emotions. The body itself is actually left in peace, and yet it serves as a means and tool upon which that beautiful art of giving form to a thought or idea can be practised.

The power for decision is a vast dimension, which is born out of a concrete thought that is free from emotion and finds its realisation through the will. If practitioners develop this power in a rational, not exaggerated, but purposeful way, dignity and magnanimity can arise. Through the force of uprightness in the primordial personality-substance, pedantic fears, misguided expectations of the body, and low desires, which plague life can be overcome. Overcoming all those feelings, which actually represent purely external forms of desire and produce unnecessary anxieties, is a task that can be clarified through the exercises and which can ultimately lead to the growing stability of *mūlādhāra-cakra*, the root centre.

Practitioners on this path study the different subtle-feelings of the soul exactly as they are set down here, and through comparisons, questions, observations, thought processes and mental images they get to know the corresponding astral region, and so they also learn to discern desire in the different ways its true, essential nature can manifest. An exercise is for them the artistic aid, or also the object through which they can measure the success of their practical, mental and sensitive study. But getting to know the astral regions and their subtle astral beings also increasingly brings about that valuable power to lead life to a higher ideal and also to a high degree of purity, and yet at the same time avoid the extreme forms either of one-sided, strict asceticism or else of a self-surrendering, emotional leaning towards the world.

If we were now to roughly reproduce the soul-life we have recognised, directly as a form of movement in our practice, we would discover a strong power to wilfully implement any activity. This power, however, is not a pure physical power that would correspond to mere muscular training, but rather it is a power that arises from resolute and concentrated thought forces themselves. A diagram illustrating this movement, that corresponds to the decisive spirit of thought, can therefore demonstrate the characteristic manner in which will-power is implemented. The centring at a chosen point, for example in the lowest part of the back, depicts the path of decisive thought. The power gathers at a point, centres itself further, and then an utterly free and light dynamic soars out of the point of concentration to the periphery. This free dynamic is depicted by the lines radiating outwards. It is a so-called vital etheric force, an etheric force of life, a very light and dynamic life-force, which unfolds out of the concentration-processes of the decisive thought with its direct centring to a point.

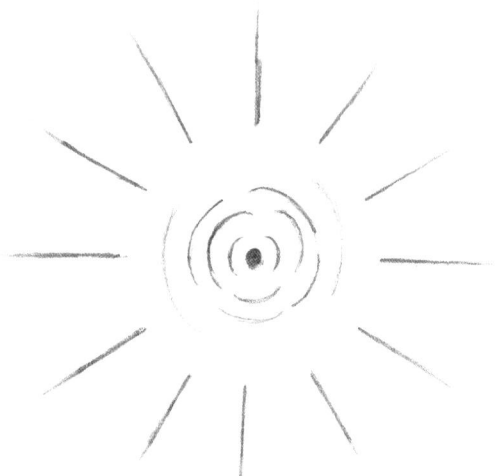

Even though this drawing is initially difficult to understand in its entire scope, it is nevertheless given a first depiction here. Practitioners dedicating themselves to the leg pose (page 272 ff), for example, will be directly touched in their experience by this form of movement. It is always a free dynamic, a free and light force that originates from practising, for the thoughts produce the right feelings and these in turn lead the power to be applied in an elegant and fluid way.

Svādhiṣṭhāna-cakra and the water element

The second region of the soul-life is encompassed by the energy centre which is located below the navel, at around the level of the small intestine, at the back on the spine. Traditionally the element of water is assigned to this centre. It can be said that in this centre, forces are active which are analogous with the nature of water. Water itself, however, is the coarse-matter and visible element, while the so-called ether, which will receive a more precise description below, is the term for the invisible and fine matter of this centre.

This region has its own soul characteristic, significant in its own right. This characteristic can be expressed in an outer, descriptive picture: In it there lies, as it were, a certain basic soul-substance, which promotes the ability to carry out a moral and good action. The more favourably this region is established, and the more individuals become familiar with this region, through carefully examining the dimensions of forces whose effects and circumstances determine, on a daily basis, human interaction in life, the more they can bring about living subtle-feelings for actions which lead away from themselves and contribute to moral and civilised good in the world. It is also the region, to put it this way, of a pedagogical capacity of subtle-feeling for action. Every human being needs a strength that helps them to step back from themselves and to give their consent to a higher feeling or a more important principle. If they are weakened in their inner constitution and in their capacity to face life with complete trust, then they will also lack the strength for an action of high moral value. If this region is developed, human beings can reflect on true and spiritually valid values and consolidate their faith in terms of trusting in these values. It is the *cakra* of trusting in concepts of moral value and this centre is like a bridge which is full of movement and yet solid, firmly anchored on two sides. Trust on the one hand accepts actual reality, even befriends it, and yet enters into its own concrete relationship to the newly arriving reality that is so hard to grasp, the reality that is described as development. These concepts of value are naturally not just those handed down by tradition and made almost into rules, but they are conceivable and concrete ideas, corresponding to a formable and practical human ideal. It is not the trust that happens in blind succession or in outer creeds that is meant here, as these kinds of faith even illustrate lacking strength in this soul region, but rather the trust that happens through belief in feasible and recognisable values and the consequent ascent of life towards a moral perfection.

This region of the soul-life is now somewhat more subtle or refined than the first region. Whereas with the first centre the question was raised of how to deal with solid structures, with the world and with physical bodies, now the question arises regarding the so-called watery element. To describe the circumstances that take place in the soul-world after death, it is helpful to use the analogy of the coarse-matter element of water once again. In the soul-world after death, everything physical is shed and that free and true form of experience ensues which originates from the inner conditions of relationship. The soul in the world beyond, which now enters into this realm, experiences the *kāma* forms, the *kāma-rūpāni*, now submerged and clothed in the essence of water, which has the tendency to flow down as well as to rise up in a mist. This water, which on the one hand wants to flow downwards and yet on the other hand also wants to evaporate upwards, almost as if by itself, should not have its nature impeded, because it works like a flowing force, just in the almost pictorial way the soul experiences it, naturally maintaining earthly life and even leading the thinking to become more animated and imaginative. This flowing force, which never stands still, but is always in motion, and represents more than just the blood or the lymphatic fluid in the body, can be described as ether force. The ether, therefore, possesses more of a subtle dimension, invisible to the eye, yet shows itself to be effective as an essential and moving force in human beings. Students on the spiritual path can imagine the ether by becoming aware that, for example, in all plants a subtle streaming and flowing takes place and yet the plant has no pump. Also, in human beings, the blood can rise up against gravity. The ether puts into effect the force for these movements in the body's fluid system. The water element is therefore the coarse-matter element, and behind it, or with it, there works the fine-matter element of ether. This fine-matter ether element is very subtle and carries within it the tendency to gather and at the same time to internalise. Thus, the ether gathers in the human body and organises next and higher forms, while externally the water in nature gathers and, probably unlike any other element, is able to form one horizontal expanse from many streams. So water is a living symbol for the ether force and carries this force, which leads to natural connections, and to forms being built up in life.

How, then, does this water and ether element correspond to the soul quality of trust and how is this trust connected with morally good action? In order to answer this question, it is important to know that this inner ether force must be left to its own natural devices and to its own inherent wisdom. The ether force builds up both the thinking and also the health of the body. The human mind should not intervene in this region, which has its own wisdom, through direct manipulation, practice techniques, or specific concentration processes. The learning step exists much more in developing thoughts in the most concrete way possible, testing these thoughts out and then, once they have been shown to be right, accepting them in trust and practising them flexibly and freely.

The facts of the soul world can best be rendered in pictures that are not only symbolic, but have the power to convey active experiences. One can picture a person standing at a fork in the road with two signposts, each containing a summons. On one sign is written: "Dare to think an ideal and take the path of your ideal delineated here." On the other sign is written: "Listen to your bodily energies and trust in what does you good." Now this person can make a decision and only take one path. The path towards an ideal starts by disregarding that tangible life energy, and demands a great basis of trust. The ideal itself leaves many uncertain questions open and there is never a worldly instance that could give assurance to these questions. The life energy on the other hand ranks among those feelings that are known and tangible and so those who choose this path can initially lull themselves into a certain sense of security with their body and mind. However, they forget that water in its alternating direction of movement and flow has a mediating task, but can only execute this task when life is given a greater discipline and clearer form by a more ideal aim. The one path is the path of trust in a next possible stage of development, which requires greater and more expansive, ideal thoughts, while the other path is one of fear, which secretly reserves a physical security with the aid of the tangible bodily feelings.

Today many yoga practitioners will contradict precisely this differentiation and introduce the argument that it must be possible to combine both ways, and that there ought not to be such a great difference between life energy and an ideal. In the soul world after death, however, this mixing up of concepts, which happens today in yoga and in many esoteric branches, cannot be accepted, because this world beyond death discerns the forms of its elements very precisely and orders them in the way they really relate to each other. The soul world after death is characterised quite specifically through its truthful order. For this reason, the discernment made here arouses a perfectly true and very common sentiment, which rests in the depths of every single mind and wants to be recognised as the determining cause of many fateful events.

The soul experiences itself, in this second region, in its strength to trust what is morally good. This strength to trust, however, flourishes and grows during earthly life to a particular extent when human beings, who are contained in a body, do not rely so much on the emotional and tangible certainties in their temperament, but duly leave these in peace, calmly observing them, while nonetheless reflecting on higher ideals and values. Through an appropriate attitude towards one's own personal life energies and in rising up progressively towards greater ideals, there is an increase in the force that can be implemented within the soul body, and so individuals acquire a greater capacity on the path of development and can live according to high moral standards and even continue to improve themselves in their morality.

Within the exercises the learning steps are to develop a flowing and unified movement-dynamic, which, however, and this is the important thing, manifests in a way that is as free as possible. The dynamic of this flowing essence, or of the so-called water element, also actually exists in the characteristic forms of movement and these pertain to the second centre. It is a movement which glides out in a dynamic strength and then gathers again in a contraction towards a centre in the region of the lower spine. In this process, however, the movement is not motivated by an energy, and above all it is not forced with a particularly intensive wilfulness or technique. Rather, it happens through releasing that characteristic flow of forces, that element which is experienced gathering from above downwards to the ground to a surface and ultimately represents the beauty of the forming and free so-called ether. This ether has an edifying effect and it is the procurer and preserver of life. The ether, however, is particularly beautiful when it can act in free availability and can take its appropriate direction on the one hand towards the earth and on the other hand towards the further build-up of thoughts.

Practitioners consciously create an exceptionally elegant relationship of tensions by paying attention to unity and freedom in the movement and by using their capacity for coordination. During the exercise, they not only leave the body with its emotions in peace, but they create a quite specific relationship between releasing, gliding and flowing on the one hand, and contracting, gathering and resting on the other. In a sense, they construct the exercise by handing the limbs over to the flowing element and producing a form, which seems to draw back and, so to speak, releases the usual, familiar emotional desires in the nearness to the ground. What now builds up in the exercise is beautiful because the body flows out to the earth and remains free, and the life-forming energies migrate unobtrusively and almost invisibly into their new gathering and centring. The movement itself displays gathering and coordination, and in this sense, through flowing freely to the earth and yet finding its way back to the centre with a greater force, it adopts the role of mediation and free connection.

This movement, which represents the flowing element, can be clarified with the following, simple diagram of lines that gather and direct towards the centre. The etheric body gathers in its flowing streams, concentrates and in this way internalises a substance. Concentration and internalisation is a particular gesture, which can become clear for practitioners, and which ultimately also takes shape in an exercise to form an aesthetic and vivid expression. This drawing can then be discovered in the exercises described later on.

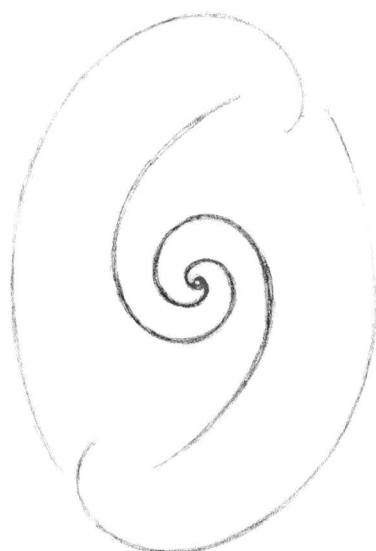

Maṇipūra-cakra and the air element

The third region of the soul-life is expressed outwardly as a sense of purpose, the capacity to want aims, to think aims, to build aims for life, and through these aims to create in life a growing expansiveness. This region, in its ideal image, is literally one of wide, opening space, a space which neither dissipates nor restrains itself in narrow confinement. Just as a plant cannot grow under the dense branches of trees, so too individuals are unable to achieve healthy progress in their development as long the determinants of willpower and conditions of societal life prevent them from receiving sufficient space. The question of space in respect to the soul corresponds closely to the question of development and the conditions of freedom that surround it. So this question of space is dependent on the freedom and expansiveness that it is possible for human beings to create in being together.

This region could be described as the centre of vitality for the astral body. It forms the strength of the astral body. When thoughts, subtle-feelings and wishes extend healthily out to others, this usually brings respectful feelings and generous sentiments. The will should not be used in a possessive, driven, harassing or demanding way to bring these feelings to others, rather the will-impulses should newly integrate themselves into an articulated order, and so with more attentiveness, observation and creativity they should produce a form that brings about connection and growth amongst people. Those people who have brought their will into this ordered articulation, that is so essential for communication and active relationships, accept others and bring a natural, edifying joy and congeniality into the field of personal, practical and societal relationships. They accept others because they feel them to belong to a whole, they respect the freedom of others because they experience themselves as being more ordered and free in their own will, and so in the depth of their soul they will experience a feeling of being accepted. When consciousness is extended to others in the right way, preserving their freedom, and consciously encouraging the uniqueness of their individuality and the versatility of life, true feelings of expansiveness along with connectedness result. The right extension of the soul's inclinations also leads to a pleasant atmosphere in being with others.

This truly expansive and free space in the soul, where healthy communication and edifying relationships happen, can be greatly developed if the learning steps waiting in the world of the soul after death are already studied now with the practice of yoga. The soul, which one day will enter into this region, experiences especially the element of air, because this soul enters into the ambiences, that took place during life in the relationship and experiences with the breath and the associated sphere of air. The air as an element possesses the property of filling every empty space by itself, and beyond this it touches, in sensitive weightlessness, all objects of this world. Being so inclined, it has the effect of bringing the most direct connection and encouraging subtle-feeling. For example, we would never be able to feel the movements of our limbs so clearly if we were not surrounded by air. Every movement in a sense cuts through the air space and in doing so it displaces sensitive substance. The air can be considered to be the substance of subtle-feeling.

The experiences after death always happen free from the body, but they happen in such a way that the different relationships which took place in earthly life become openly present as an immediate and direct truth. The soul, therefore, experiences the relationship that it had to the surrounding and pervading sphere of air. Usually the action of breathing involves a hidden process of feelings and will, and so during life the profound effect of the breathing in determining the entire development of morality is not recognised. But now, in the life after death, the soul experiences this encounter with the vast nature of the air space intensively and genuinely, and with that it experiences the circumstances of its own will. If this air space has been fostered and left open for work to happen freely through one's own will, so that there was a place for all human beings, this space opened up during earthly life now benefits a person's ascending moral development. The air is like a vast, sensitive cloak that wraps around the earth and in this sense it is an expression for the arrival on earth of the astral body itself. Its dimension is vastness and freedom. The air also gives fulfilment, closeness and touch. When it is possible for people to order and articulate their will, they soon become familiar with the wondrous shaping-force that they can introduce into the spacial sphere of air. The ability to articulate the will also means clearly attuning the wishes of one's personal life to external circumstances and to others. As long as a wish is bound only to the bodily world and as long as it is motivated by undifferentiated wilful impulses, we speak of impulsiveness. But from the moment the consciousness brings the will-impulses and wishes into a natural order with external life, these impulses and wishes acquire a constructive and beautiful structural form. Impulsiveness is transformed into rhythmic shaping.

The exercises should serve to develop the so-called *maṇipūra-cakra*, the subtle-matter centre located approximately level with the stomach, on the spine. This is the centre of great dynamic strength or of burgeoning activity in the will. However, this dynamic strength does not develop by managing one's forces in a bound, vital way, rather it develops out of a differentiated and articulated approach to movement. All these exercises apply the principle of free, natural breath and of openness to the vaster space of air. Even in the most strenuous and challenging exercises, the will does not lose itself in the body, rather it continues its constructive work of shaping, and maintains an articulation between observation, relaxation and exertion. It remains free from the hidden intentions of physical, impulsive egoity and in this way encompasses the individual with a whole. Thus, it preserves the air space as a vaster social space. The two photographs of *cakrāsana*, the wheel pose, on pages 52 and 53 illustrate how the high level of activity in the limbs and will-forces can be combined with a feeling of the articulation present in the body, and with a sense of etheric lightness.[6]

The activity of the thoracic spine seems important for the third centre. In the example of the wheel, this activity in the middle of the spine prevents compression in the lumbar spine. An insightful exploration of the third centre best starts with the discipline of observing the mobility of the thoracic spine as it is moved forwards and lengthened. Practitioners wanting to develop this centre always keep aims and objectives in mind, and develop an aesthetic sense for different physical postures or for an aspirable, good posture in life. The reason this exploration with objectives seems so important is because all the aims that people plan hold a force of attraction from the thinking for the future. The will-life, which is what the *maṇipūra-cakra* is about, always tends to introduce a next possible and greater future achievement or advancement into life. The will-life with its inner, hidden drive, forms the vision for the future. A will-life is never oriented to the past and it is not even anchored in the presentness of life. This is why it seems so important that aims and objectives are clearly formulated. They give one's temperament the necessary strength and form, so that ultimately the will can naturally enter into the potential of a free space and a released creativity. Those practising the exercises in the later sections on the third centre can discover the simple form of articulation illustrated in the sketch, and this sketch could also be applied to all the pictures. The three moving lines illustrate the essence of rhythm in the life of subtle-feeling. On the one hand the three lines show a clear articulation from each other and on the other hand an intrinsic, growing reach outwards. Through their inherent rhythm they integrate into the space, and through their articulated disposition they give a feeling of generous openness without demanding specific dimensions or spacial conditions.

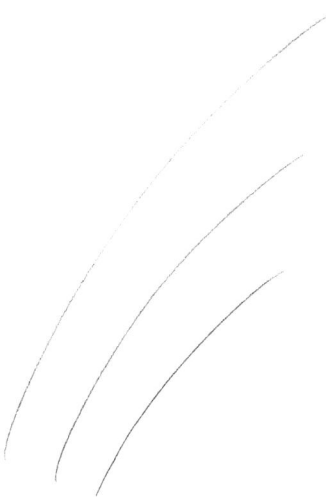

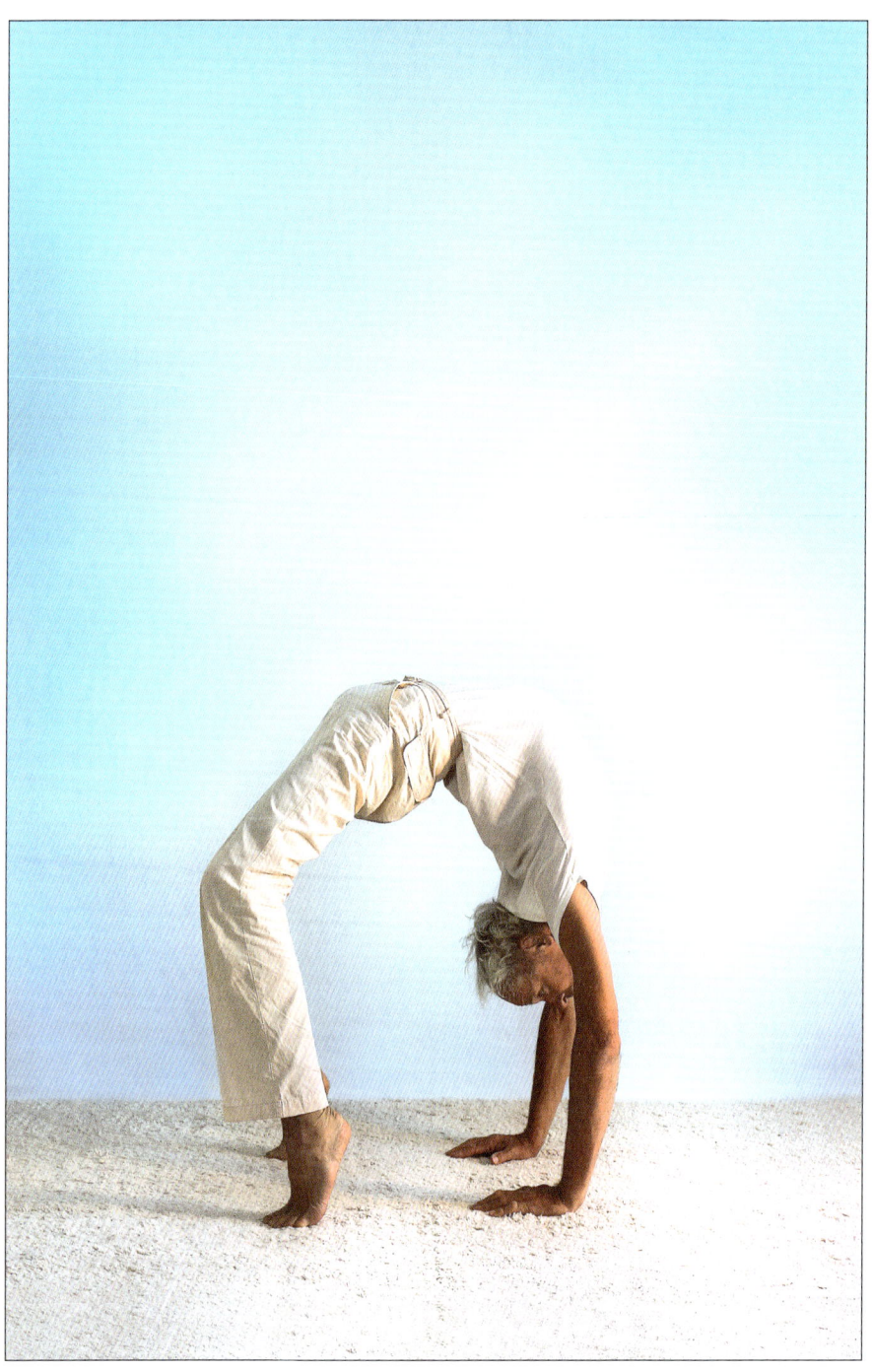

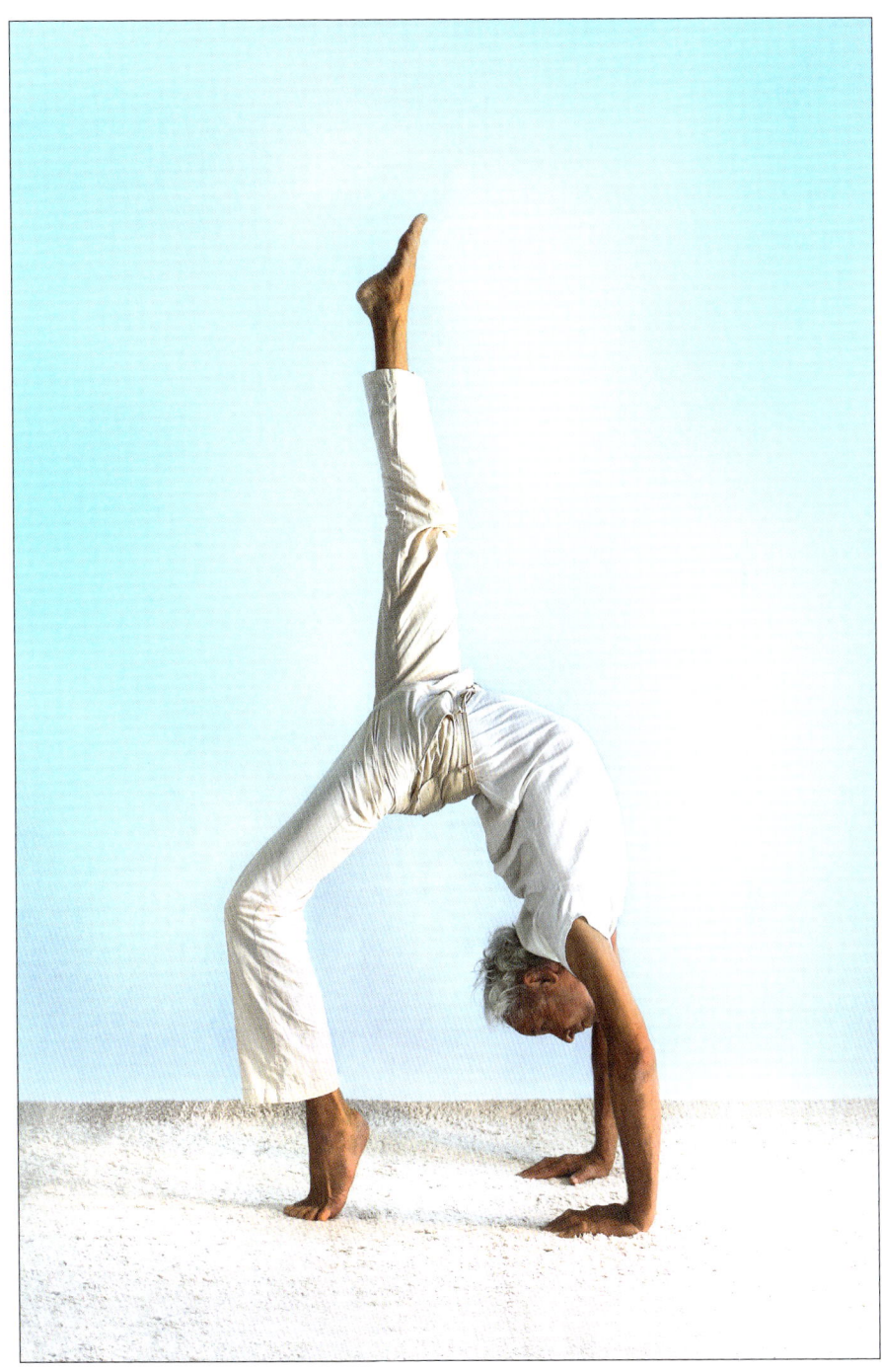

Anāhata-cakra
and the warmth element

The next region that needs attention is the so-called sun-region of the soul. It is localised in the astral body through the *anāhata-cakra*, the centre level with the heart. The heart is generally connected with warm-heartedness and feelings. In this region of the soul, however, it encompasses far more than heart-felt feelings and their connected emotions. This centre is the inner resting pole of human beings. It occupies an exact mid-point, a mid-point between three higher centres and three lower centres. The true and right feeling of the heart has the character of sensitive inwardness and silent centring, and so in its true and healthy nature, this heart is anything other than emotional.

The element of this centre is fire. This is a far more profound and subtle element than the others. It can be said that fire, or warmth, is invisibly immanent in universal creation, and through its particular spirituality, this warmth fully and continuously transforms substances. The property assigned to fire is transformation, or the alchemy of substances, the power to turn one substance into another. We can picture how fire needs a material basis in order to carry out its alchemical work of transformation. However, this substance, this matter, must not suffocate the fire. One can say: Either without any material basis, or with too much substance the fire goes out. The element actually represents an active and at the same time also a balanced, progressive process of creative development through transformative activity.

Drawing an analogy with this progressive process hidden in the heart with its element, the question arises as to where the fire itself comes from, or what inner nature it possesses. Fire ranks as its own spiritual, original substance, higher than the astral body or the cosmos, and so this fire-essence represents the human I. It is active in the heart. But this human I also needs a concrete definition and a clear position in relation to the whole of human development. Although the I represents the original, pure spirituality and therefore constitutes, as it were, a dimension without space or time, there must nonetheless be a manifestation or a concrete definition that seems to represent this I.[7]

The spirit is a reality and the I is also a reality, and they would not be reality if there were no such thing in life as the phenomenon of content. A content always has in its source a fire, an actual spirituality, a basis for creating, an idea, and in this sense it forms a silent and unseen mystery of reality. Therefore, the spirit expresses itself in life through varied contents with their changing and developing forms. For human life, content is indispensable, for it is the nourishment that delivers the material basis for all warmth processes. However, it is not the external world, other people, the various state systems, or even the entertainment on offer that should provide the content for human beings, but rather they should learn to encounter life productively, to take up ever more content through being consciously active, and to incorporate this content into life.

The heart centre is the place where content is given shape, the site of the ability to face life on the one hand with calm, but on the other hand with a high level of activity. The heart centre is like a sun that silently bestows the harmonising and calming warmth for existence. To give life appropriate, spiritual content, or even ideals, enables human beings to live with more freedom and order in all their relationships, to find harmony in the balance between their inner feelings and outer needs of existence, and ultimately to contribute to life from a growing and greater spiritual ideal. It is a task that fosters the mediating position of the heart centre and keeps the physical heart organ healthy. A balance between earthly heaviness and spiritual lightness, through a relationship to life shaped by content, leads to the sweet-sounding tone that could be detected in the heart by many yogis in their meditation.

The sun itself reveals the active shaping-force of life. It is the ether-source, the life-source, the creating-source for earthly existence. In its crystalline rays live the thoughts of universal creation and in a transferred sense they give human beings content. For those wanting to progress on this path, an important challenge is to get to know the difference between the active form-building forces of thought, and the passive, imitative, consuming feelings of human nature. The soul itself can become a sun if it becomes conscious of this difference at the very depth of its nature and in the deepest layers of its will. A consuming orientation shadows the sun-like consciousness-sphere of thought, and over the periods of development it leads to a great many unnecessary forms of material compensation, and ultimately to egoistic ways of behaving. It must be overcome, right into every unrecognised depth of the will, and it must be surpassed through a productive, thinking, form-giving and concrete, mental, sensitive and active building process, while the soul-forces become more and more articulated.

A sun-like life emerges through socially integrative spiritual activity. Those who aspire towards this integrative, connecting spiritual existence need, in order to shape contentful forms through their activity of consciousness, a clear, concrete agility of thought directed towards ideals, which flows together with processes of dedication to societal and earthly life based on healthy perceptions. From this synthesis between thinking and perceiving, a so-called mental picturing activity develops. Life becomes experienced pictorially.

In relation to the exercises, the learning steps consist in developing a practice of shaping content, which specifically puts in first place the pictorial mental involvement, but at the same time also cultivates a healthy perception of societal life. One should never succumb to the error of thinking one could reach the heart centre by means of particular feelings or through building up energy emotionally. Without the sun, the earth itself would be mute and gloomy. The sun, however, resonates, and shapes forms. In the same way the heart centre, even the physical heart too, reacts to the aliveness of a well-ordered, creative mental picturing ability, which ultimately works itself into the practice in a kind of pictorial, calming thinking activity. It is not the body that should dominate, it is not the body's energy that should be the yardstick for success, rather individuals should add meaning to the practice through their alive activity of thought, their perceptive activity of feeling and through their pictorial way of thinking, for only then do they begin to lead the consuming behaviour with its lack of content, over to a process of shaping and forming with content. The conscious giving and shaping of meaning, which happens through one's own thinking, and develops its order in pictorial, calm experiencing, raises the path of training to its relational and warm expression that is representative of the heart.

Once again, this discussion of *anāhata-cakra* can be rounded off with a picture, which at first is not at all easy to understand. Like all the other sketches, this one too is to be understood in a meditative way. Its meaning can be discovered again in the exercises. One can probably picture tangibly that every content that is thought vividly will, in its course, also enter into the higher worlds.

At the same time, a content leads to relationship with earthly existence. Chosen harmoniously, held in thought with sense and empathy, a content creates a clear order and calms life. However, if the thinking and picturing of content is missing then, perhaps not always consciously but nonetheless on a subliminal level, human beings inwardly experience life like a cross. In other words, they experience unconsciously in themselves a horizontal, earthly plane and a vertical, spiritual dimension, which do not meet each other harmoniously, but in the truest sense cross in a cross.

Through shaping life by thinking content, on the one hand people are centred inwards, and yet through the consciousness which makes real mental pictures they are elevated to a freedom. Through appropriately formed mental pictures, arcs emerge in people's aura, circling them harmoniously and at the same time centring them.

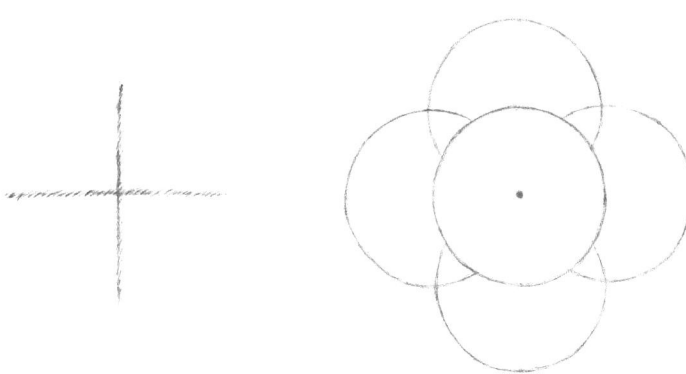

Viśuddha-cakra, and learning to differentiate between a consciousness free from the body and a consciousness bound to the body

The fifth region that now follows is the region of clear consciousness itself. It is the region of the clear light of the soul, *jyotirloka*. The term light, which is often used thoughtlessly in esoteric language, should not be confused with the emotional feelings belonging to life. Although light in its essence can certainly be very closely related to feelings, the feelings must always be discerned from the thoughts. It is the thoughts themselves that are denoted by the term "light of the soul", for if there were no thoughts then no development would be able to take place in human life either, and every feeling would fall into a bodily attachment and with this into shadow. The existence of the thought therefore provides the *jyotis*, the light for the soul.

To date very few spiritually true ideas exist about the processes of neurotransmission that take place via the peripheral and central nervous systems. The conduction and electrical transmission of impulses is known. As a rule, science thinks of consciousness as being bound to the brain and dependent on the brain. Following this logic, a thought would be a product, an expression of brain activity. But the thought itself is a high, creative existence, which is received via the nervous system, but is not produced by the nervous system in the way usually imagined through hasty conclusions. Thinking can happen free from the body, for it is luminous activity itself and only needs the brain as a place of reflection. Like the light that shines onto the earth, that is how the thought is, which glows in the space, already existent. Therefore it originates neither from the earth nor from the brain, but it becomes discovered through human beings and then, being freely available, through the consciousness it can also be thought by human beings.

The learning steps in this fifth level, the level of the light of consciousness, are to develop a differentiation between a consciousness dependent on the body and a consciousness free from the body. Students on the path of yoga can now learn to understand the law of consciousness and enjoy a greater openness. The fifth level is characterised by openness in a very concrete and self-aware form. When practitioners devote themselves to an object, a matter or a task, they will become increasingly conscious that any correct perception, recognition, exploration or experience is never based on repetition or on identifying the object with old, familiar thoughts, patterns and feelings, but is created from an actual, active, open, conscious new experience, and this requires a conscious activity of thought. This openness in the consciousness illustrates a courageous attitude, which requires a certain degree of alert and evolved self-awareness.

In all conversations, all forms of relationship, in all exercises or activities, the consciousness is literally released in its nature from the old, familiar forms, and through the existence of the thought or even, to put it another way, through the existence of light, it wants to acquire an experience that goes beyond the old form. A free human encounter, or the establishment a free, objective relationship, is actually only possible when, through its own individual rightful activity, the consciousness shifts itself into a process of activating mental pictures and thoughts. In consciousness itself, in the so-called *cit*, in an inner and hidden way lives the eternal process of release, which is connected with an eternal new beginning. From this true working of consciousness, the manifestation of light comes about.

The level of learning that can begin here, both through exercises and also through a proper exploration of the given content, becomes clear when that soul plane after death is once again considered carefully and precisely. In this plane of the afterlife, human beings become increasingly conscious of the real, inwardly existing duties for which they are responsible. Once they reach this place, they can no longer be excused if they have followed perhaps a false master, bad worldly wisdom, inferior yoga or even a catholic church doctrine, because having entered into the light spheres they will be most clearly and unmistakably corrected with their own self-awareness and now in *jyotirloka* with the power of courage. In this world after death, in a sense there is no longer an outer teaching or manuscript, a book or a creed. Instead the human soul receives its own rights, and even more than these rights; it enters, or wants to enter, with the most sincere desire, into its rights, and these are the right to establish the truth and to rightly picture truths.

But now it can be the case that during their physical embodiment, human beings had devoted themselves to rules and teachings of life, or to religions, more for the sake of their own security or even for the sake of belonging, and thus denied the real and true right of their soul. This denial of the right of their soul itself led them increasingly to close themselves off in life and ultimately (to state the facts as they really are) it even led them to cowardice. Their self-awareness, however, should have wanted to grow through their own thought process and through the courage for this thought process, and they should have scrutinised the life-teachings, the religions, the traditional doctrines, as well as the people who advocated these, and they should have classified, identified and evaluated them according to their correctness or incorrectness.

Upon entering into the plane of *jyotirloka*, students practising yoga cannot make any excuses, saying, for example, that they had been instructed in the rules of their faith and therefore were innocent of the error. The immortal soul world now reveals to them this beautiful and high sense of consciousness of their self, which means creating mental pictures out of thoughts of life experience and out of what is communicated in texts; mental pictures that can ultimately be verified in their truth. Students on a spiritual path must to some extent carry out this luminous and creative activity right from the beginning. Courage and openness are therefore necessary prerequisites, which ultimately lead life to an appropriate, independent attitude and make possible for human beings both their duty and their right together.

In relation to the exercises, a first learning step now consists in the observation and perception of the act of breathing. The breath should become freer from the thinking and freer from feelings and emotions. This development of a free activity of breathing is directly connected with openness and also with the courage of consciousness. In all exercises, individuals should develop a form of practice in which the activity of breathing remains free, and neither the thinking nor the feeling become bound to the energies of the body. In some exercises the free movement of breath is easier to feel and therefore these exercises can be representative for the fifth lotus flower, or *viśuddha-cakra*, but basically the whole way of practice is linked to free breathing. Free breathing actually indicates the possibility for free thought activity. It is a basic requirement so that the consciousness can work to develop mental pictures and content, which can ultimately be verified as to their correctness.

This thought activity can indeed also be interpreted as an activity of observing and picturing. While a mental picture is being created, aspirants can observe the form of this mental picture more and more, and furthermore they also learn to perceive the relationship-direction into which the thought processes move. So, with the free activity of breathing, the thought activity becomes released from its emotional binding to the body and is articulated into thinking, perceiving and observing. Those practising in this way therefore learn to examine and correct themselves. The free breathing activity leads to a freely observable thought activity.

This plane sees the emergence of the practical ability to detach oneself from old emotions and half-formed ideas, and in a concrete, open way to adopt new thoughts, impressions and content, and create mental pictures from these. This independent work of consciousness, in the sense of an ability to release oneself from previous habits and form new ones, and with this to encounter every human being with consciousness and animated, thoughtful exploration, is a task that practitioners learn at this stage of soul-quality development.

Finally, a picture can meditatively characterise the experiencing of the soul as it happens in this thought-led practice. The arcs create a connection between above and below, between a freer soul space and an earthly sphere. In this sense an arc supports, protects and connects. When practitioners form very clear and good mental pictures, they create spiritual forms that correspond to the arcs in their direction of movement from above to below. In *yoga mudrā*, in the fish, *matsyāsana*, and also in the half moon, *āñjaneyāsana*, these beautiful, protecting arc forms emerge. However, they emerge in the sense of a spiritual movement of thought and can only be recognised in a supersensible way.

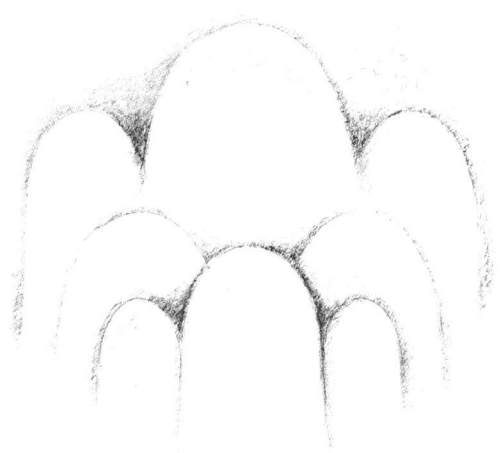

Ājñā-cakra
and the development of a freely creating power of thought

The sixth region is the direct region of fire and force of the soul-life itself. This region is located in the head with the so-called *ājñā-cakra*. *Ājñā-cakra* means much the same as "the uppermost place of command" or "authority". It is the place where concentration is formed and the place of true calmness, the region of the direct, fiery power of the thought, which moulds itself out of the fire of the spirit. The mid-point that lies between the eyebrows can also be designated as the place of the free and creating thought and this would be a practically accomplished and existentially developed meditation. So with the transition from the larynx to the head, a new plane is entered, which can be called *satyaloka*, a plane of truth, the plane of the active and actually existential thought in its unfolding concentration.

Practitioners learn now of the magnificent shaping-force that lies in the thought-life, and they learn that this thought-life can only be existent when they themselves create it through their own individual decisions. Furthermore, they differentiate the thought-life from mere intellectualism or from a thinking blanketed by emotion. Finally, they soon sense the great incompatibility between a so-called projective thinking and a quite differently positioned, creative, concentrated thinking. By getting to know and experience this region of the soul-life and developing it through an appropriate exercise-discipline, they can practise for example the yoga positions with an even greater freedom from the body, and with the power to mould and shape with guiding overseeing and watchful intensity. This moulding, freely creating, mentally concentrated creativity out of the thought is the task, now in the sixth region of the soul-life, that practitioners incorporate into their lives.

One might think that a plane of creativity and formation, or development of a meditation, would always have to be unfurled out of one's own personal inner space. However, particularly the usual ideas that are often formed too rashly about soul and spiritual reality can lead to misunderstandings and not seldom to serious errors. In the soul world after death, which has an important role here for establishing the path of practice, now upon entering *satyaloka* a most fascinating and clear reversal to earthly reality appears. It is not, therefore, possible to draw direct conclusions from earthly experiences for the soul world after death, for this soul world almost always appears as if opposite, and thus often in a new and higher, yet real, logic. When someone wants to acquire an authentic experience of the plane of *satyaloka*, of the sixth region of the soul realm beyond death, the experience must be gathered from this region itself, and conclusions reached from the personal mind must be rejected.

In the sixth region, into which the soul will enter after some time following its earthly embodiment, the soul experiences significantly that the thought wants to penetrate into the earthly world, and exercise there its shaping activity. But where is the place of the thought? It is always situated outside the person, in a sun region, and from this region it generates its effects for the shaping on earth. In order that the thought can work, it must not be brought by the mind too much and too quickly into a bound sphere of emotion or of will. The thought works all the more intensively and freely the more it can be left in its freedom and in its sun-like field of influence. If the thought remains in its expansive and free availability, it works naturally and securely to build and create forms. The secret, however, is that this thought must really exist as such.

A small example can facilitate a pictorial understanding of the experience the soul will one day have in *satyaloka*. There is a great difference between creating a thought by thinking it, or avoiding it through unthinking omission. In the first case the thought is raised to a state of existence, while in the second case there is no existence. For example, a person thinks a triangle and keeps it in mind in its form, its appearance. Through this thinking activity, the triangle also exists in the form exactly commensurate with the way it is thought. The thought itself leads the object into its reality of being spiritually existent. Thus this object becomes a thing, it becomes *sat*, which means that it receives an existence of its own. Through the thinking, it becomes raised to *sat*, to a state of being. The triangle therefore exists as a true reality.

This activity of thinking raises the human soul to its potential, spiritual, creative power. Thus thinking becomes a self-aware and true basis of being human. A critic might say that with this activity of thinking and creating, human nature can fall into an absolute temptation, for it would be seemingly possible, through the thinking process, to lift into being all sorts of negative contents and ideas, thereby having a destructive effect. However, precisely the opposite is the case in the most eminent sense, for when people refuse this thinking activity, and this applies particularly in mature adulthood, then their minds are taken over by all sorts of foreign influences and unseen desires. The activity of thinking, as an existential discipline creating out of spirit, connected with the development of concentration, and with meditative observation, provides an exceptionally stabilising and formative force for human beings, both for their physical health and also for their emotional and mental disposition.

When a person thinks a triangle, then the triangle is present as a spiritual form, which corresponds in size and regularity to the nature in which it was thought. However, a square will not be present when a triangle is thought. In this same sense, a human ideal exists when human beings themselves bring it into being by thinking, but this ideal does not yet exist if people only read it or only wish for it as a formless and vague feeling, without the activity of thinking. The productive power of thinking cannot effectively think up and generate negative forms, but only forms that are edifying and good. Negative influences take people over because they so often fail to get to know this discipline of productive thinking activity and are therefore unable to practise it either. Those who unfold their thinking activity through sincere questions and conscious, objective relationship to the external world, were they now to create a contrary, negative thought that could work destructively, would also directly notice its destructive effect and they would as a rule find this intolerable. For this reason, real thinking activity only gives rise to constructive and supportive spheres of action and destructive influences can very quickly find a healthy elimination.

In this kind of thinking activity, represented by the sixth centre, lives the sustaining and good strength of mankind, which in Indian mythology is connected in the broadest, most complete sense with *nārāyaṇa*, the protecting and sustaining divinity. However, when this thinking is not sufficiently taught and trained, it can naturally happen that someone takes thoughts from a book but does not independently bring these thoughts into being once again anew through the thinking process. Then the will does not really take up what has been read by independently and authentically forming the reality of the thought, and projections rise up out of the mind and take over this sunny sphere. In these hidden encroachments of will or mind, which so often take place within human nature, the thought in its natural creative power can no longer penetrate the earth and edify it. The thought should therefore come into the greatest consciousness possible and at the same time should not be plunged by projections into the bound earthly world. The consciousness leads the aims, and forms the thoughts, but leaves them in their free sphere of activity, and so they provide a fire, which ennobles and enriches life.

So when practitioners obtain an idea of this region of the sixth soul realm, they get to know the place out of which they must work with their own responsibility and their independent awareness. They work therefore not out of the midst of their body, their will or their mind, but they begin to take up a thought, at best a valuable thought about spirituality, and think it in its actual true nature, until it is ripe to express itself in its contour and in its content. The will for implementation, which follows this process, for example in the form of a practical realisation, now remains essentially freer, as through the individual thinking activity the thought too has developed to a free dimension.

Now those who have projected a lot in a lifetime will not come upon an open door in this soul region. Access to the blissful substance of *satya* will remain barred to them, for they will notice that the true effectiveness in their whole personality is missing. Those, however, who were able to discover this shaping-force out of the thought itself and also put this to use by developing concentration, enter into a unified, soulful atmosphere with a happy self-identity.

In the practice with the various physical positions, practitioners now learn to create the images of the content they have read and absorbed in a very independent and individual thinking activity, and then to lead this content as a basis of reality into the ensuing exercise. They learn to bring the image into a form that is their own and yet meets the guidelines given, and at the same time they retain a free and alert overview over the whole practice process. With this discipline they develop an expansiveness in their thought-life by learning to retain the thought for longer, and only once it has been solidly brought into being do they introduce it into the willed practice of the exercise.

In comparison with the expansiveness corresponding to the third region of the soul-life, this expansiveness, which arises through the generative, creative force of thinking, is born directly out of the head and lives out of the thought in a sensitive availability of concentration. While in the third realm of the soul-life concentration is established in a targeted, still more vital way, this sixth region now bears a far more delicate consciousness oriented towards the thought itself. True development of concentration, without reaching back onto the bodily energies and onto projective forms, which in reality come about because the lower regions take over the thought, provides a stabilisation and a sense of reality and truth for the whole of life, and when implemented this would always be connected with an increase in morality and development.

This thought-building process is outlined diagrammatically and practically in the following drawing. The crystal is permeable to light and thus is an expression for a form created out of the light. Its structure is exceptionally regular and therefore it remains transparent for the light, or one can say it remains faithful to the light. Foreign structures have not yet penetrated into it. The thought becomes a super-sensible eye as long as it remains pure. Thus the pure thought and also the pure crystal exist in a noteworthy analogy through their affinity to light. The spiritual world appears as if unified in connection with this thought, and the earthly world presents itself receptively like a bowl. If the thought were now to rid itself of its truth, blend with projections or unsound feelings, it would also resemble a fallen crystal that collects foreign substances into itself, and these no longer allow it to appear translucent.

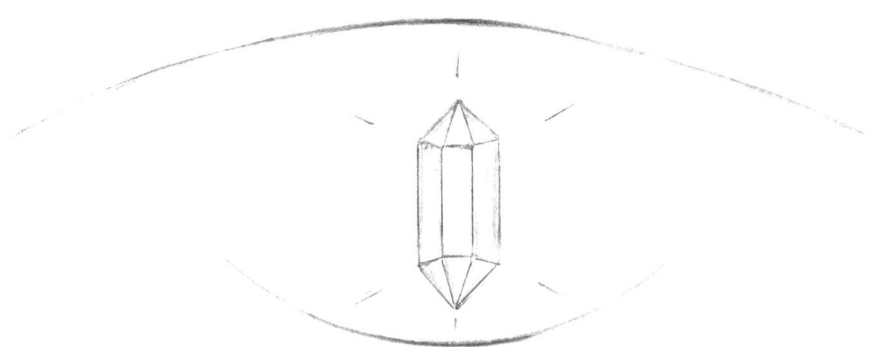

This image of the translucent crystal can be recognised meditatively and specifically in the later chapters on the *āsana* exercises relating to the sixth centre. In principle, however, the structure of the *āsana* should always display a tendency towards pure crystal clarity, and should avoid emotional envelopment as well as clouding of the consciousness through lacking alertness or inappropriate ideological thinking.

Sahasrāra-cakra and experiencing the meaning of soul content

The seventh and last region of the soul-life now manifests in the form of yet another new and different characteristic. This region is the mysterious and wondrous world of the planet Saturn who, from an astrological perspective, is generally regarded as the harsh master of the ascetics. Saturn also represents the old, the past, and also the law of life. Those who speak of Saturn literally feel the stern expression of his face and his menacing call for freedom from the worldly desires that are so addictive and constricting.

In fact, those who, after their earthly incarnation, enter into the sphere of Saturn, feel in a particular way the substance of desire as a power that binds earthly life, thus leading to suffering. Desire for the world causes attachment and suffering, and ultimately destroys people's nervous health and also their morality. This observation and perception describes one aspect of desire that everyone can become acquainted with in their life through careful observation. The other aspect of desire lies in that mysterious depth, which can only be discovered when we adequately form the concepts and perceptions suitable for the inner circumstances of the soul. Desire is a basic force of divinity in the soul, and in reality this would be bliss, that so magnificent, glorious, pure force of heaven, *ānanda*, that so indescribable dimension of the higher worlds, which like the finest fall of dew descending from intangible, other-worldly spheres, can moisten the soul and the will. In the purity of the higher worlds therefore, desire would be anything other than suffering. Both the yogins and also the Christian mystics of old therefore turned away from the world, and with their many ascetic and sometimes even brutal seeming penances, sought the aim of unification with God by attempting to enter into this pure sphere of desire with its bliss.

How can it now be that this desire, being made of astral substance from the highest spheres of bliss, *ānanda*, falls so deeply into the claws of the world, so that it can no longer manifest in its uplifting and joyful nature, but rather in its aspect of pure suffering?

Enjoyment for its own sake, when elevated to a life principle, without any greater question of meaning and without further spiritual exploration, leads sooner or later no longer to development but rather to forms of suffering, which either impact on one's own life or express themselves in the surroundings of others. As enjoyment similarly represents an attachment of desire to the world, it produces a specific feeling for the soul, and the soul can either make itself dependent on this feeling or not. The soul can acquiesce to the enjoyment, accept it, and recognise it as a brief and passing trait, or without further efforts for an advancing development of morality it can subscribe to this enjoyment fully, as its life content or even soul content. So when the soul subscribes to enjoyment, a cycle of desire comes about, which the Bhagavad Gītā describes with the terms *kāma* and *krodha*, with desire and subsequent anger, which then leads to delusion, *sammohāḥ*, and finally to loss of memory, *smṛti-vibhrama vibhramaḥ*. However, usually it is not only the individual person that is weakened and ruined on the basis of these desirous forces towards the world, but rather with this person the surroundings often begin to suffer much more. The astral substance does not usually remain with a single individual alone, but it also radiates in a particular and intensive way over onto other people and carries these people, in their healthy mindset, into the depths: *haranti prasabhaṁ manaḥ*; with literal force, desire tears away the healthy feeling of the soul (Bhagavad Gītā II/60). Desire in this sense is a great and mighty force, which can contribute both to the forming and development of the soul as well as to passions, violence and destruction.

When those who will enter into this sphere after death look back upon their lives and upon those they have left behind, they experience suffering no longer as suffering, but they experience it as the shadow of bliss. All suffering, seen from the sphere of Saturn, is a form of purification for the development of blissful happiness. In the essence of suffering there already lies the seed of bliss. The reason for this great difference is that during earthly life, enjoyment is submerged in attachment to the world and can remain hidden in its true binding nature. Through this lacking development of insightful knowledge, which today sadly is also to be found in psychotherapy, enjoyment and also emotion seem to be worthwhile life aims, and those who stop at these aims and acquire no higher perspectives fall back and do not perceive the true might of heaven in its real joy, but in its shadow image, suffering.

This region of the soul-life can be explained using the Sanskrit sentence: *yad bhāvan tad bhavati*, which means much the same as: "Whatever the inner state of being, that is what a person will become." The individual human being is born of God, created out of ideas, woven out of the substance of spirit. This spiritual substance is in reality nothing other than thought itself, it is the fire substance of heaven. All the appearing forms of the earth and of humanity are manifestations coming from thoughts, which ignite from a divine origin or from a spiritual force of creation. Here on this plane of the soul-life the difference should now be recognised as to how on the one hand it is the thoughts themselves which create life and visible, earthly existence, and how on the other hand the substance of desire in its astral nature gives rise to unending movements, and these movements now either lead to attachment and to suffering in the world or, through a suitable form and through development of consciousness or, to express it in still more concrete terms, through a positive asceticism or through a form of suitable renunciation, they can rise up to their true, joyful and vivid nature. *Yad bhāvan tad bhavati*, the inner state of being will at some point express itself in its outer form.

In this seventh plane of the soul-life, which is related to the *sahasrāra-cakra* or the thousand petalled lotus at the crown, practitioners get an idea of the transcendent experience of the thought, and at the same time, however, of the nature and laws of desire. Desire certainly carries thought within it, although often unconsciously and therefore without form or even manifestation, yet this desire will attain its precisely determined form and eventually express itself in its manifestation. Human beings will become what they develop in their thought-life, or they will also even become what they do not develop in their thought-life, but what is conveyed in the subconscious through desire. The body, the psyche and even the surroundings become a precisely determined imprint of a subliminal consciousness, for desire produces its results, and if individuals do not assume the responsibility of discerning the true and deeper motives, and also do not want to get to know and observe the higher laws of existence, this desire ultimately leads to fateful misfortune and forms of suffering.

At best practitioners get to know this so very subtle and mysterious region of the soul with a few practical criteria for discernment using the practice of physical exercises. Through active exploration, with the activity of thinking and the development of subtle-feeling, practitioners now learn how they can bring the wished for expression into the exercise through an activity of concentration and consciousness. They learn to transfer the content meaningful for the soul onto the exercise. This content meaningful for the soul is truly a soul content and is dependent on a concrete consciousness. Their body, or their activity is transformed into an expression of this concrete, meaningful content, which is characterised by a thought or a mental picture. The thought shines through the body and leads this body into a growing transformation and with this into a new, wished for, soulful expression. The soul content of an exercise is ultimately expressed directly via the subtle-feelings and radiations of the body.

Just as in the sixth realm of the soul's experience after death, the thought becomes experienced in its potential existential reality, so now the importance of the significant content, being soul content, makes a very vivid impression. A soul content is, however, only soul content if it can mould the development of human existence in a positive and ascending way. Not all feelings and impressions that exist in life, with its thousands of faces, warrant the declaration of soul content. It is even better to say that soul content is rare and can certainly not be conveyed through customary utilitarian texts.

However soul content is experienced quite particularly in its supportive nature, as it possesses the power to reject in a positive way an attachment or a suffering in life and to present a truly concrete reality. The concrete quality of soul content expresses its liberating validity both in the physical and also in the soul and spiritual world. A soul content is always concrete and it can be formulated into a clear and vivid ideal, it can even be portrayed pictorially, down to its very principles, whereas unformed desire possesses the human will like a driving force, and tears this will away, both in oneself and in others, into an illusory existence. When the Bhagavad Gītā speaks of *haranti prasabhaṁ manaḥ*, then figuratively speaking it means that it really is a case of tearing away concrete reality and also of destroying *manas*, which formerly did not represent only an intellectual dimension but a deep and true world of subtle-feeling. To a certain extent the way of practice also involves a kind of aesthetic activity of giving form, as students now learn to discern conclusively whether they are placing a thought and a soul content into an exercise or whether they are taking for themselves, out of the exercise, those energies that are so easily noticeable but always remain unconcrete, and in doing so are building up indulgence for themselves. Consciously thinking the soul content and applying it to the exercise demands in this sense the greatest possible concretisation and at the same time always a rejecting of the bodily energies. Those who apply their practice in this way will soon become conscious of the important significance of building up soul content and implementing it.

The seventh region of the soul-life, which is governed by Saturn, can be described as *karmaloka*. *Karma* means work and at the same time in its comprehensive characteristic it embraces the so-called law of cause and effect. In this sense it becomes true that all the thoughts and feelings which a person sows have a consequence, and human beings will become in their *karma* whatever they have carried into their lives by way of content. This seventh plane reveals to individuals the necessary criteria for discerning the situation of their own soul, and so it rejects everything that is detrimental to the development of the soul or harmful to the life of the spirit. Those who now endeavour to bring soul content into life – and soul content belongs more to the plane of the sun, as already described in the chapter on the fourth centre – and those who make careful endeavours for the correctness of this soul content, will also eventually be accepted by Saturn. Otherwise Saturn, the conscientious ascetic, literally hurls people back and does not allow them to enter into their blissful fulfilment.

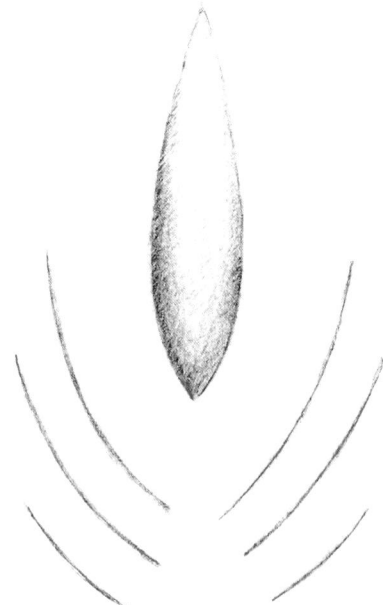

The exercises, which are described in the practical section of the book, bear a characteristic feature of lightness and generation of warmth. This warmth is produced from an intensive centring, which is acquired from the surrounding influences. Thus the picture shows the form of a flame in a high and ascending gracefulness. The flame is warm and desires the spiritual world. It wants to purify all that is low. The image of a receptive capacity to absorb from the surroundings, which brings about that free, unbound flame, burning as if without substance, characterises the plane of Saturn.

If individuals seek to expand their experience, these seven regions of the astral body, and the vivid soul experiences living within them, can be reflected upon, inwardly felt, and built up in pictures into authentic insights. Practitioners discover some most important depths of their own inner life, and approach the soul worlds as they are according to their cosmic laws. These laws usually exist in an as yet unformed way and therefore they remain unidentified in the very innermost realms of human existence, and yet they exist as a greater reality and after the physical demise, when the soul sets foot into the cosmic space, they will ignite in their truth with still more extensive and alive forms.

Attention, Concentration and Relationship

There are a great number of physical exercises presenting varying levels of difficulty and different challenges. These exercises in particular offer a good, aesthetic opportunity to identify and compare the various features and qualities of the soul to be developed. Alongside its technical perfection, every exercise also has the meaning and thought activity that is put into it, giving it its own specific expression. This language, this expression, is an important element in this yoga. In the practical steps that follow, those interested in the New Yoga Will presented here should learn to read in a particular way the different expressions that an *āsana* can offer. The expression is related to the life of the soul, while technical perfection relates more to individual skill.

In most yoga approaches, the *āsana* practice gives rise more to relaxation, calm, and generally to a more profane experience of the oneness of intellect, feeling and body. Practitioners are usually looking for the energy that is released through a pose, and use it to strengthen themselves mentally or to develop a more intensive power of concentration. However, as already mentioned, this route from the body and its energies to the consciousness seems very questionable because it does not train the qualities and sentiments of the soul directly through independent activity of the consciousness, and this results in subtle dependencies on the body and on the practice itself. Practitioners then make themselves dependent on the determining information in the genes they have inherited and thus on the deep hereditary factors stored in their cells, and in their concentration and meditative feelings they experience only a reflection of their inner existence up to now. In a sense they experience only a repetition of something that already exists, a passive, energetic reproduction of what was stored up in them through an earlier life, and of the fruits of development already formed deep in their innermost physicality.

However yoga as understood here, with its artistic and soulful forms of expression, is not intended to lead to a reproduction of the knowledge and feeling previously existing within the body, but rather to liberate the soul from the body and deliver a creative new beginning with clear, open, expansive perceptions that come from the independent present moment of the situation itself. This requirement can be given the name a New Yoga Will.

Practitioners who develop their attention in the way that has been newly formulated here, acquire a direct activity of consciousness, and more and more they encourage the creativity of their will, their feeling and their thinking. The consciousness becomes self-active and forms its possibilities in terms of attention, dedication and relationship to the various areas of the body and to the thoughts belonging to the *āsana*. Here it should be noted that the term "attention" should never be understood in a passive sense as a pure sensory process. Attention is sooner a productive and constructive process of consciousness, which starts with sensory perception, but never gets lost in sensory perception. In this way of thinking, the attention organises the senses, shapes the process of sensory perception by adding a mental picture and with a further natural act of memorising. Therefore, the senses do not lose themselves outwardly, but together with the consciousness they enter into a process of shaping and forming.

The consciousness itself, amidst the process of sensing, becomes the shaper of forms. In the *āsana* exercises this relationship of consciousness of the activity is expressed in a way that is quite easy to understand. For example, after a relatively short period of training, practitioners start to experience their own bodies as the manifestation of a process. The body is what has come into being, and therefore comes at the end of a preceding movement. Practitioners look at their own limbs, their spine, their head pictorially, like a replica. This pictorial experience of the bodily conditions is the result of a preceding thinking process that has been able to reconcile itself with the earthly world. By expanding the perception of the earthly reality with a clear conceptual picture, the pictorial observation comes about that allows one's own body and the physical circumstances to be recognised like a calm replica of a greater whole. Experiencing the body pictorially gives calmness and a natural freedom. It should not be interpreted, in the way some critics do, as being hostile to the body, rather it is an ordered and very healthy experience, for it allows the senses and the processes of perception within the physical world to remain very free and yet integrated.

Corresponding to the three great components of human existence, spirit, soul and body, in analogy to these are the thoughts, which are directed towards the physical world through the stream of the senses and, from these senses, they form the consciousness. The consciousness, in its soul foundation, then in turn experiences all physical appearance as something that has come into being, a manifestation or a kind of picture. The reading of expression therefore needs both the thought and the ability to perceive the physical structure, and lastly the soul's pictorial observation as a final component. For example, the extent to which the meaning of an *āsana* has been understood, absorbed and experienced can be read in its expression. Even after a relatively short time those practising in this way can get a sense of the different qualitative and aesthetic forms of soul-life, for they learn to observe pictorially, and to think in a way that is guided by a thought, and so they learn to transform the feelings, which usually have an outer character, into deeper subtle-feelings.

The sensory process, organising, with its inherently productive and growing attention, should never be confused with using and thus materialistically capturing the object to be observed. The senses neither lose themselves externally, nor deliberately capture their object, rather they joyfully induce the consciousness to penetrate, with creative thoughts and expanding perspectives, into the world sphere, ennobling this sphere in a lighter action.

For example, those who develop a sense for this contentful shaping-force, that exists in the growing attentiveness to the objects and observations of the world, and who realise the potential of guided consciousness, will further an ascent in the soul on all planes of life and will soon themselves become testimony to a productive life in the soul. This is the context in which life in the soul takes effect in a oneness. *Yad bhāvan tad bhavati* says the wisdom of yoga: "That something, which lives by way of thoughts and feelings in the soul, or to which the soul adds, which the soul takes beyond the normal habits, that will become the authentic state of being in life." The life of the soul, with the attention that is formed, brings a growing and congenial development.

The kind of attention, the way it is structured and formed, and the thoughts that accompany it and the processes that orient it, form a first step, which is absolutely necessary in this way of practice. Aspirants must not indulge in an exercise out of habit, routine or on a whim, rather every time they must confront themselves specifically with the right choice of content and set themselves aims, and in a process that shapes consciousness they must apply these contents and aims to the exercise. An alertness to the present moment and a mental agility are necessary in order to distance themselves from automated patterns of habit, habit for example of how sense-life is dealt with, or how routine behaviour is rushed into with the will without perception of the external world. Distancing themselves from this habit enables them to becomes free from the emotions dependent on the body. They should therefore dedicate themselves to the individual exercises, and also to the forming of thoughts and subtle-feelings each time with new intentions, in concentrated mindfulness and calm overview.

In their daily practice, practitioners will first of all develop a natural, conscious relationship between their own I and an object to be observed. The act of experiencing is firstly split into a subject and an object or, in yoga terms, it is born within duality. Duality is called *dvaita*, while non-duality is called *advaita*. Although, according to the general principles of yoga, the intention is to overcome duality, at the very start of every observation and dedication to an object, a conscious situation must be created that enables a concrete order in the relationship between observer and observed. It would be very detrimental for the consciousness, and for the healthy development of a so-called I, an overseeing I, if practitioners were to adopt the so frequently used saying: "All is one", and in doing so did not become sufficiently conscious of themselves as observers in relation to the observed object. By differentiating between these counterparts, an I and a you, a self or another object, a healthy duality emerges, and this then promotes a healthy overseeing I.

Individuals should not merge too early with the objects of their observation into a so longed for, seeming oneness. To be precise, they should not merge at all into a oneness between their current being and the outside, because in any case this oneness only exists in the outer feelings and is devoid of any real wisdom. Any experiences of oneness acquired too prematurely are almost exclusively only of emotional, bound significance and obstruct the true work of consciousness. Through very clear, ordered attention, turning to the object in a concrete way, and through lively activity of thought, the feelings assign themselves to the object anew and only with this form of organised attention do the favourable relating-conditions for the further development of soul qualities come about. The self, the *jīva*, the observer, remains organising and attentive, it consciously experiences itself in the process of the exercise. It thus experiences its own thinking, its own feeling and acting in a conscious and forming activity, and it notices in what is external, or in the counterpart, a growth that faces its sensing and its thinking with a relationship of its own.

Only by adopting this impartial, unemotional, yet clear and independent relationship in a concrete form through attention and dedication, can the new impressions develop of the exercise and of its meaning. Learning becomes true openness for the object of learning. The thoughts can develop more freely through the alert consciousness. From this lively activity of thought, a far deeper joy in subtle-feeling develops, which then no longer depends so much on the body and on emotions, but bears the stamp of the true, authentic impressions which enter in in the shaping process. The life of the soul acquires its own light joy and its own clear order. The aura, in other words the practitioner's subtle radiation, can develop initial crystal clear rays, as opposed to a woolly, cloudy envelopment.

A practical example for attention

The organising activity of consciousness, which acts within the sensory process, can be most easily understood by means of a comparative example. The observation of a natural object, like a plant can serve this purpose. Practitioners direct their attention to a lavender plant flowering in early summer and with uncomplicated and yet very conscious participation they observe the forms of the flowers as well as the stems and the shapes of the few leaves.

For this observation practitioners should neither lose themselves in rapturous feelings nor observe the lavender plant according to its usefulness. Both ways of forming a relationship, that of losing oneself without thoughts or further ideas, and that of utilising and therefore wilfully grasping the object are unsuitable temptations, which do not lead to the adoption of a true relationship or to a soul-consciousness for nature.

It therefore seems necessary to find a third form of observation, which is as effortless as possible and yet concrete and invites relationship. This third form happens by simply creating one or a few mental pictures to add to the sensing process. For example, during their observation, observers picture the lavender flower specifically in the first half of the summer with its beautiful, luminous, blue-mauve colour, flourishing to its highest radiance and fragrantly emanating itself as a plant essence. This way the picturing activity recreates the perceptible sensory process, and leads this process into the human memory. The picturing activity, through the additional thought, organises the attention and lifts the experience, received into the senses, to a created image. The outcome of carrying out the thinking, and perceiving the object, is to elevate and manifest the pictorial form of soul experience.

Now observers can leave their attention with the lavender for a few more moments and even picture that its delicate, bluish flower-form will transform, and towards late summer and autumn begin to wither. The flowers fall from the calyx in which they are held, but the leaves remain and retain their form. The flowers preserve their fragrance to a certain extent however, and they now conserve this fragrance internally. Those who now touch the dried lavender blossom, and this is how the thoughts can be pictured further, actually open again, with their touch, the inner floral and fragrant life of the plant.

With these observations, observers become more conscious both of themselves and of the object, and at the same time they notice how it becomes possible for them to avoid that utilitarian, wilful assault of materialistically grasping the plant or strenuously, thoughtlessly looking at it, and to establish an alive and productive relationship with the object of observation. In the images that arise there breathes the sentient soul. This now newly developed relationship opens to them subtle-feelings for the plant essence and, through the mental pictures they have created, it even prepares them to develop those more subtle impressions which correspond to the soul and which gradually pave the way for a higher capacity of perception.

In this process of attention lies an organising activity of consciousness, which protects the nervous system from exhaustion and organises into the body those health-giving, so-called etheric formative forces, which naturally supply life with an influence of light.

Those who practise this form of attention in relation to the physical yoga exercises, as well as to the most varied sensory processes of life, notice very quickly how they naturally become more independent on the one hand and more inviting of relationship on the other hand. It is the soul which creates images and which, in these processes of sensory perception of the earth, achieves a relationship, and with the thinking preserves an independent and sustained freedom.

The beginning of a path of consciousness to develop the soul

The word *āsana*, which describes the physical exercises of yoga in general, is classically translated as "seat". In the earlier form of yoga, sitting itself was a basic posture which would not have been comprehensible without dedication to a cosmos or to a higher world. The seated posture describes the calm, meditative position that symbolises a perceptive state of consciousness of oneness with a whole. The *āsana* therefore used to have a different meaning from the one it adopts in yoga courses today.

Now in the generally known yoga approaches the *āsana* does not reveal only a specific seated posture of meditation, but rather an especially selected position of the body, which can become either easier or more difficult and thus also all the more unusual. Here, however, in this entirely New Yoga Will, the *āsana* takes on the role of art. As already mentioned, it is not the body that serves as a means to develop an ascent of consciousness, but rather it is the soul-life itself, via the thinking, feeling and willing, which is led to a differentiated expression and which ultimately seeks its affirmation in the art of leading the body into a particular, aesthetic form.

Practising with the body can be considered as natural study, inviting subtle-feelings, for which the student must procure the relevant literature on the soul foundations of yoga and must make time to practise and explore. Both a mental and physical discipline provide a good basis for a noticeable, progressive development. It is good if the practice of exercises finds its expression in rhythmical, regular forms and in this the consciousness becomes conscious itself of the creative development possible. A rhythmic practice-discipline leads to an inner-bodily order and promotes the calm of the soul-life.

None of the exercises should be practised in combination with music, not even with meditation music, for music leads into too subjective, dreamy a world. It is very important to see a discipline of visible learning, of concrete, calm attentiveness, of sensitive dedication, of a joyful search for insightful knowledge in the practice, and to practise with natural ambition, without compulsion yet with the aspired wish for success in developing a more intensive soul and moral life. Also, the aim should certainly develop for more beautiful and complete physical exercises expressing suppleness and harmony. The exercises can be practised at any time of day.

The etheric body is a subtle body, which organises the life forces in the physical body and stabilises the power of thought. Regular practice and occupation with the body of thought of this yoga is very helpful, as through the repeating exploration in a rhythmic sequence it forms a healthy etheric force in the personal sphere of thought, and through this one more easily finds one's way to the deeper subtle-feelings. The repeated, active occupation with these thoughts about the soul world, followed by the practice of exercises, attunes the etheric body and strengthens the life forces. Along with health and well-being, the strength of the psyche increases and a natural, gentle light of radiance develops; that is a light that, via the aura, emanates health to others. The attunement, activation of the inherent ether through developing thoughts and subtle-feelings brings about a first enlivening of the soul-life.

In our Western, consumerist culture, a discipline is normally only practised for as long as it promises noticeable results and advantages. If after some time of practice, the pleasant, conducive feelings and enlivening energies, which result from the fascination of the new, diminish, most practitioners start to doubt their discipline. However, precisely these fluctuations of the noticeable and exploitable, material or health results should not be allowed to distract practitioners, as in order to attain a deeper tuning in the soul it is necessary to bring about a certain sacrifice of work and of abstention, so that those boundaries are finally overstepped that are necessary in order to penetrate from the surface into the deeper feeling-world of true soul existence.

Practice should never become a compulsion, as compulsion is a quality of the bound will, and once students have arrived there they cannot find success for the soul. It is not wilful, fixed practice with dogged study programmes that can secure success for the inner life of the soul. It is far more the persistent, calm, attentive, repeated, rhythmic and dynamic fostering of the thoughts set down about the yoga of the soul-life, and the recurring practice, that give success for the inner experience. In patience, and in a positive, expectant hope with alertness and recognition towards the spiritual worlds, the right feelings and insights out of the invisible heights begin to develop in the soul. The thoughts, the attention and the will can only be steered onto the discipline of study through repetition and without compulsion. The success that is granted from these efforts is ultimately a matter that will be answered through the work of the higher hierarchies, in other words through spiritual forces active in the creative world.

In cases of anxiety or other health problems, those interested should not practise the exercises without clearing it with a competent teacher or doctor. A schooling path of this nature requires on the one hand resolve and enthusiasm, on the other hand however, all rational criteria and necessary precautions must be adhered to. Nevertheless, these cannot be delineated in the most careful detail for every single exercise, as they are also dependent on each person's individuality. Just as a mountaineer can sprain an ankle, so too with unsound practice someone can naturally exacerbate a spinal problem through the exercises. Exploration of the circumstances in which an exercise brings an improvement in the body and when it might represent a danger must be an independent responsibility. It is the consciousness that is addressed at the heart of the schooling, and in a healthy and rational way this should arrive at greater activities, inner possibilities and meaningful steps for expansion. Although studies of this nature can offer very valuable help in illnesses and afflictions, it is helpful if you clarify the individual possibilities and precautions with a competent teacher and develop the courage to judge your practice independently and responsibly. Generally the studies are suitable for all adults, nevertheless an individual adjustment in the time duration and specific objectives can be factored in.

Studying the soul-life can be compared with designing and building a house. In order to plan a house in its architecture, it is necessary to observe various laws and acquire ideas about the construction. Practitioners enter into an intensive social process with a teacher or also with practice-guidance set down in a book. Practical ideas can only be acquired, however, if the architect is clear in his consciousness and capable in his field. The architect must nevertheless adhere to the prescribed guidelines and logically developed measures, as otherwise his planning becomes fantasy. The architect gives the specifications, and in the same way this book is like the description of a possible architecture for the life of the soul. It falls short of being a finished and complete guide, as through the process of development and through reflections on the part of the practitioner it can certainly be led into a further improvement. Some initial and possible suggestions and inspiration are nonetheless expressed and relayed as well as possible. In this sense, practice combines a living, a spiritual and a social process.

The life of the soul, to repeat this once again, has very little to do with fantasy and mystical states of immersion into subliminal, unconscious existence. The right ideas develop through repeated study of the thoughts about the life of the soul, and by and by, through these thoughts, the individual building blocks develop to bring into being the expanded soul construction within. On days affected by illness or other interferences, workers on the construction site will not overexert themselves and so on days of exhaustion they will not wear themselves out further through an overstretched discipline. With common sense, dedication and perseverance, the individual steps of development flourish to a deeper responsibility and wisdom, and a joy will thrive, silently accompanying life. Practitioners will notice after some time how their inner life shines more abundantly and how through their foothold in life they receive confirmation that they are on the right path.

The two pictures below show less the technical detail of the exercise, but rather the attitude of consciousness itself. The eyes are open during all the exercises, for as soon as they were to be closed practitioners would all too easily also lose the overview over their body. At the same time, the sense of sight encourages the possibility of an edifying and constructive attitude, which is always involved in the practice of an *āsana*. To a certain, very finely attuned degree, the eyes construct all those thoughts that the practitioner thinks.

Using its capability for perception, the consciousness observes various parts of the body. The following exercise, presented in two pictures, is *eka pāda paścimottānāsana*, the head to knee pose over one leg. Practitioners become centred, for example, in the leg region and in the lower back and with their arms they glide far out forwards. Their head and their visual sense always remain free. These do not get involved in the exercise while, however, the will needed to execute the exercise, through repetition and rhythm, gradually comes to build up in the appropriate way.

Practice that is free from compulsion and yet motivated with a good dynamic strength, leads in this sense to a natural self-responsibility and ultimately also to a better self-evaluation.

*eka pāda
paścimottānāsana*

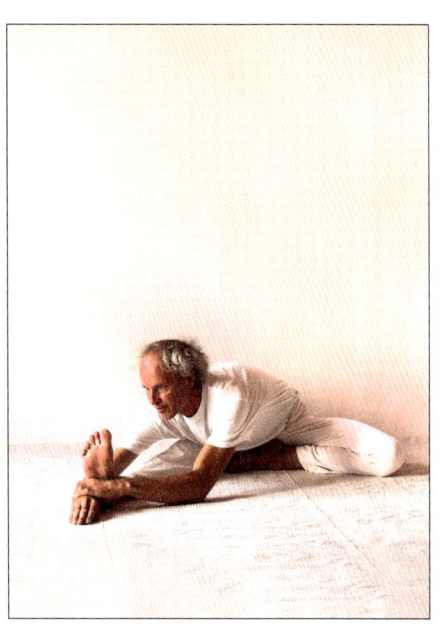

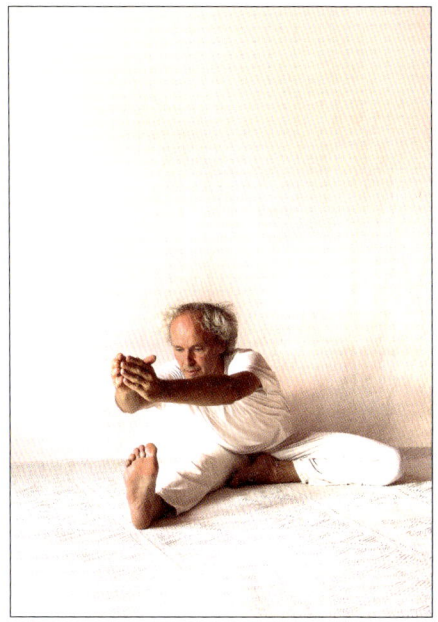

*Beautiful and light forms of
expression come about when the
consciousness leads the body.*

The different energies in yoga, three different radiations of the aura

Portrayed simply, we can distinguish three fundamentally different forms of energy. This distinction is quite basic and important, and follows the simple system of body, life and consciousness. Efforts to distinguish between these energies can help practitioners on the path to avoid wrong spiritual interpretations and to assess their personal experiences better.

The energies of the body, which are probably familiar to everyone, usually result from the unconscious drives of desire and they are generally described by the words "lust" or "longing", which have more negative connotations. In Sanskrit these energies are called *kāma*. Passionate lusts, as long as they are not derived from a natural, existential need, come about through unrecognised dependencies and internalised psychological trauma. They also commonly come about through a weakness in personal strength or through superficial life-habits. The tendency for *kāma*, for desire, also comes about through anxieties that are taken on from society and they increase further through giving up oneself and through states of weakness. The forces of *kāma* must be brought to recede on a path of spiritual training, as they would stand dramatically in the way of a wisdom-filled and devout entering-in to the inner world of the soul.

At the beginning of a path of practice it is certainly difficult to see the different radiations of the astral body or the soul body and a long period of exploration is therefore needed to build up a discernment between the energies. Basically, however, practitioners acquire first experiences and notions, and thus soul perceptions via the soul-body itself, and on this basis they notice different radiations. These radiations belong to the so-called aura. The desirous aura, determined by the body, is undifferentiated, without boundaries between the body and the atmosphere, as if red or dark; it acts like a bundle of vital energy, demanding space, intrusive, coarse, insensitive and usually restless, driven. People who move in social circles where these energies predominate usually find little space for clear thoughts, ordered relationships and therefore cannot easily put themselves in an independent and yet socially capable position.

Nevertheless, forces of desire must be distinguished from natural needs. It is very important that practitioners who are treading this very specific path of yoga do not renounce the natural needs of their bodies and life situations, but make efforts so that all those drives and forces which hurt others or contradict an aesthetic way of life recede.

A next and different form of energy corresponds to the etheric body or belongs to natural and clear thinking. This form of energy is generally known by the term *prāṇa*. *Prāṇa* literally means "life energy". In human beings this life energy is always mysteriously interwoven with the thoughts. This life energy, which is connected with the thoughts, might be stimulated more from the bodily aspect, from the radiation of the blood and so from the forces of *kāma*, but then in the long term it is not really an energy that builds people up, but one that disguises and shadows them. The *prāṇa* energy, which constitutes the actual energy of yoga overall, needs today to be motivated from the aspect of the thought-plane.

In the favourable sense, a natural *prāṇa* develops from people's alertness, joyful relationship and natural, objective outward orientation. However, if it is motivated more subjectively from the body, this *prāṇa* energy is overshadowed by all the bodily forces of desire. This is why it is so important to discern whether a build-up through *prāṇa* originates from the will and emotions or whether it arises from the aspect of concrete thinking and picturing, and therefore produces a natural and free life-force. The most common temptation in yoga is that practitioners devote themselves to set phrases and forms and in so doing never notice the *kāma* that emanates from the body, and so they enter the path of practice with a confusion that has serious consequences. However, if an exploration is led to develop in a natural way through involvement with others, with the outside world and with the various questions of interest, and if it is strengthened in a spiritual process that is really comprehensible, as well as a subsequent social process, then the life of thinking and picturing usually gains an edifying and shining intensity and the *kāma* recedes.

This discernment is so significant because in the yoga exercises this life energy, which is rooted in the life body, is addressed anew from the astral body and stimulated to a more intense dynamic. Through the various stretching, lengthening and relaxing exercises, through taking up various positions for a period of time, through steering the attention and through observing the free flow of breath, on the one hand the blockages in the physical body dissolve and furthermore the congested energies in the life body begin to move more intensively into a flow, and therefore energies that come from below or from the physical body mix with those that come from the thought-life to shape the form. Therefore, practitioners must not practise a path of yoga without building a clear discernment and without a thought-based and creative mental forming-process, for they would plunge into an unconscious depth which would overwhelm them with its obscure forces. Yoga would really be harmful if these distinguishing criteria were not observed.

For example, someone who takes up the shoulderstand for a few minutes in calm perseverance, observation and silence, feels afterwards how the life energy gathers in the heart. Each individual position increases the *prāṇa*-energy in the corresponding energy centres, but this increase will also definitely come from the body. Now it is the highest and most important duty that practitioners bring their own soul activity into the exercise, and lead into a formed expression those wisdom-filled thoughts which lie in the meaning of the exercise. With this personal activity they overcome the rising physical energies of *kāma*.

For our practice it is therefore decisive that practitioners do not allow themselves to be influenced one-sidedly by the forces and energies of the physical body, as is generally the case in the various approaches to yoga, and to use the energies, which can be sensed so very quickly, for indulgence, for egoistic purposes or for hasty, subjective immersion into the unconscious inner world. It is much more important to observe these so easily perceptible energies, recognise them in their flow, and then with greater wisdom of thought guide them in their appropriate direction. The energies which arise are then differentiated and they can ultimately be of value and support in developing concentration and healthy harmony in life. However, even when a positive and good *prāṇa*-energy is involved, this should not become a medium with which a spiritual result is intentionally generated.

In those who experiment a lot with these energies in yoga, the aura is cloudy, enshrouding, sometimes dreamy or trance-like. But when practitioners do not use these exercises for their own mystical immersion, but create them as aesthetic forms and so bring into being a natural *prāṇa*, the exercises serve them harmoniously and a greater purity and wisdom can be developed. Then the cloudy entities of the aura lighten and acquire a sympathetic and more regular form.

The third form of energy comes about through the active participation of the consciousness itself. This is a deliberate activity of the consciousness which can be described as *buddhi*. *Buddhi* means "wisdom". It refers to the inherent wisdom of human beings in the consciousness. Through developing alert activity in the consciousness and through developing ordered thinking, profound feeling and sunny-warm willing, through clear interconnections and concrete working steps on the spiritual path, the inner *buddhi* is brought to intervene meaningfully into the overall bodily structure. The *buddhi* should learn to steer the forces of *prāṇa* and to reject the tempting powers of *kāma*. The unfolding of the right *buddhi* within, of an alive vision and dynamic based on wisdom, through the life of thought and subtle-feeling, is part of the activity of this new yoga and leads a soul-life of higher quality to develop.

For our path of practice, it is useful to learn to distinguish those three forces *kāma*, *prāṇa* and *buddhi* from each other. If the higher force, that is the *buddhi*-force, is brought to intervene over the other two planes, the soul-life is purified, the pressing forces of the body are released and the beauty of a crystal clear radiation, an aura exhibiting beautiful colours and shining out without demanding space, soon develop. *Buddhi* is that dimension of consciousness which can no longer be felt in the form of energy, as it corresponds to light, and usually only over a very long period of time does it want to be furthered towards its crystal-forming aura through exercises.

Different demands in the exercises

The physical, technical difficulty of an *āsana* can be mastered in very different ways in the practice. Almost all physical exercises can be practised from an initial, simple elementary form right up to one that is acrobatically advanced. It seems worth noting that even in their initial stages all exercises contain the subtle-feelings of the soul to a sufficient and discernible degree.

Nonetheless when practising the individual *āsana* it is very valuable if practitioners pay attention both to physical progress in giving the poses a precisely shaped form, as well as to the mental attitude emphasising consciousness. Practice represents a discipline on the physical level in that practitioners are persistently countering certain feelings of lethargy, which are called *tamas* in Sanskrit, and furthermore are curbing their restless nature, known as *rajas*. On a soul level, practitioners become acquainted with various new subtle-feelings, which constitute not only bodily feelings, but actually essential, connected perceptions concerning human integrity, and with these perceptions they develop a greater span in their societal and interactive life. On the spiritual level, the perception of self with respect to the transient feelings of the body is ultimately strengthened, and so is the ability to add to life new contents of consciousness and more noble feelings.

The bridge, *setu bandhāsana*, is one of the basic yoga positions, which requires a relatively demanding dynamic, as well as a pre-existing flexibility in the back and in the legs. The initial practice can be built up in various stages of shaping and training, which are necessary to achieve the perfect end position. There are systematic and meaningful demands on both the body and also on the consciousness in these preparatory steps, which precede the final position, the actual *āsana*.

The demand on the consciousness in *setu bandhāsana*, for example, is specifically that practitioners do not force themselves into the end position too soon, but develop the dynamic, preparatory phases adequately and with this they work step by step towards the aesthetic far-reaching movement. While dynamically stretching out in the bridge they do not fall down to the ground onto the foot, but rather with careful observation they lead the

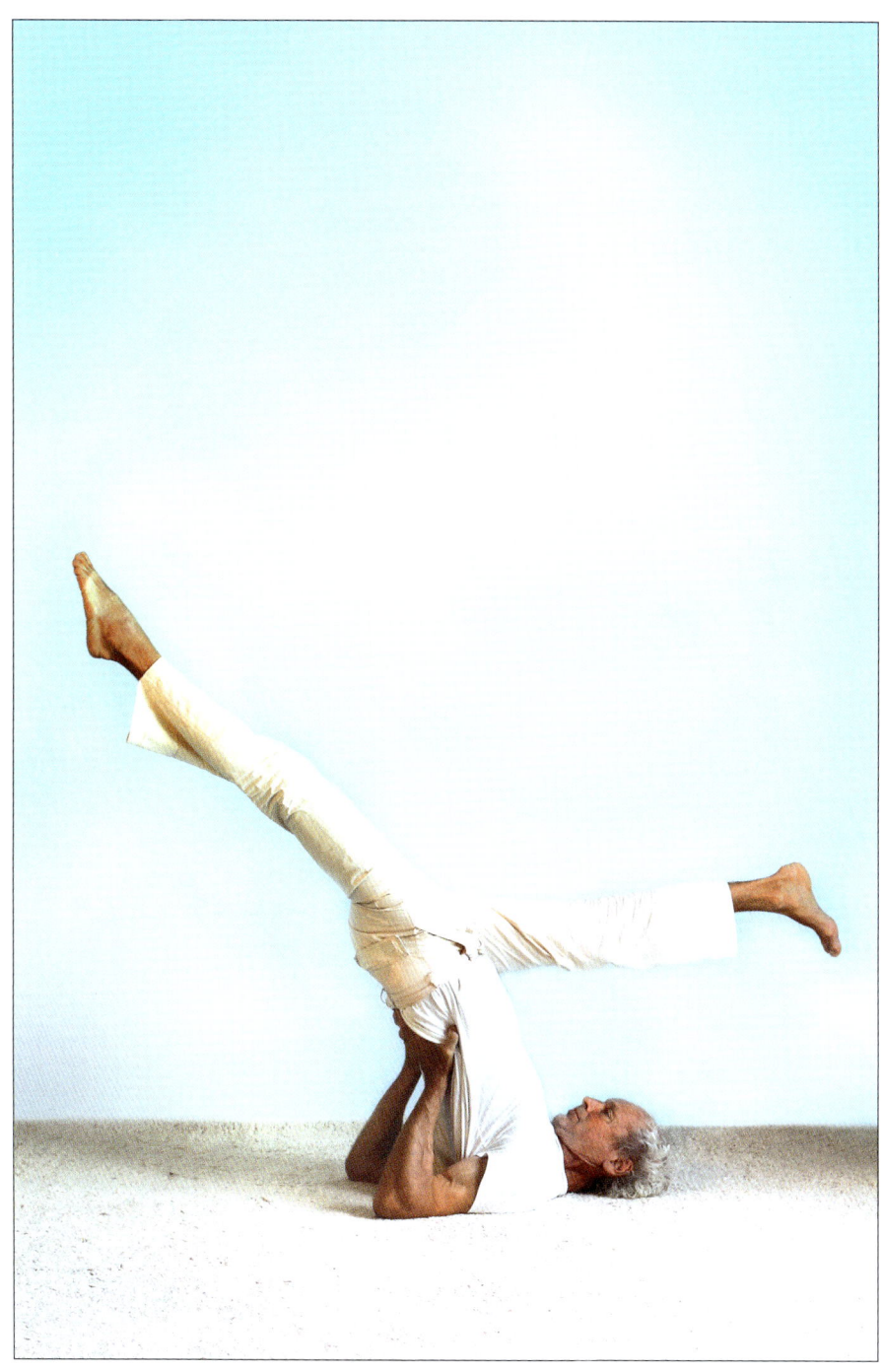

movement through the air until the whole arc can stretch out far enough like a smooth, old drawbridge. Practitioners have the far greater challenge of an intensive, dynamic play of movement, which involves holding the torso and at the same time drawing in the base of the pelvis as they glide out into the expanse, so that in the last stage, seamlessly, with a gentle touch, one after the other the feet reach the floor. The exercise can be assigned to the second centre.

Right from the start, practitioners experience in the play of the leg movement, the characteristic contracting force, which always represents a kind of holding back. The dynamic, in the way it can be set in motion and experienced already at the beginning, is described in the chapters on *svādhiṣṭhāna-cakra*.

The pictures are intended to portray how a movement is shaped in the stage of its dynamic preparation. The end position carries in its subtle-feeling ultimately the sum of all the preceding dynamic movements. Particularly in the preparatory stages, the practice can be developed in a sound way. For this reason, many relatively difficult *āsana* are also suitable in the early stages of practice.

This *āsana* can be practised in its initial stages as a complement to the shoulderstand, *sarvāṅgāsana*, or also the plough, *halāsana*. The far-reaching play of movement of the legs gives an aesthetic grace and practitioners can feel their way to the maximum possible boundaries of their movement. They should perceive, and at the same time lead, every step, both consciously as well as physically, so that a premature, interruptive leap does not cause the movement to slip out of control onto the ground.

The bridge in lotus is shown here in addition, in order to demonstrate what possibilities there are to build up the movement and to play in coordinating the individual sections of the spine. It is one of the most difficult backward bends as it requires not only complete flexibility but a most intense, skilfully applied spiral dynamic in the back. Those who are very advanced can try this position in its beginnings, starting from the shoulderstand. This position challenges practitioners to precariously feel the limits placed by the balance and dynamic strength.

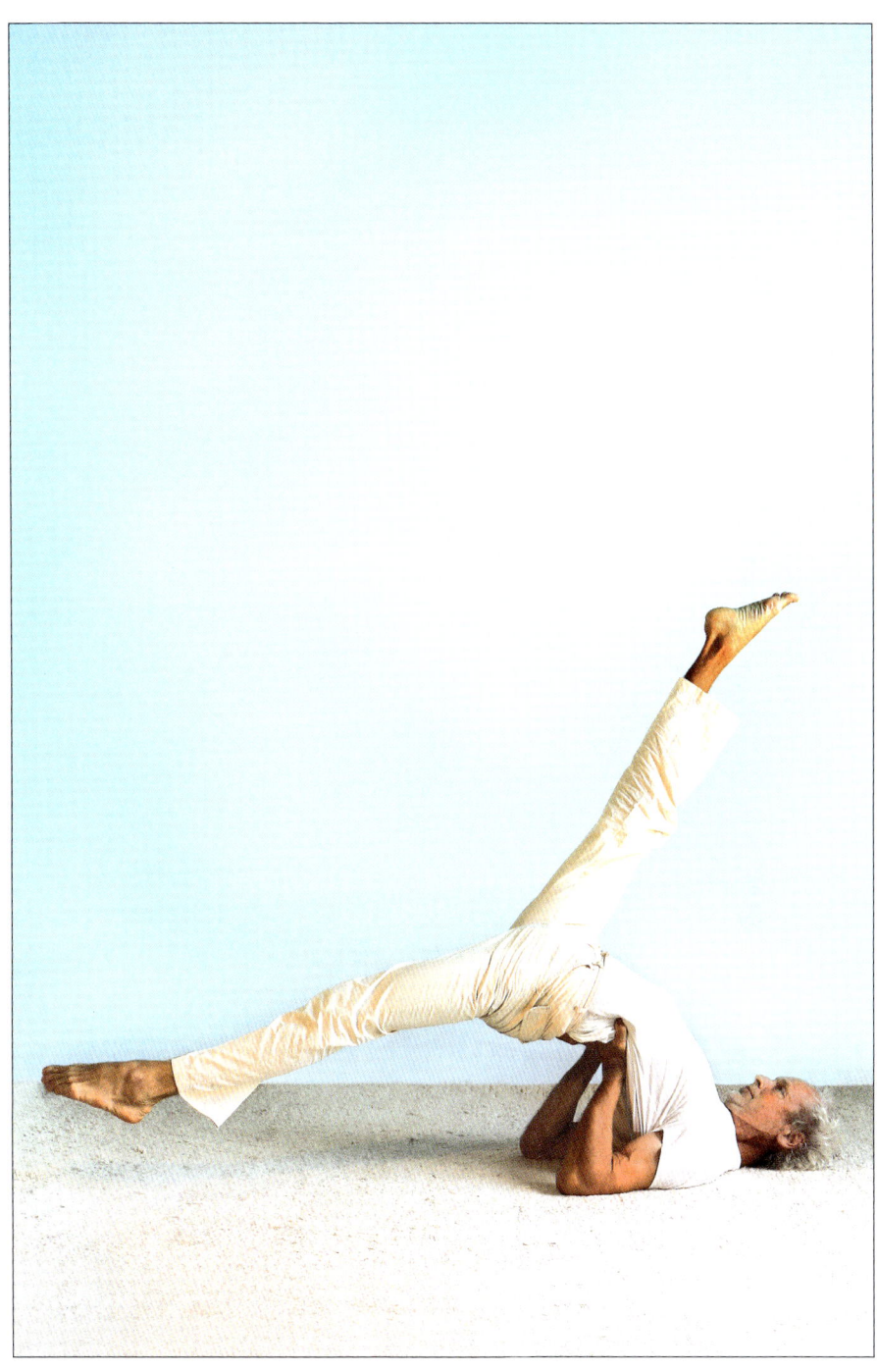

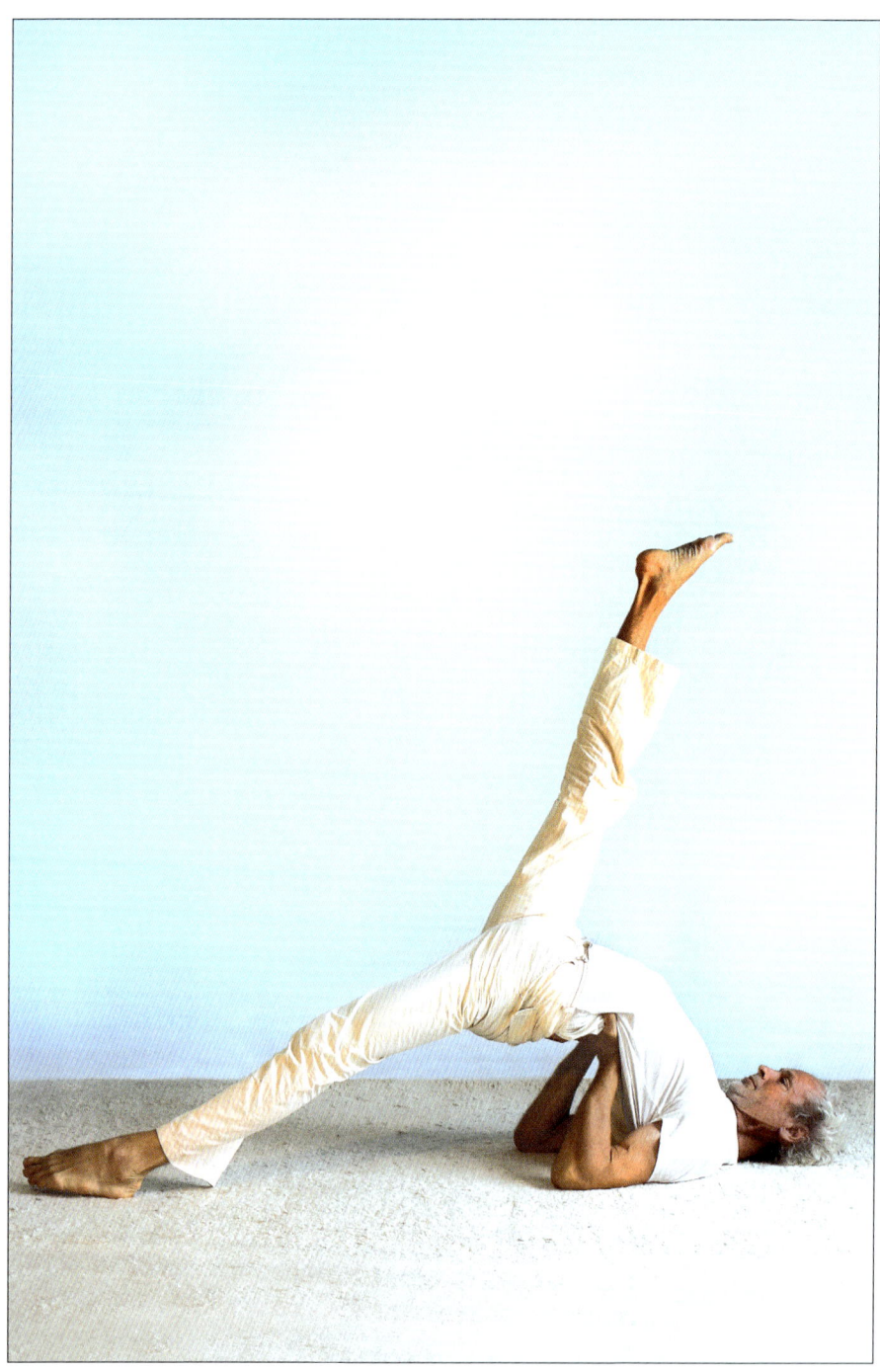

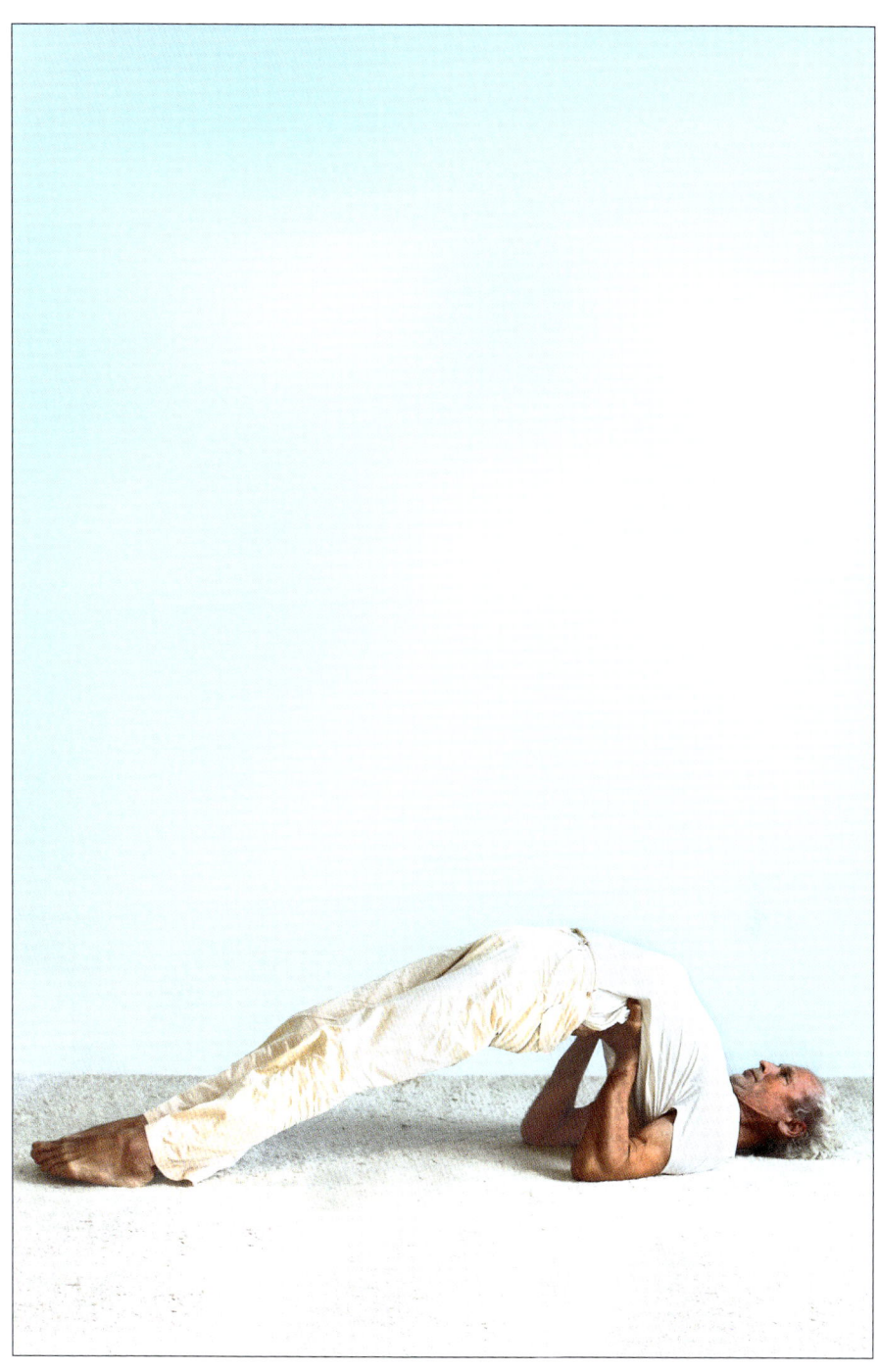

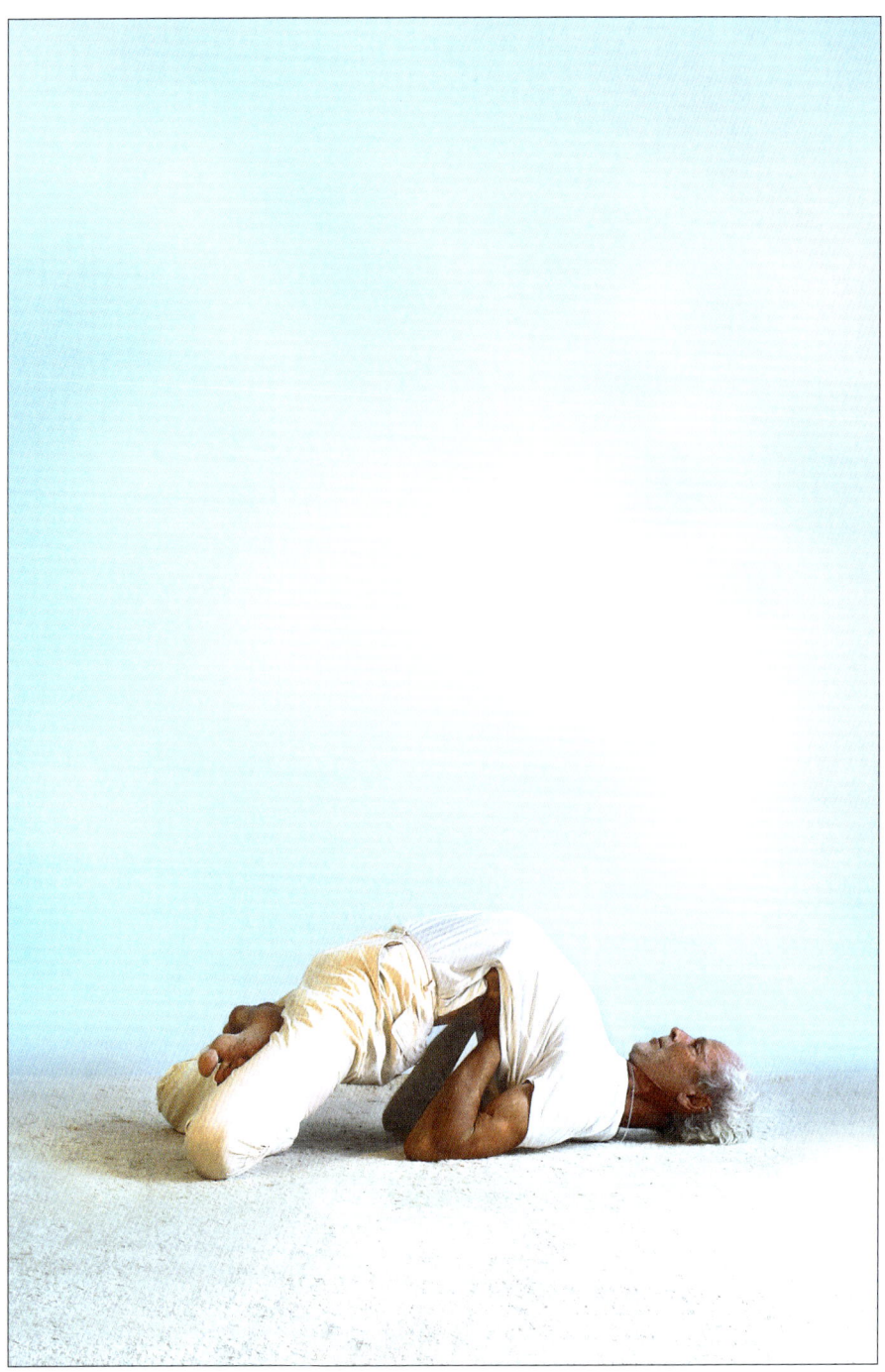

Rhythmically building up an exercise and developing yoga out of the social context

An exercise does not lead to escape from the world

When observing a yoga-*āsana*, a typical physical exercise, the particular calm and inwardness that it usually radiates is apparent. Particularly in the meditation posture in lotus, this almost self-contained oneness of the personality with one's own body seems striking. From the impressions that can be gained from yoga, one could think that this kind of practice does not lead into the world and into societal life, but rather withdraws from life and directs all its attention ultimately towards an individual and personal experience of harmony.

In the soul dimension of yoga, however, this impression should not guide us, for the whole way of practising is developed out of the social context, out of the human capacity for encounter, out of empathy and perception of others, and ultimately it also builds up not only the individual personality, but a communal whole and an actually real and true feeling for the conditions within human relationships. The technique is not the starting point for the discipline of soul yoga, for without a broader view of the order within human souls and relationships, this would only produce a reattachment to physical existence. Through observing the soul and spiritual conditions, and through the possible shape-giving forms of consciousness that come from a growing inner human poise with its aesthetic and its wisdom, its sensitivity and vital creativity, finally the starting points for the practice emerge, and they bear the aim not of throwing human beings back onto themselves, into their closed-off calmness and isolated meditation, but of lifting them up and furthering them to become more mature human beings in their ability to relate, both in their receptive perception as well as in their capacity to communicate and react.

The body is a precisely measured expression of earthly existence, through which a transcendent and cosmic wisdom shines, illuminating it with life and soul. The body itself, however, is not spirit or soul; through it there shines, in an individual way, a universal spirit and a cosmic soul. The way of practising with the soul aspects of yoga is not therefore oriented or even fixed to the exercises with the body; rather it develops a lively and communicable awareness, which can then take expression in a dimension of existence with expanded relationship. The physical exercise, the *āsana*, never therefore seems like a self-contained, stand-alone exercise, in which practitioners enter into an exclusive world. If it were a stand-alone world in this sense, it would even be contrary to soul and spiritual development.

An *āsana*, a physical exercise, reveals the specifically developed thoughts and feelings and also communicates these outwardly, for it is not at all so much a pure physical exercise, but rather more a sensitive exercise of subtle-feeling, in which the subtle-feelings become experienced and conveyed in their expression more and more as creative forces and also as real forms of consciousness that invite relationship.

In movement, in the rising and falling of the limbs, in the dynamic interplay of stillness and motion, there breathes an inner feeling, which always streams out, in its soul-origin, from the light of the cosmos, although at first it is not recognised as such. By studying the movement according to its inner soul-content and hidden subtle-feelings, practitioners now experience this movement no longer only as physical vitality, unconsciously and non-specifically, but rather with specific subtle-feelings and effects on the soul, and with this they notice that these subtle-feelings and effects possess a higher and thus cosmic origin.

Every single *āsana* can develop an easier or more difficult expression, from initial, awkward, stiff hints of approaches to the movement, to a flexible, masterful completion. In the expressive and pure perfection of an *āsana* are expressed the wisdoms of higher worlds, which practitioners have recognised through laborious study, and when these are right they also work outwardly, can be communicated and related to by all outside parties. The aura becomes experienced like a joyfully communicating radiance.

The cosmos is always present, and so its influences likewise at every moment have an effect on the human body. However, as long as the subtle-feelings are not thoroughly formed, practitioners cannot really feel themselves as a component part of the cosmos. Individual human beings without specific development of the soul are literally like a global bundle of thoughtless mechanisms and unconscious or half conscious feeling-reactions. They lack the real and true receptors, the astral organs, which would be necessary to filter out the deeper subtle-feelings from the global and much too unconsciously functioning, complex will-reactions, and thus to order and experience these reactions in the consciousness. By now dedicating themselves in a detailed and differentiated way, with thoughts and subsequent subtle-feelings, to the contents describing the meaning of the *āsana*, they order the non-specific action of the consciousness, which originates from the cosmos, lift it out of its complexity, give it a specific form, in this way animating the latent soul-life within, and can thus discover themselves again in a cosmic connection.

Rhythmically building up an exercise in three phases

An *āsana* is always a motionless movement, a form that has come into being, into which the body is led in a very conscious way. The *āsana* is built up, however, according to a rhythm, for it is preceded by a dynamic phase and also followed by a concluding phase. Seen in this way, every *āsana*, every physical exercise of yoga, consists of three very clear and consciously experienced individual steps: the initial phase of the movement, the still phase and the returning, concluding phase.

This way of yoga attaches particular importance to building up all the exercises in a rhythmically shaped way. Rhythm is always an expression for a superordinate activity of soul-forces. A rhythm lives in the stars and in all movements of human existence. All forms of consciousness are built up in a rhythmic interplay of thoughts, subtle-feelings and willed actions. Rhythm is a world force and in the practice of yoga it should receive particular consideration.

The initial phase in the practice of physical exercises happens through specifically planned, pictured and activated movements, and leads the limbs, or the body in general, into a particular, specific form. The hitherto habitual and comfortable posture opens up into a next and new dimension, which is formed through the dynamically effected movement. A new relationship or a new expression is sought. The body and its limbs could be said to move forwards into the next possible position, which is usually also more difficult. It is not that the posture of an animal is imitated in a certain gesture, as is often believed in yoga, but rather a form is sought, which represents a new or different order and which thus brings itself in a concrete

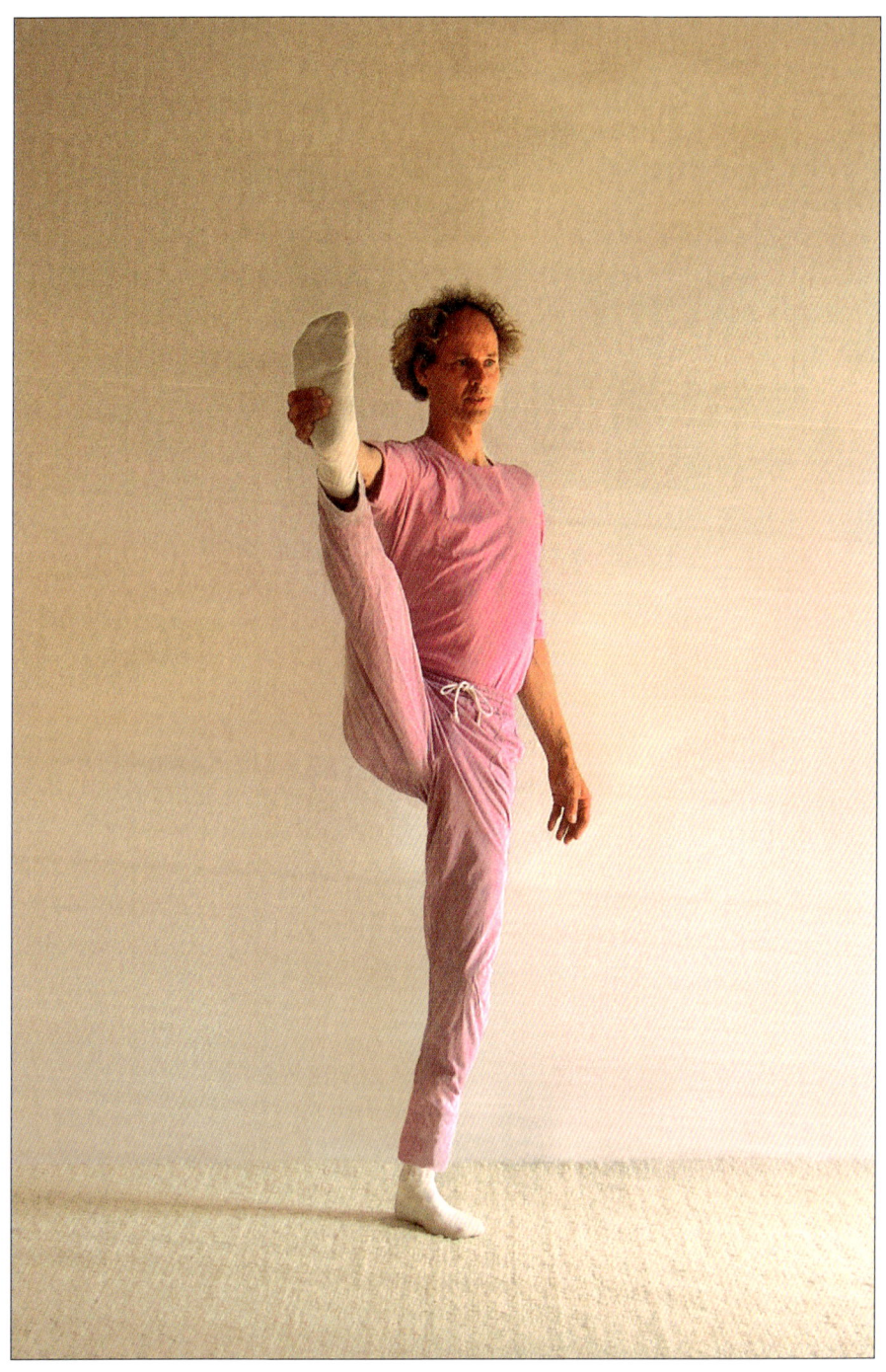

and conscious way into relationship to a whole or, to say it another way, to a cosmic and universal light.

This first phase of dynamic movement, led by thoughts, takes up a heightened and new relationship to a developing form. It never becomes bound back into the pure subjectivity of a sunken state more in the body, it is far more a phase of building up and shaping a next possible experienceable order, and a state of consciousness linked to this. In this sense the dynamic phase speaks to the so-called astral body. This astral body, as already mentioned, is the carrier of desire and it constitutes the forces of the soul-life. Through seeking a next order and state of consciousness in the movement, the astral body with its thoughts, feelings and impulses also transitions into the forming of a new, aimed-for consciousness. The astral body in this sense, with the help of the movement, seeks a new form of relationship. It fulfils itself in its desire to take up relationship through the well-formed and conscious development of a new form.

From the dynamic movement, there now follows the static phase of stillness which, in a completely focused and conscious way, is held for some time. This time varies, depending on the difficulty of the *āsana*, from a few seconds to a few minutes. Overly short or long holding times are not recommended in this soul-based yoga. For example, there are reports that the headstand can be held by advanced yogins for up to three hours. If it is held in this way for such an extremely long time, it leads to a very great inner calm and at the same time also to maximum stability of the consciousness. However, this stability based more on the body, achieved through discipline, is very difficult for the soul-life to use, for it does not build the ability to communicate and empathise, and it does not shape the consciousness in a way that is sufficiently flexible and open. Too strict a discipline with extremely long holding times would not be helpful in this kind of yoga practice, which aims to create a forming of the entire being of the soul. By way of practice, nevertheless, an exercise like the headstand can certainly be held on occasion for ten to fifteen minutes.

It seems very important to understand that an *āsana* in its still phase describes nothing other than a form and an ordering of the so-called I. It is a specific dimension into which practitioners move. The more difficult the end position is, for example the king cobra or the full sitting twist, the higher is the order which practitioners occupy with their I as they pause in the still phase. Also, by remaining so still, practitioners experience on the one hand the body in its form and clear earthly order, and they observe on the other hand the external space, contemplate thoughts and notice the feelings that belong to these. They do not digress outwards, but remain in the intended thoughts and observe the sentiments and feelings. The consciousness is active in all phases, but since the body has now arrived at a really still, even silent phase, practitioners experience themselves not only as alert and actively forming with the consciousness, but they also experience a great overseeing in their thought-perspective. They experience the thought as thought, as the body is silent. The thought is now no longer sunken in the body, but becomes perceptible for practitioners themselves to recognise. The I is addressed in this dimension. It becomes furthered to its greatest possible, thinking overview, wisdom, and in its function of body-free, insightful knowledge.

The exercise has a different effect on the I, however, if practitioners do not develop a soul-activity of forming in thoughts and feelings, and if they sink into their subjective world. It must even be said that the I gets lost, so to speak, if the *āsana* becomes closed off during the still phase. Unfortunately that is the case in most yoga approaches today. An *āsana* only has an edifying effect on the whole human and socially-capable consciousness when it is incorporated into that thought-based, subtly-feeling and integrative forming-process, and thus, in spite of the still phase, conveys the impression outwardly that it remains open and able to communicate.

The final and closing phase of the exercise is the return to the normal starting position. In almost all exercises it is best if the movements are led back in the same way in which they were started. Step by step, practitioners release themselves from the still phase and, maintaining consciousness and guidance, lead the movements smoothly back to the starting position. This closing phase is also very important for the entire rhythmic process of forming the consciousness, for, in a very careful and strengthening way, it now addresses once again the so-called etheric body. By leading the individual movements back carefully, with natural consciousness, the motion-sequence ultimately engraves itself more deeply into the memory. Practitioners therefore make an effort, for example, not to leap carelessly out of the headstand, but in a similar way to the initial phase they lead the limbs back again into the starting form and release the position in this way, with conscious perception.

It is even advisable after the *āsana* that practitioners think back over the completed exercise and mentally reconstruct the individual phases of the exercise they have just done. Half a minute is usually enough for this concluding, retrospective overseeing.

An *āsana* therefore describes a rhythmic cycle, which begins with the extension of the astral body and its joyful inclination to form the movement; in its middle it adopts a concentrated and calm ordering with oversight and clarity of thought, and finally, with a movement guided carefully back, it finds an end. The exercise begins with a thought or a mental picture, which practitioners decide upon, and so right from the start the I is active. In activating the movement, these thoughts are now led into a next possible order of relationship and so in the first dynamic phase the astral body is shifted into activity. When this dynamic phase moves over into the calm *āsana*, the static position, the thought or mental picture is now experienced most noticeably as if outside the body and therefore this still-standing phase of practice most clearly characterises the I. Practitioners experience the still-standing body like a picture, calmly in the light of the thought and in the subtle and free touch of the sensory stream. The thought literally seems to the outsider to be tangible, existent, like a light that wants to communicate, and therefore the *āsana* never appears as a closed-off, stand-alone reality. The last phase now leads naturally back out of the *āsana* to the first phase. This closing dynamic phase happens consciously, for now in a pleasant way the etheric body is addressed in its function of rounding off and integrating.

The *āsana* is therefore led by a very open and clear activity of consciousness in rhythmically built up phases, and although it uses the body it does not see the aim in the body but rather in an aesthetic and comprehensive process of building up, thus contributing to a growing willingness to make connections in the whole of life. Practising an *āsana* is therefore not to be banished solely into silent chambers or placed in the solitary site of a monastery, it is much more to be integrated into human encounter and communication and should also be informed through reciprocal reflections.

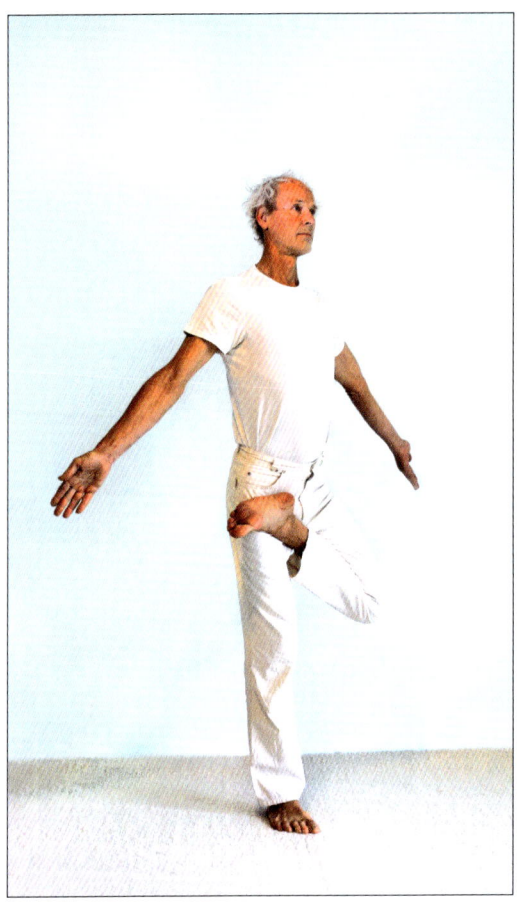

The initial dynamic phases as well as the closing phases of an *āsana* always bear the associated soul feelings.

The tree, *tāḍāsana*, both at the beginning and at the end, activates various movements with the arms.

The soul feelings of an inner centre in the heart and an open connection outwards can even be intensified in these moving phases.

Inner calm and relaxation

People usually assume that for any meditation or high level mental activity, first of all some composure and calm is needed. Although inherently this assumption is not wrong, it seems very helpful for the description that follows if the essence of inner calm and its real meaning are precisely presented in a specific and articulated way. Inner calm can be established in the best and most exemplary way when it is characterised within an entire process of natural soul-lawfulness and soul-development. Calm and relaxation develop out of a lawful course of progression.

The opposite of calmness is fear and this seizes the body, penetrates and encloses it. It is as a rule like a dark power. When we become conscious that fear and unrest are two unmistakable brothers of earthly existence, we can build up a very significant and exemplary image: Someone is in a dark room, fearfully and clumsily groping with their hands from one object to the next. A shiver floods through them as they do not know what dangers await them. But suddenly someone kindles a light and illuminates the structures of the room. At that moment, when the light illuminates the walls and objects and the sense of sight can orient itself, the breath relaxes and a natural calmness sets in.

Similarly to the way the event described in this image can be understood, the relationship of the soul to the body can now be explained. As long as human beings are thrown back onto the body and their own perception, they are in an inescapable state of tension and unrest. But if a light hastens towards them, illuminating the surroundings, the state of being constricted and thrown back onto the body recedes and the natural calm and confidence emerge.

So we can say: As soon as human perception enters into a natural and realistic relationship to an object of the external world, the bodily nature recedes slightly. The object gains the attention and with this the interest. The bodily situation can now be forgotten. People feel secure in a safe space through the illumined situation of the external world and this bestows upon them the relaxation they need.

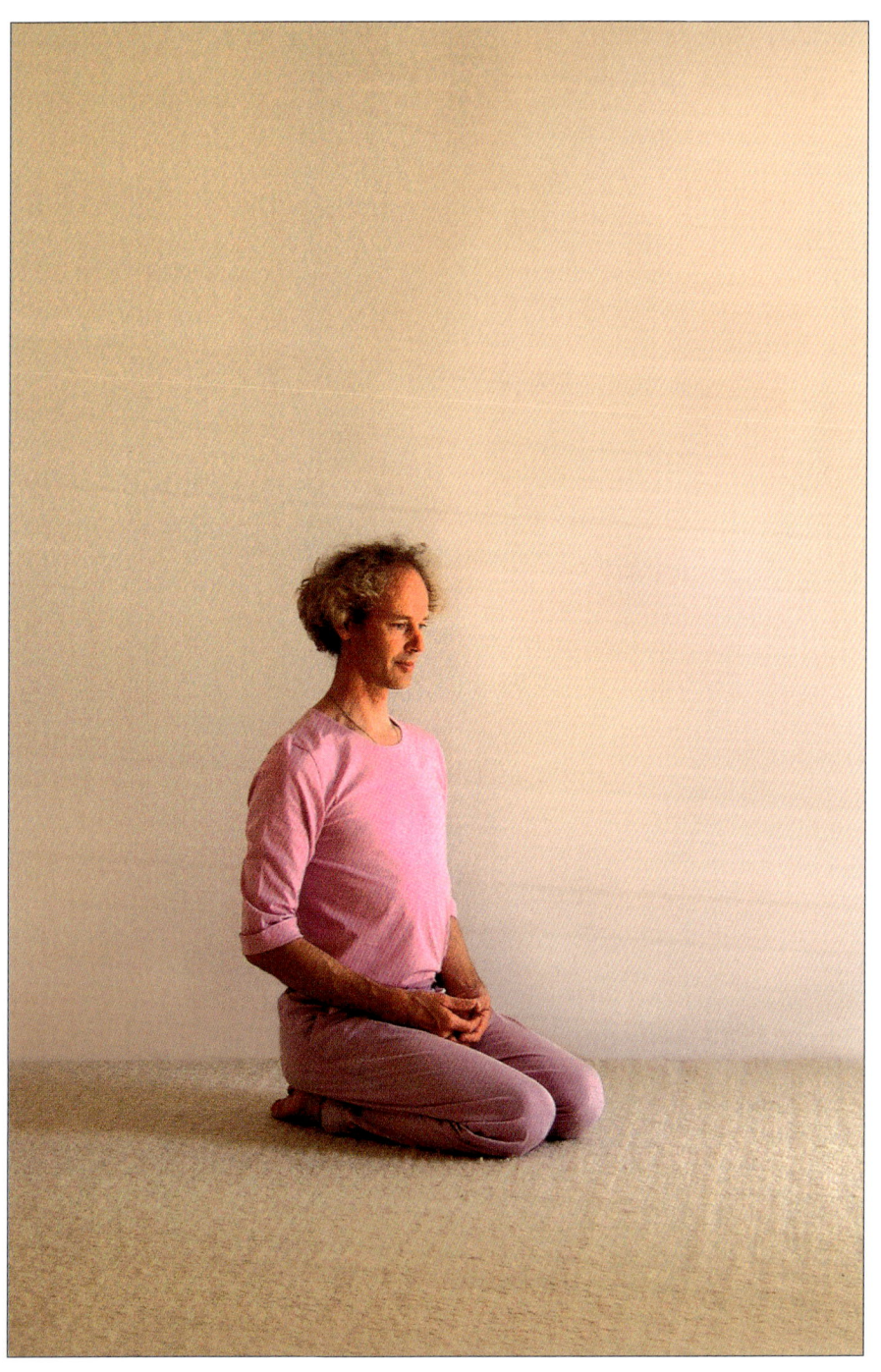

Now this comparison can be applied to the practical exercises. For this it is helpful to sit on the floor, for the sitting position on the floor, in contrast to sitting on a chair, more easily provides a natural orientation towards matter and more easily allows conscious feelings concerning the body. Sitting on the ground, practitioners feel closer to life. However, it is important to note that when they adopt the sitting position practitioners do not instantly draw back into the close feelings being set free and signalled to them by the body, but now establish a clear, thoughtful relationship to an object. The first foundational step of the practice starts with a few minutes of attention to the existing conditions and to an object that they take for contemplation. This relationship to an object may well be their own body or an object in the external surroundings or also the observation of their own thoughts and passing feelings. Preparing to mentally picture the exercises also opens up a suitable, thoughtful relationship to an object.

The sitting position should give rise to as little strain as possible. However, if it is too difficult at the beginning of the practice, practitioners can also start by lying on their back and adopting the position known as *śavāsana*, the relaxation position lying on the ground. In this position some tensions are released and the joints and muscles can relax. However, it is important that this position is not experienced passively as a resting position, but rather that practitioners endeavour to achieve a clear relationship to an object.

In this relaxation position the body rests flat on the floor, the hands face upwards, the eyes are closed, the consciousness is directed to the individual limbs of the body with alertness, observing them and experiencing them closely. Now the individual limbs, the back, the shoulders and the head can be experienced in the way they gently touch the earthly ground. The consciousness experiences the individual parts of the body with more differentiation and sensitivity. This experience of an articulation, of a loosened singling-out of the parts of the body, as if the arms, hands, legs, the head, the neck and the hips drop entirely into the state of differentiated, motionless matter, arises particularly through the fact that the position lying on the back enables maximum contact between the body and the flat ground, and the body is perceived as a material limb belonging to matter. The back itself represents an important, very sensitive region of the astral body, and when this region is noticed it enables a natural sensitivity for the whole body. Experiencing the back leads to relaxation.

However, experiencing a rhythmic sequence of mental images is also a suitable way of generating a natural calmness, as every rhythmic development of thoughts leads to an ordering within the body. So the limbs should not be experienced in a jumbled way but systematically, in sequence, for example from top to bottom, from the forehead to the back of the head and from there to the neck, then to the collar bones, the upper arms etc. This rhythmic sequence of conscious processes of perception and mental images also leads to calmness through the process of giving attention.

This form of rhythmically sequenced feeling and picturing develops out of a conscious activity. This should not be confused with auto-suggestion directed to the body. Any rhythmic, active action, connected in a natural and concrete way with an objective and imaginable reality, leads to a receding of the body and with this to calmness. When auto-suggestion is used, this activity of consciousness with a concrete relationship to an object does not occur and that is why it is not employed in this yoga.

After lying on your back, a posture in the so-called cross-legged or half-lotus pose, or most simply kneeling on your heels, is nevertheless indicated once again. A rhythmic and articulated observation can also take place in the sitting position. For example, practitioners can carry out a sequence observing either objects in the space outside themselves or perceiving their own limbs. The ordered sequence and the concrete, thought-based relationship to an object are very important for these ordering steps. Practitioners do not sink into their own world of calm, do not daydream, but maintain the mental activity and lead the consciousness in a systematic and ordered way from one image to the next.

Another possibility that deserves attention is the observation of the breath. During this yoga activity the breath is left free in its rhythm and intensity. According to whether a strenuous or a relaxing activity takes place, the free flow is always granted to the breath and so it can adapt itself to the corresponding conditions. On this basis of free breath, a natural relaxation develops more easily and the life of thought and subtle-feeling can enter into relationship to objects in a concrete way.

The thought-life is actually like a light and when the thought moves objectively into observation, the body's states of unrest recede. Practitioners become conscious that their active thought-life always works back onto the body and also onto the life energies. They now become conscious of this and recognise in this way a lawfulness that exists in their life. As soon as a thought is perceived in a direction that really relates to an object, a calming, luminous process comes about, a kind of I-process, and the body recedes. This basic condition describes the fear-free and natural human self-awareness.

By establishing this all important awareness of their own thoughts through conscious observation and perception, perhaps culminating in a rhythmic ordering of these observations, practitioners of this yoga can now recognise the many other coincidental, automated and constantly fluctuating thoughts and emotions as disturbances, and through observing them allow them to come to rest. Probably at the beginning of this path, and perhaps even as it progresses, these many unconnected and unrelated ideas and impulses, which slip through the mind, will not immediately be brought to dissolve, but through specific observation they can now likewise be viewed objectively and with this rendered ineffective. This attitude of observation and relationship to an object will ultimately lead the body to calmness and prepare the consciousness for a freer activity. It can be described as *sākṣī*, the witness state.

Working at inner calm leads to a first concentration and also permeation of the thought-life with light and to a purification of held feelings. The body recedes in a first unnoticeable way. That which is essential, that which is to be aspired to, or the mental pictures to be developed, can now move in an unrestricted and pure way into the light of contemplation, and all inessential and emotional preoccupation, all everyday cares or passions recede from the stream of attention and the activity of practice.

Once, with a few minutes of preparation, practitioners have adopted this attitude of concrete relationship to an object, of rhythmic ordering and of observation, *sākṣī*, there follows the first practical step of shaping an exercise. While carrying out the exercise, vivid feelings and perceptions can be allowed amidst the observation, but it is important that the consciousness does not slip in or down into the so-called inner world, and with this into the bodily feelings. Although it is more difficult to retain a certain degree of freedom from the pleasant feelings, which very quickly set in in the yoga exercises, and therefore to hold the consciousness in an objective and

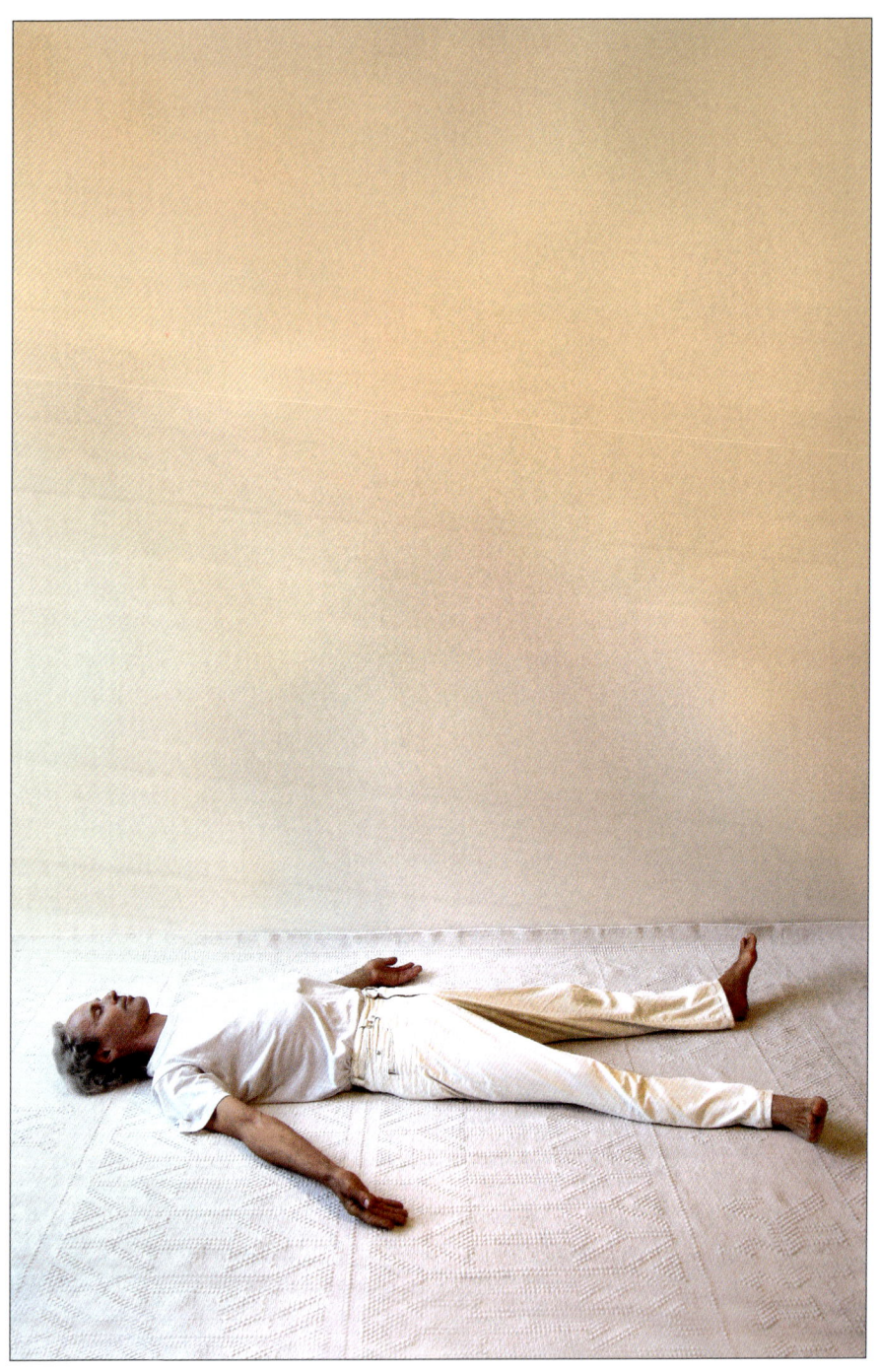

concrete relationship to reality, it is now nevertheless in the long term a great advantage, as on this basis the forces of the personality are strengthened and the soul's true forms of relationship develop.

The development of the soul-life takes place in three steps

1. An alert and actively held perception in relation to an object or theme is always the initial step.

2. From this a subtle-feeling develops, giving calmness, and enriching the life of the soul in a sensitive and pleasant way.

3. Active implementation finally follows on from the mental picture, and the exercises activate the further development of subtle-feelings for the chosen theme.

Shaping life with content
anāhata-cakra

The first exercise recommended, aims to develop a feeling that the heart represents the centre of the feeling of self. This focus on the heart centre happens through conscious, productive work of shaping the exercise with content within the practice. It is not what individuals take from the exercise, what they can gain for themselves from the exercise, but rather the strengths, the attention, the dedication and the content-filled consciousness that is put into the exercise, which comes towards them as success and ultimately also as the true force of the heart. Just as the sun cannot obtain its light from the earth, but sends out its rays unconditionally, independently and unreservedly, in the same way the consciousness should become conscious itself of the productively active process of shaping and working, and see in this the required step. The success of the practice, the outcome to be obtained, results from assigning the exercise itself its ordered place. Fire represents the I, it is the uppermost element and it leads to the ordering of the other elements as well. There are three limbs that should come to develop equally in the practice of shaping with content. These are active thinking, which should flow together harmoniously with the sensory processes and with perceptions. From this ordered synthesis, ultimately a pictorial experience of one's own body and of the world should result. To calmly experience a picture would neither be possible without thinking nor without perception. It is an expression of heart-feeling. With patience, calm and a natural, expectant hope, the most astonishing and beautiful experiences soon open up, and ultimately enrich the life of the soul from above, or from the spirit. The results are like the most subtle and unnoticeable constructs, which form an etheric heart [8] and are bestowed upon practitioners, but cannot be forced or claimed.

For all exercises, and quite particularly for the exercises to develop a conscious heart centre, practitioners direct their attention to a theme or to a thematic connection. For example, using the text they have read, they develop a mental picture that is as authentic as possible, and bring this picture into the practical exercises, or they direct their attention to a specific part of the body, observe this part, explore its connections, and in this way they get to know for themselves the feelings that are developing. At no stage should students lose the independence of their consciousness; they are always present in their work on the theme, and involved in the process of shaping forms, and through this they order their thoughts and feelings in accordance with the theme and the evolving processes.

Although a silent stillness, a deep contemplation, an absolute calmness are important for the free and new experiencing that opens up in an exercise, nevertheless the aim of practice is not to immerse oneself in this calmness as if mystically, maybe even to fall into a trance, or to savour these rapid feelings of mystical experience and see them as the benchmark for the state of awareness to be attained. What is far more significant, and transcends the calmness, is the aesthetic shaping of a higher sense through the exercise. The thought that exists in the mental picture should develop in the *āsana* through the right kind of self expression and should create itself into a work of art. The calmness that can be observed serves this heightened work of mental picturing and the awareness of subtle-feelings. In this way, the experiencing becomes a sun-like shaping-force, and individuals experience a link from their thinking to their feeling and finally, on this basis, a close connection to their own body again. It is order. The body is harmoniously experienced in the direct field of expression of the thoughts and subtle-feelings. This harmonious experiencing corresponds to a sun-like consciousness, which is expressed in the middle of the heart as a still feeling of self.

The discipline of the consciousness that brings about the unfolding of the heart centre can be summarised as follows: It is not a method of mystical immersion, not an emotional, rapidly achieved feeling of unity with God, humanity and the world that should be the benchmark for development, but rather an animated, theme-related, mental, ordered exploration, which does not suppress the thought but even trains the thinking and brings it to life in the theme, and from this thinking experiences the divine wisdom of creation. This exploration is what leads to the true feelings of the heart. This process of activation in the theme through the thinking, not by intellectualising but through animated, thought-centred, spiritualised and pictorial thinking, bestows a process of being born anew in the etheric heart. With this unfolding of a so-called spiritual-mental discipline, students experience the love of the creative spirit as a centre of feeling-of-self within them.

Exercises for experiencing the spine pictorially
pārśva parivṛtta trikoṇāsana

The limbs, in comparison with the spine, are the younger or more subtle parts of the anatomy. They are situated at the periphery, while the spine forms the centre or the personal axis of self. The limbs are geared towards possibilities for expansion, while the spine has only limited potential for movement and its task is geared more towards stability and centring. This spine is the product of many streams of thought and ways of feeling. The vertebra itself is the archetype of bone, a typical picture of something solid. The spine is the most compact, solid part of the body and so it also symbolises the being of self in mortal life, or being placed into mortal life. Through the fact that the spine can now be experienced pictorially from above to below and from outside inwards, people experience themselves as being formed by the thought and anchored in the will.

Experiencing the spine pictorially bestows a natural ordering and calm. The body can be experienced as a pictorial imprint of a greater process when the natural perception through the senses is combined harmoniously with a thought or concept. Those who experience the body as a picture, have a notion that this body is the product of a soul-spiritual process and thus the body represents the end and not the beginning. A natural calmness and centring in the heart can result from this initial closely felt insight.

In the four short exercise cycles that follow, the spine is experienced in its own dynamic potential, and in its inherent, central, stabilising function for the body. In particular, the upper section of the thoracic spine should find its way into a first gentle activity. With light arms, shoulders and neck relaxed, practitioners lift themselves up either into a twist or into a natural, straight line, and then in the final stage they become calm. In so doing they feel both centrifugal and centripetal forces acting in the middle of their body. The consciousness, which is perceiving the spine, acts from above to below, and the will-activity acts from below to above. With light breath, the limbs and upper body rise almost like the air itself.

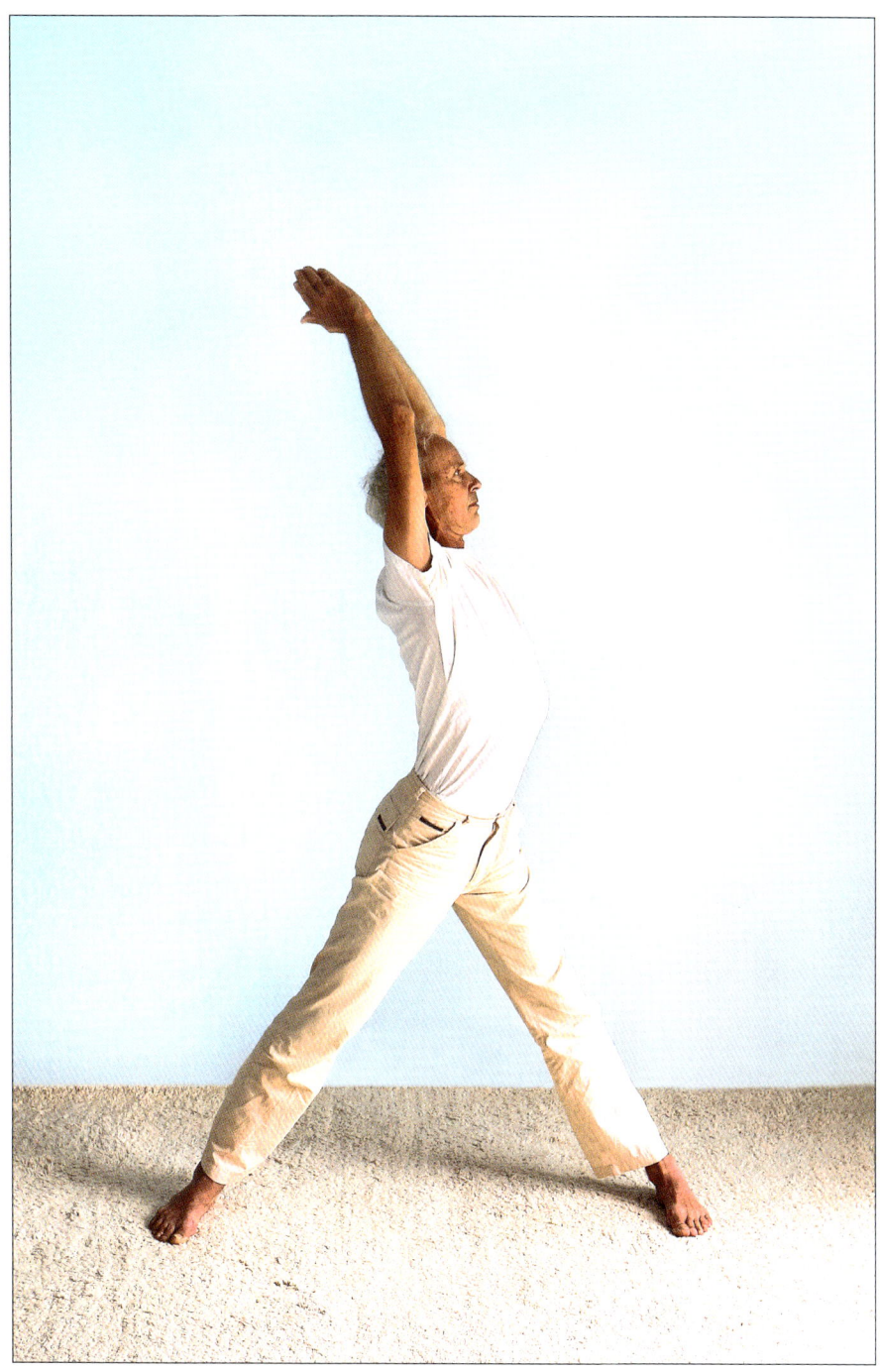

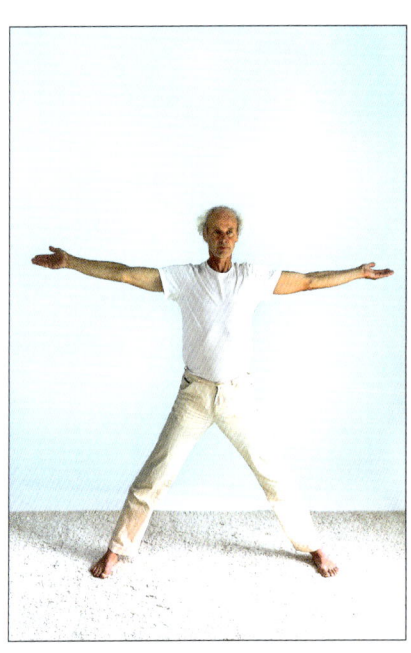

1ˢᵗ cycle

The positions start with a harmonious triangular base. Take your arms wide out to the sides and even stretch your shoulder-blades outwards in this lateral position. The collar-bones and the uppermost thoracic spine are lifted lightly upwards right from the start. Always breathe in a free and easy rhythm. By opening the palms of the hands upwards, the impulse to lift the chest almost seems to happen automatically.

Then, while gently lifting your spine, take your arms up until the hands meet. Your eyes look upwards and experience the vertical line that ascends right up to the fingertips. Hold this position for half a minute and then return again with a lightness in the arm movement. The act of feeling the spine as the central axis moves into your awareness, and the lifting gesture promotes an initial dynamic in the thoracic spine. Through feeling the lifted spine, a perception of self comes about, which is an expression for the heart centre.

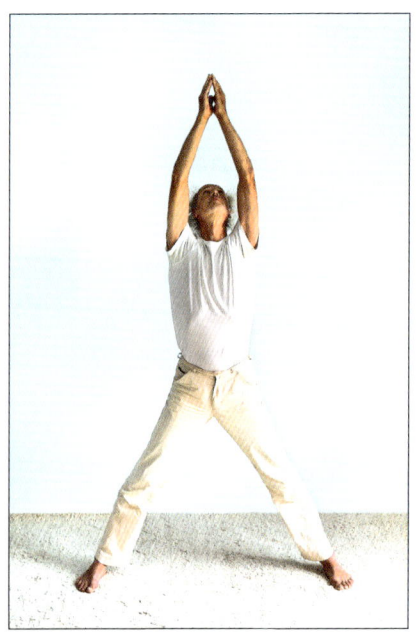

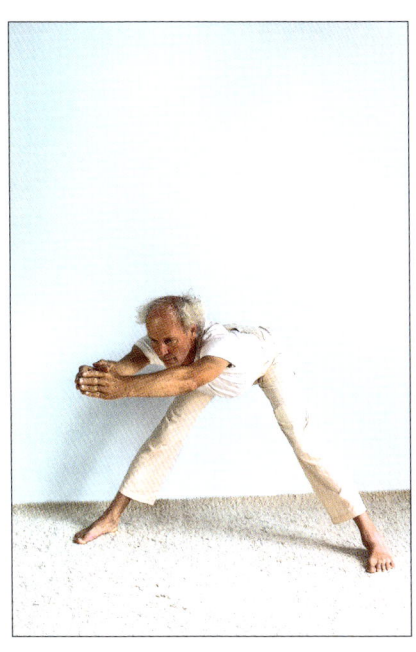

2nd cycle

Once again the triangular base is adopted. In a fluid movement, the upper body glides out forwards horizontally and the thoracic spine experiences quite a powerful pull. Move round to the left over your left leg. Relax your neck throughout the movement. Observing the movement stretched horizontally out in front gives the feeling of a pulling force that approaches the body from the outside.

Because this movement demands a relatively great amount of physical effort and precise contraction in the upper back, it is particularly important not to tense up the breath, but to let it flow so that it is freely available. After holding the final position for a few seconds, return to the middle again and repeat the exercise on the other side. At the end the body straightens up in the middle (see p. 116). The attention should be directed once again to the upper spine.

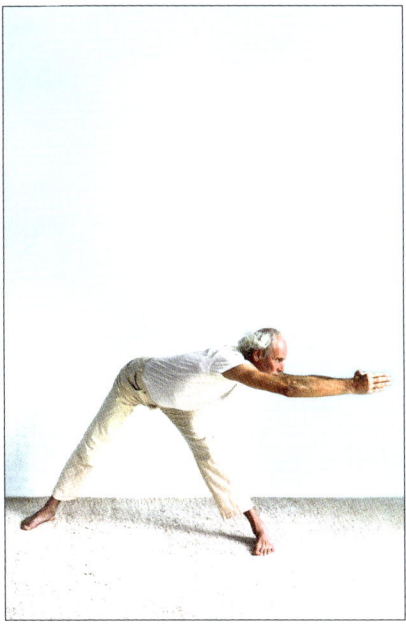

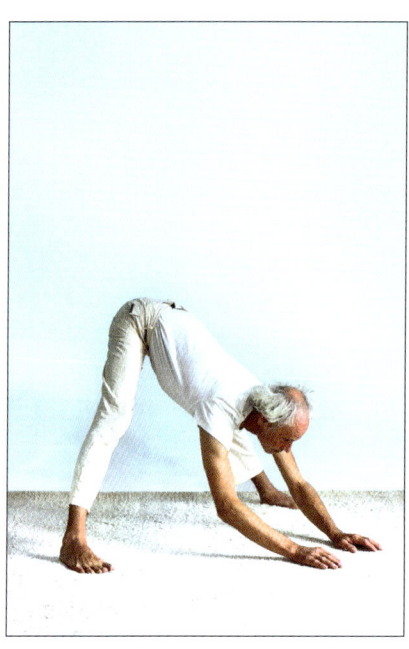

3rd cycle

Glide forwards towards the ground with your upper body and let the breath flow completely freely. In this initial stage of the exercise the back, shoulders, neck and face should remain naturally composed and relaxed. A strong stretch should never be forced at the beginning of this cycle. The body seems to glide out forwards as if out of itself.

Now rise up fluidly, as if in a big breath, letting the neck relax again and lifting the thoracic spine farther and farther up, until it curves backwards slightly, through its length. The lower back should not sink into a lordosis and should under no circumstances be painful. The lifting happens exactly from the middle of the spine upwards. The position is held with this dynamic of the upper back and at the same time with the stable base of the triangle for about ten seconds. After returning a kind of centred flowing can be experienced in the upper spine.

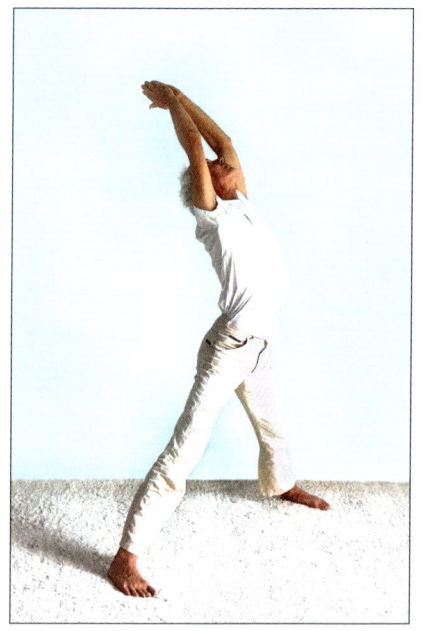

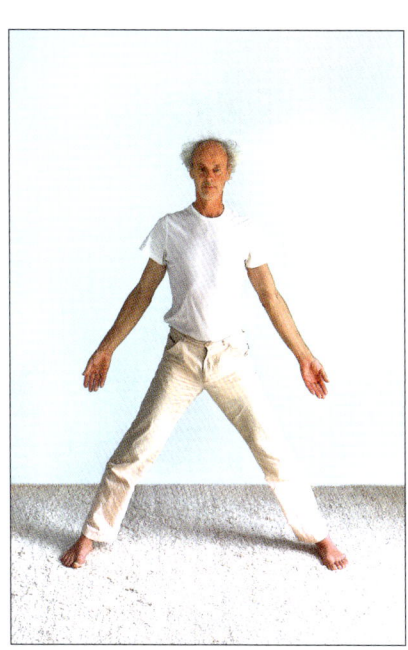

4th cycle

Once again the exercise starts in the triangular base with relaxed arms and shoulders. In a wide movement the arms are raised up and the body twists immediately to the left until a half-moon shape is eventually formed with the back and arms. Once again the thoracic spine is in an active dynamic. Weight is taken off the lower back through the lifting and shaping gesture of the upper body.

After holding the end position for about fifteen seconds, the arms are brought back down. The movement is then practised on the other side. Each of these individual short cycles can be practised on its own a few times. The freely flowing breath, combined with the centred dynamic in the thoracic spine, and the alert awareness of the different distributions of tension, promote a natural flowing of energy from above downwards and from below upwards, which penetrates in the form of a sensitive and alert centred-feeling of the heart and thyroid region. It is a relatively large and stretched out form that is achieved with the short cycle. Practitioners experience themselves wide open in the space.

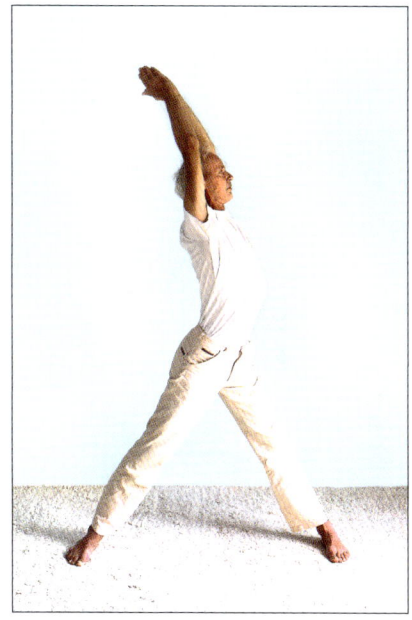

The tip-toe pose
pādāṅguṣṭhāsana

The picture and the meaning of the exercise

Balance is a symbol for harmony between an upper and lower pole, and for equilibrium between extreme opposites like joy and sorrow, success and failure, hope and despair, and so on. The heart is the organ hallmarked by contented equilibrium in earthly existence. However, the heart is not a static place that would always keep the same position once a mid-point and a harmony had been found. The heart constantly wants to experience a new building-up of ether, as during the different, active processes of unfolding it wants to attain an increased inner feeling of self and awareness of an I. Therefore constant, progressive processes of development are needed so that the heart can be built in its sun-radiant and harmonious force and healthily represents the human feeling of self. In the heart there lives the personality's healthy feeling of self. Balancing exercises represent a contemplative pause to build up calmness in the heart.

This building-up in the heart centre can be facilitated by a vivid experience of this centre's connection with the spine, which wants to be experienced in the region of the back. The heart, actively unfolded, grants a released thoracic spine, and this in turn grants a feeling of inherent uprightness with concurrently persisting inwardness and a first feeling of independence from external influences. The feeling of a long back is identical to a lifeful, burgeoning, virgin feeling of self. This virgin feeling comes from subtly feeling that through the thought, a constant, etheric building-up takes place in the heart.

The building-up causes the establishment in the so-called etheric body of a first feeling of self. It promotes a naturally close subtle-feeling towards one's own body or towards one's own feelings. It is in feeling the gracefulness of this building-up that this exercise has its meaning.

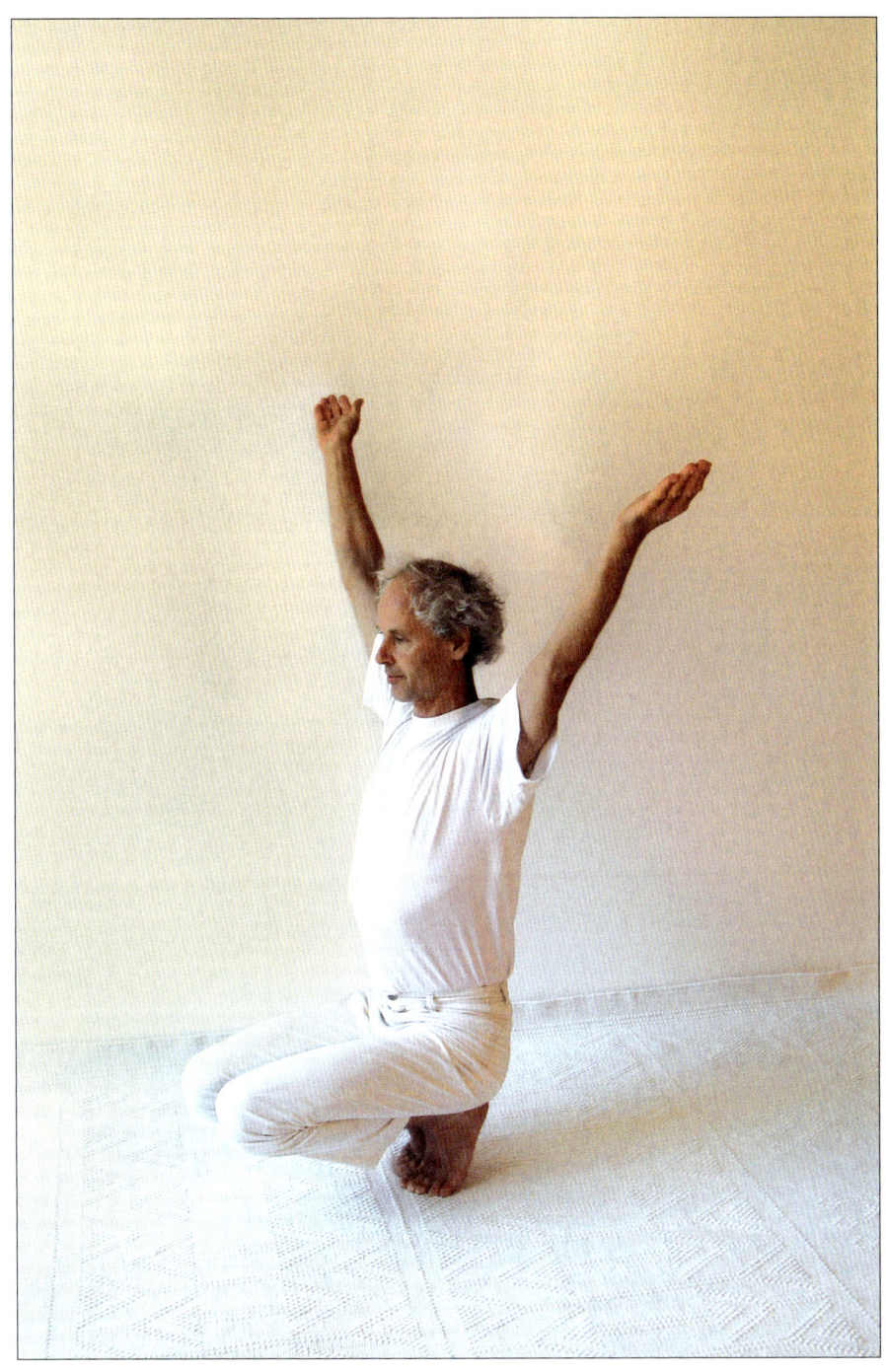

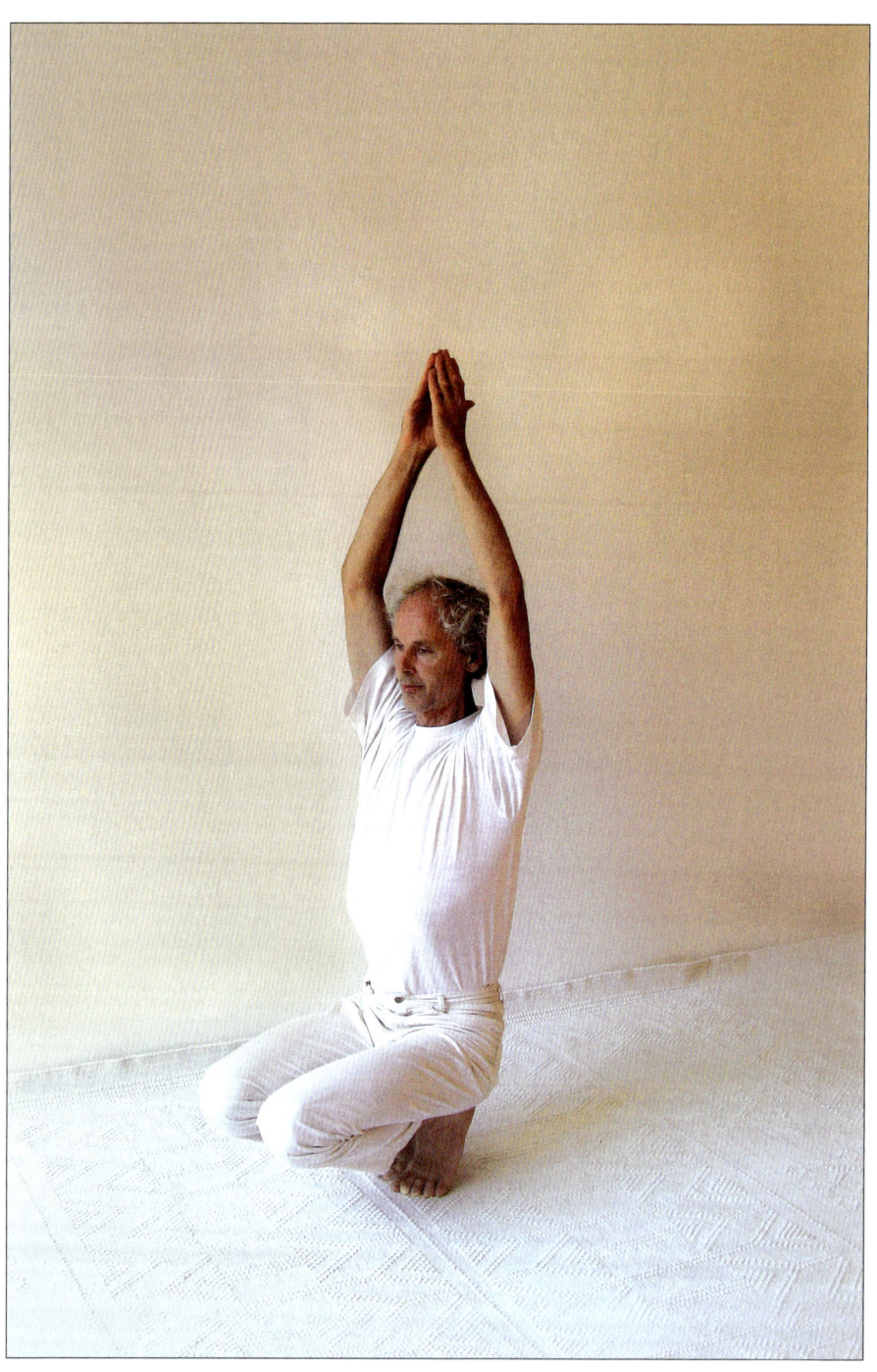

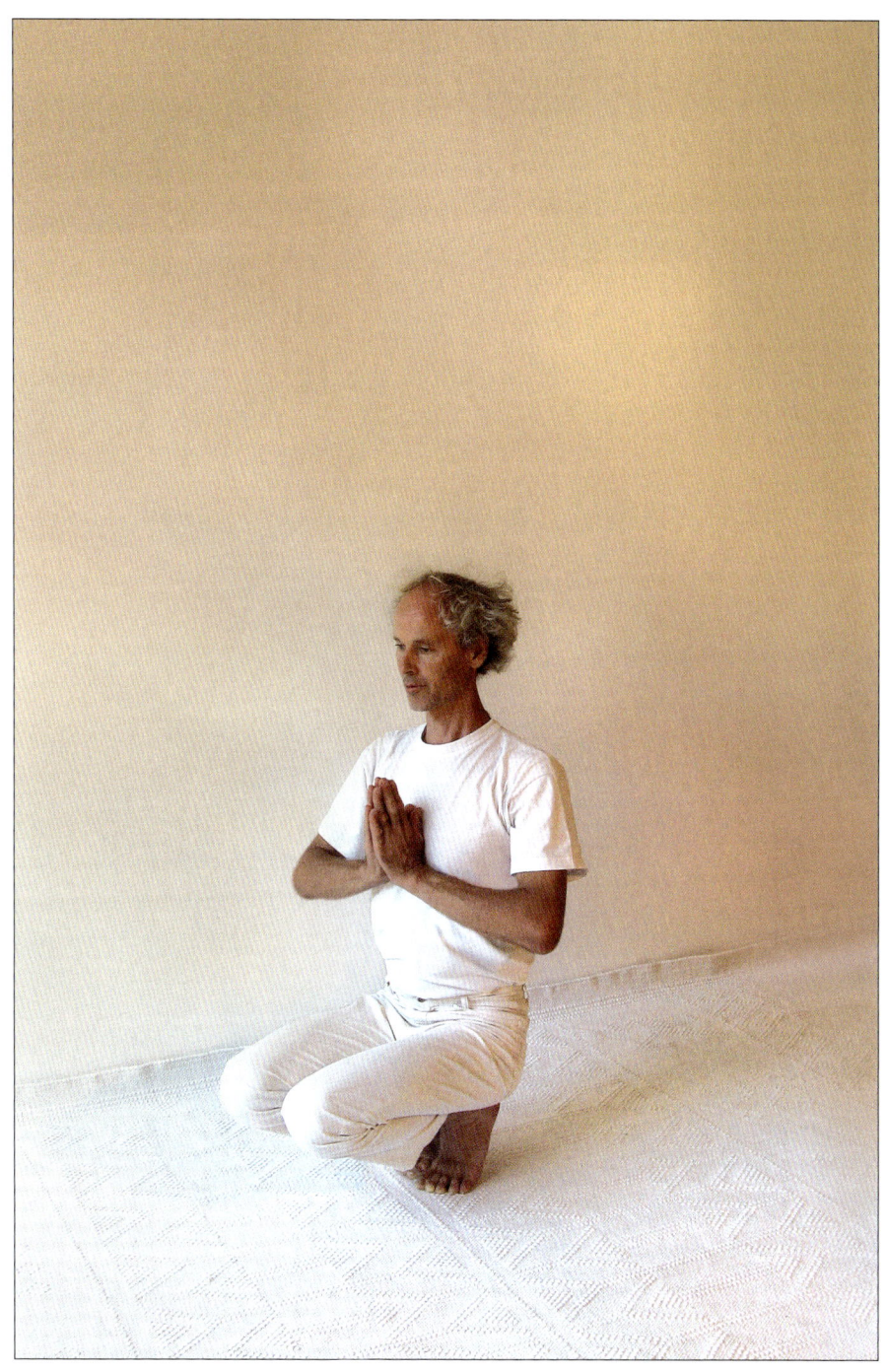

To practise

With closed legs, come onto your toes in a squatting position. Straighten your spine gently and vertically upwards. To start with your arms and hands point down towards the floor. They can be used to keep your balance. The head is also included in the vertical line of the spine. Relax your shoulders.

Now the hands begin to leave the floor and the body remains in a calm, sensitive balance on the toes. The arms now glide slowly up in a big movement to the sides, and in this upwardly aspiring movement the spine is experienced rising gently higher and higher. The spine is actually now experienced in a weightless, lengthening growth. It even becomes longer and a feeling of being subtly, subjectively liberated from the body opens up. Finally, the hands come together above the head and the arms are straightened up above the body. The spine remains "etherically light", vertically upright but without over-stretching.

In the last stage of the exercise the hands are lowered and form the so-called *ātmāñjali-mudrā* at the heart, the gesture of unification. The centre in the heart is experienced along with the upright spine. A sensitive influence of the surrounding space is noticeable.

During the exercise, pay attention to the vertical line of the spine, which can only be achieved in the squatting balance if the knees are directed forwards, closed, and the thighs are exactly horizontal. The thought that is thought builds the ether within.

Experiencing the upright spine, and at the same time maintaining the calm balance, gives a feeling of inwardness and linked to this a pleasant sensing of self, located in the heart. This is an etheric sensing of the heart, and it gathers and centres a free view, forming a sensitive counterpart to the thinking and the outer emotions that clothe the space. This act of sensitively feeling, in awareness of a counterpart of thoughts in the space, represents a feeling of self, or an I.

The tip-toe pose is performed in an ordered and inwardly experienced sequence of movements. While turning to their own bodies with a pictorial perception and, however, at the same time maintaining an alert consciousness for what is external, there arises for those practising a natural perception of outside and inside. This is usually experienced as calmness. At this point, however, it is also worth mentioning that every exercise completed not only has an effect for one's own personal life, but beyond the personal realm it releases an effect into the surroundings and towards others. This radiating aspect of the effect seems very difficult to observe, as it can only become experienced through super-sensory perception. An impartial observer can certainly establish that an exercise practised in a pleasant way emanates calm or grace outwards. The effect of the tip-toe pose in the external surroundings is very sensitive and ordering. Outside, metrical structures develop, like a square. However, this square does not just remain a square, but builds itself more and more, via an octagon to a sixteen-sided and eventually to a many-sided form. This gives a sense of how the astral world outside reacts with metrical forms to the successful practice of a pose like *pādāṅguṣṭhāsana*.[9]

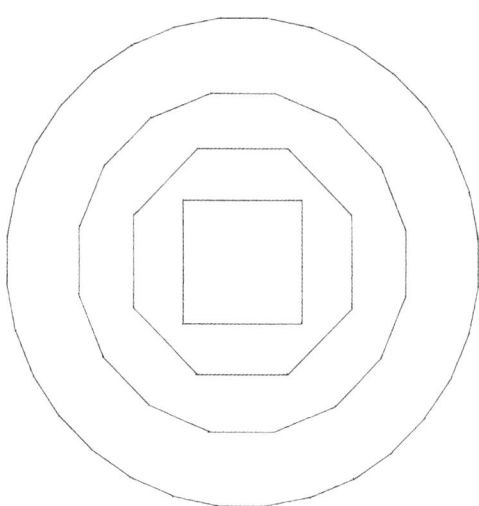

The tree
tāḍāsana

The picture and meaning of the exercise

In *tāḍāsana*[10] practitioners stand balancing on one leg and bend the other leg into the groin in half lotus. They are upright with the head held high and they also experience themselves in this state of standing upright. The eyes are open during the exercise and keep watchful control over the balance. The exercise points to the human sense of the I, which exists precisely through being upright in standing. However, this standing is not fixed, static or unshakeable; it is a standing which, through control in respect of the outside world, must constantly be held vertical. While practising the exercise, practitioners should not sink into a dream, they should not close their eyes, but must remain alert to the spacial dimensions. The I is performing its role when practitioners continue to remain watchful, ordering and adjusting within their state of relationship, and leave spaces for development open. The experience of actively performing this role of the I is the meaning of the exercise.

At the same time, practitioners experience the meaning that a first, simple form of concentration has for the soul. In the usual kind of everyday awareness, the senses brush past the objects of the outside world, jumping around without control or content, as if lost. Because of this superficial state of everyday attentiveness, people no longer experience the value of adopting an independent relationship towards the world. This general state of openness is represented by the wide-spread arms in the preliminary stage of the exercise. But then the consciousness takes a more centred form, the body holds the balance and the arms and hands move to the middle, gesturing composure and awareness, and form a centre in its own right, an I.

Moreover, the tree is one of the most excellent exercises to demonstrate the experience of time and its effect on the ether that is centring and forming within. The body and one's whole personal nature are a product of the course of time; for example, youth produces a different visible character from old age. In the tree, practitioners now experience, for a moment, time as the always present reality, which flows into the ether of the inner realm and of the heart.

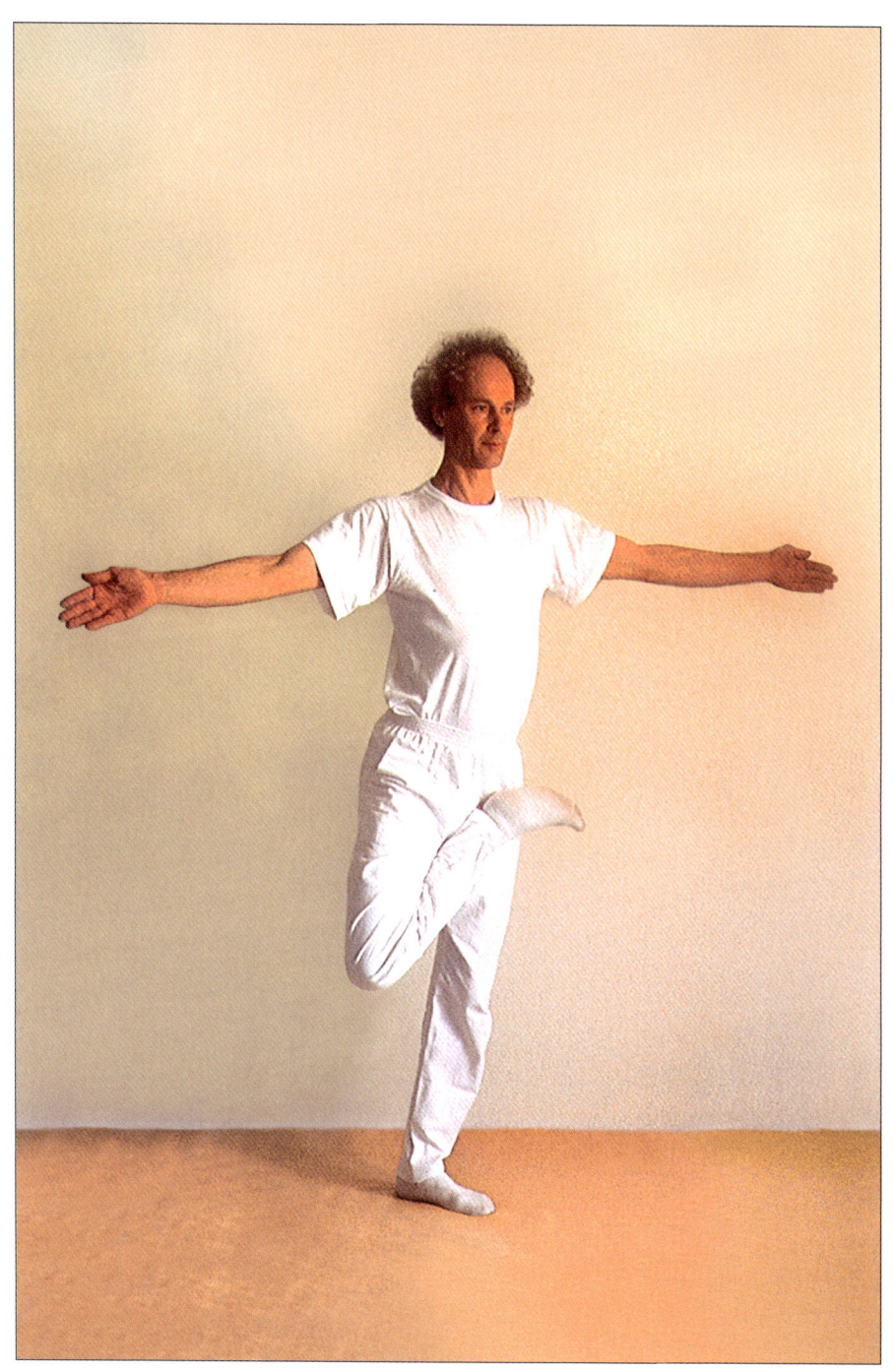

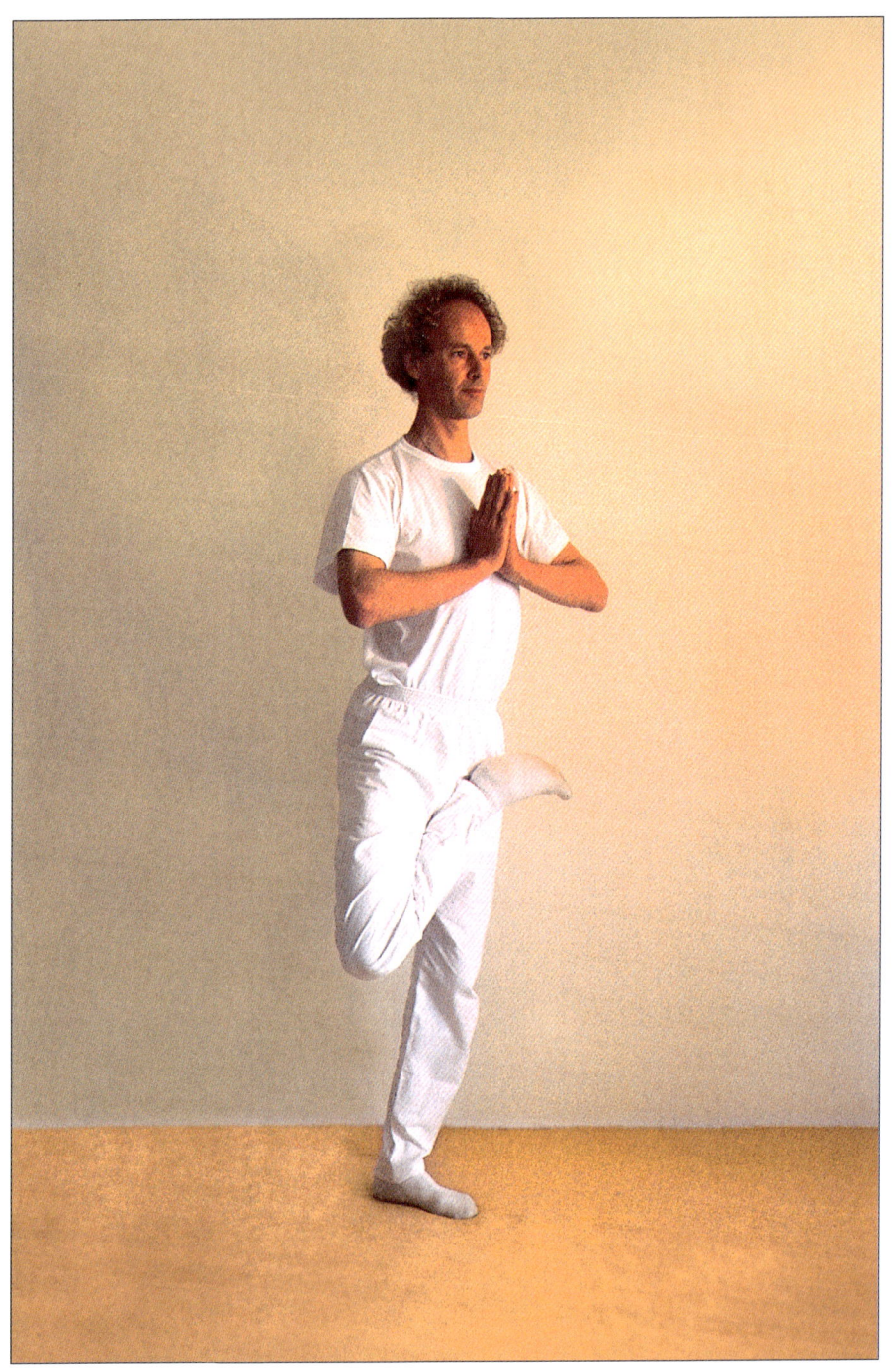

To practise

Stand with your left foot firmly on the ground and bend the right foot into the groin so that you are then balancing on one leg. You can place the right foot lower down if this is easier for you. What matters is that you adopt a balancing position on one leg. Relax the shoulders, straighten up your back harmoniously, and take your arms right out to the sides so that you sense the feeling of "being watchfully integrated into the space around you" (picture p. 127). Then bring your hands together at heart level to *ātmāñjali-mudrā*, forming a closed posture. Remain for about a minute in this standing position with open eyes and an awareness of the body's uprightness. Breathe freely, gently and observe the heart region. The heart is the organ of inner balance between above and below, between left and right. Then change legs to the other side.

The tree can best be combined with the St Andrews cross, as both exercises demonstrate a very similar theme and complement each other. With these exercises both the thought and also the faculty of perception are present with particular consciousness. Through the meeting process between perception and thought, the body is experienced pictorially. This pictorial experience opens up the sense of calm in the body and gives a notion of spiritual, acting surroundings.

An advanced variation can be developed from the tree by stretching the arms up, then coming down into the forward bend, and finally bending the standing leg to balance in the difficult tip-toe pose on one leg. Then take your hands in front of your heart again and hold the balance for a few seconds.

A particularly pleasant experience is opened up when this position is led back in the same way to the starting position of the tree. Straightening up into the standing position encourages the ability to perceive the centredness in the back while carefully maintaining awareness of the surrounding space. The outer space of thought always becomes an inner space of balance and this forms the I in the human being.

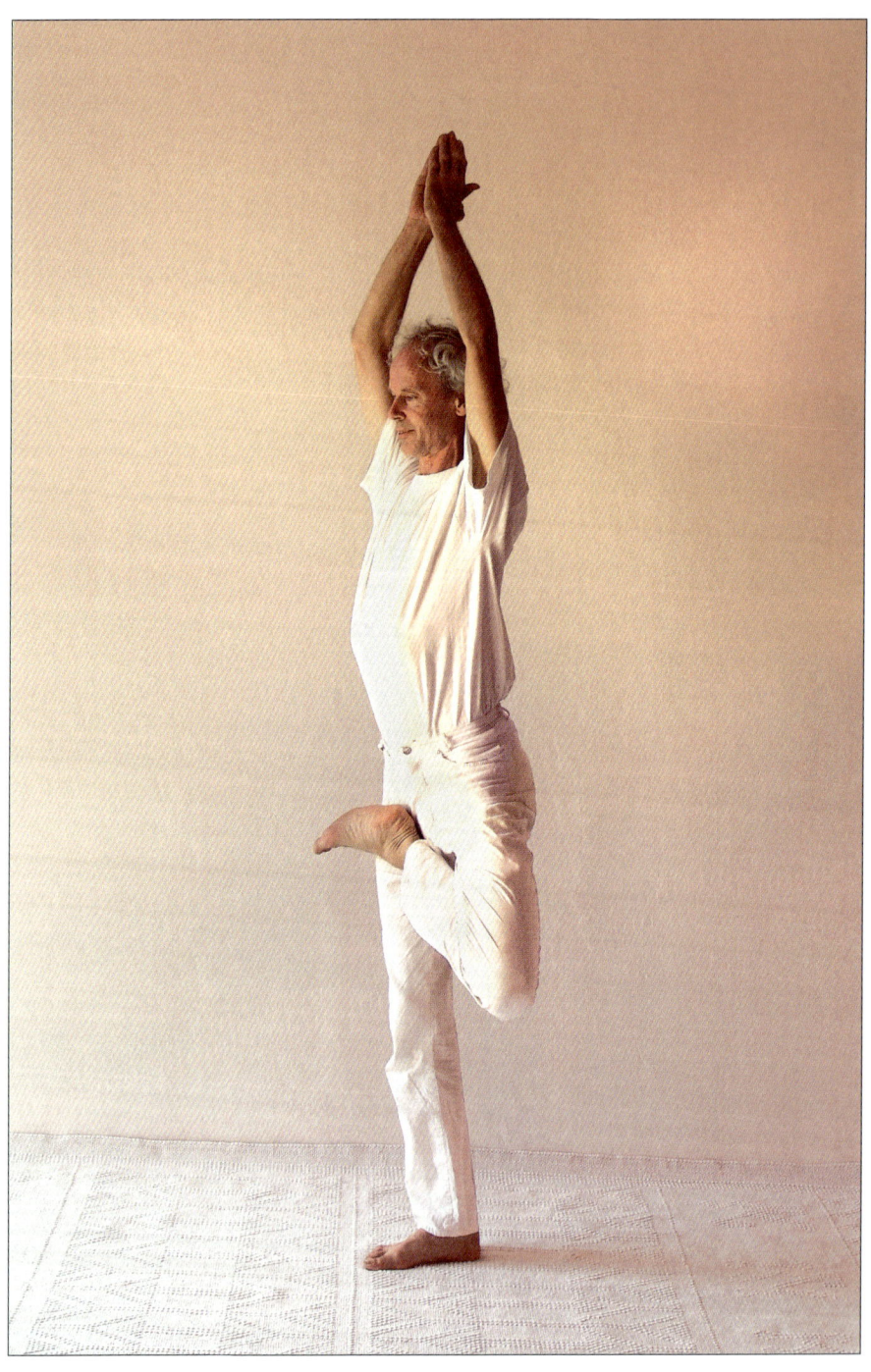

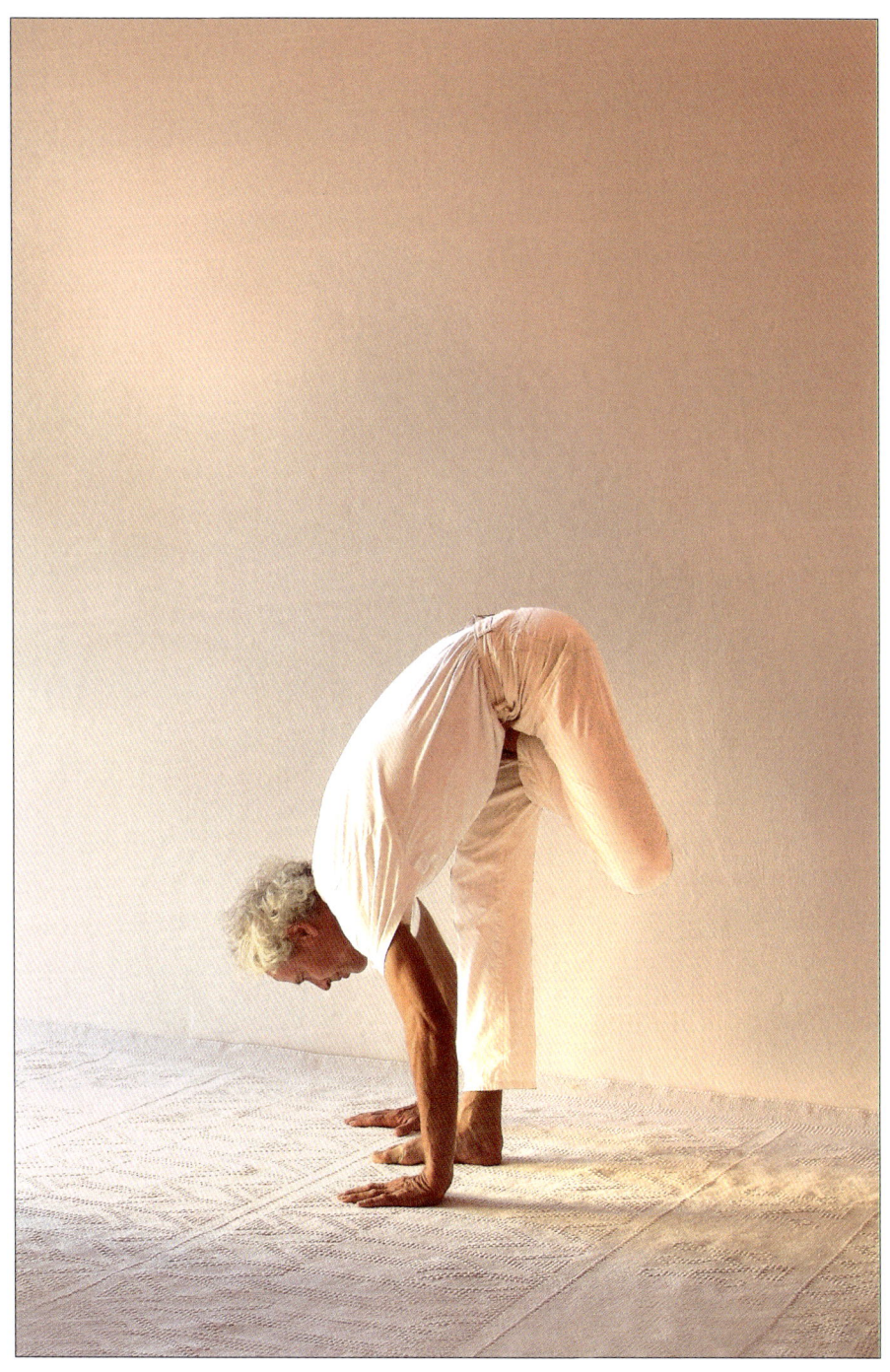

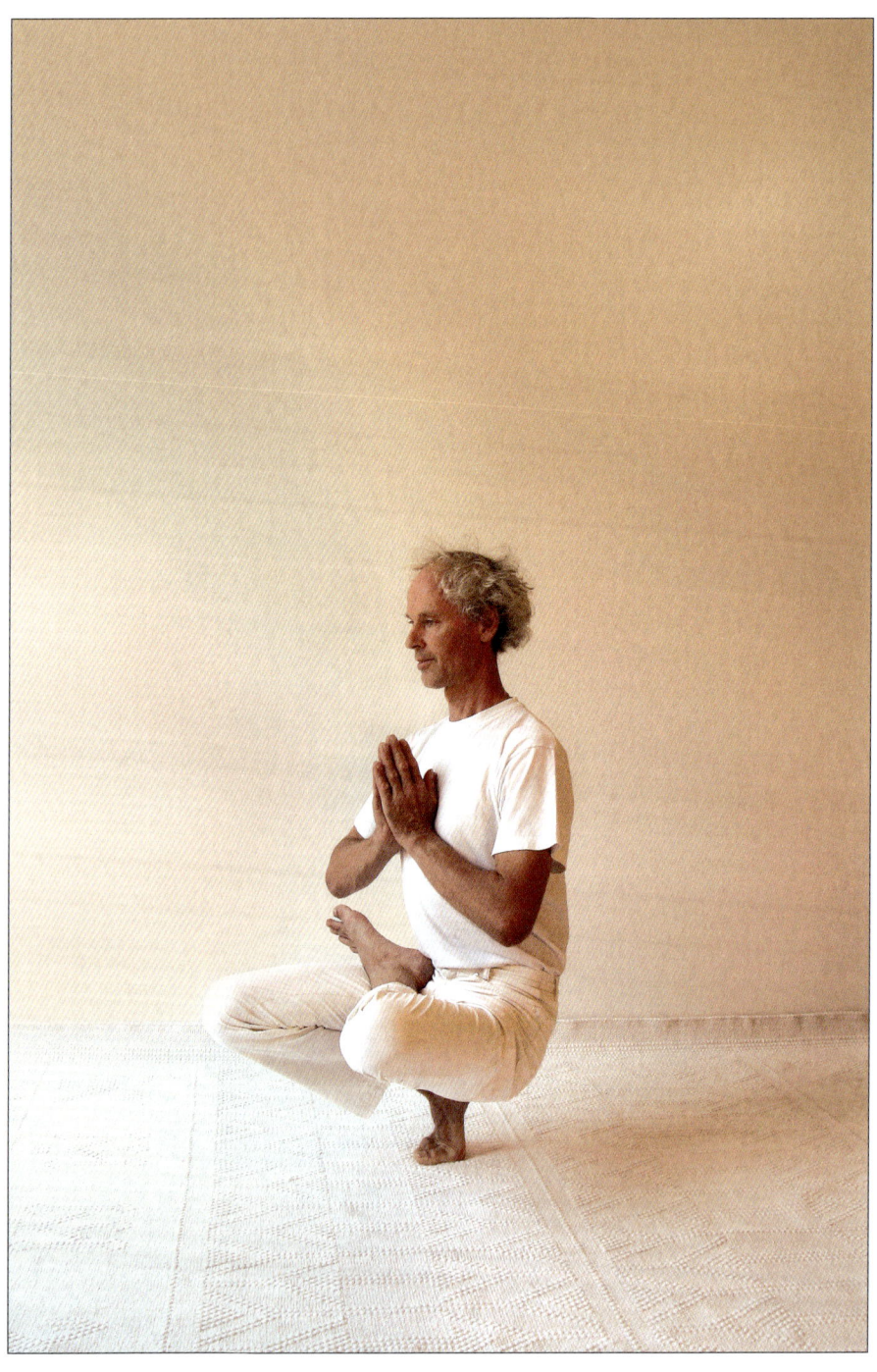

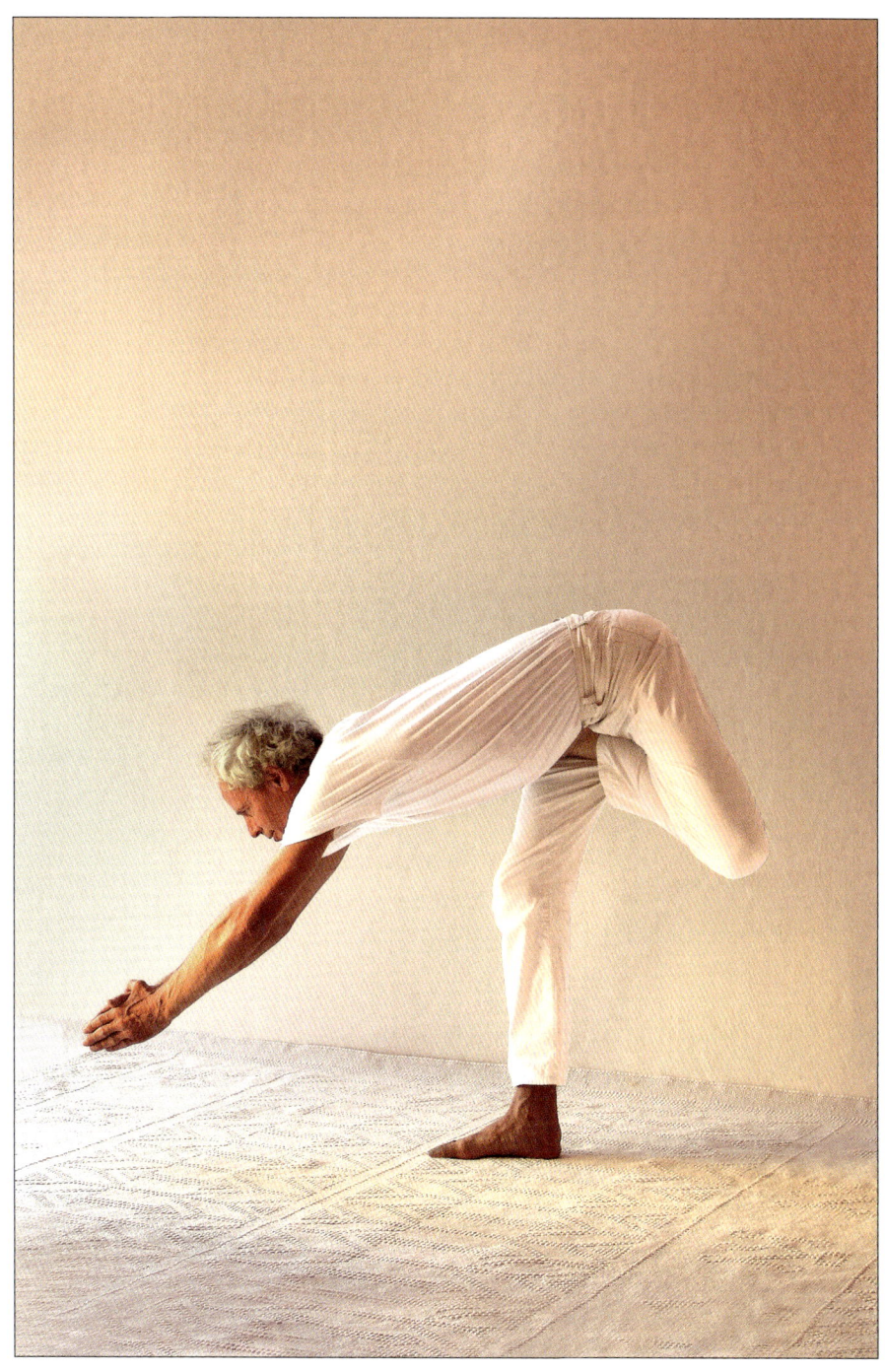

The St Andrew's cross
saṁdhisthāna

The picture and the meaning of the exercise

In a way similar to the tree, with this exercise there is an experience of space outwardly and space inwardly. The space outside, that means the milieu, the surrounding atmosphere, the forces or influences from the surroundings, determine our inner state, while our inner state also exerts an influence back onto the outer surroundings. A feeling for the outside can be sensed pictorially through the limbs, which point into the surrounding space like sense organs. In the St Andrew's cross, individuals experience themselves initially in their own general feeling of self by producing a centring inwards through the gently receiving gesture of the arms. The arms and legs form the shape of a cross. The intersecting point of the cross is between *maṇipūra-cakra* and *anāhata-cakra*, between the third and fourth centres. These two centres become harmoniously coordinated. By experiencing the outside with the long, feeling arms, while the space atmospherically affects the inside, practitioners can dedicate themselves to the idea that all thoughts and all feelings that are thought fill the space outside, and now form a mid-point within, and thus in the etheric heart. Practitioners experience their personality in its deepest state of incarnation in the crossing point of the inner space, and they experience this as the result of various thoughts and feelings coming over them.

To practise

Stand with your feet around three-quarters of a meter apart. Raise your arms taking your hands the same distance apart. The body forms a cross. Then turn your palms to face backwards and come up onto your toes. Your attention goes calmly into the space outside and calmly back in, to the central crossing point. Picture the space around you not as merely empty, but even as being formed by existing, and actively thought, thoughts.

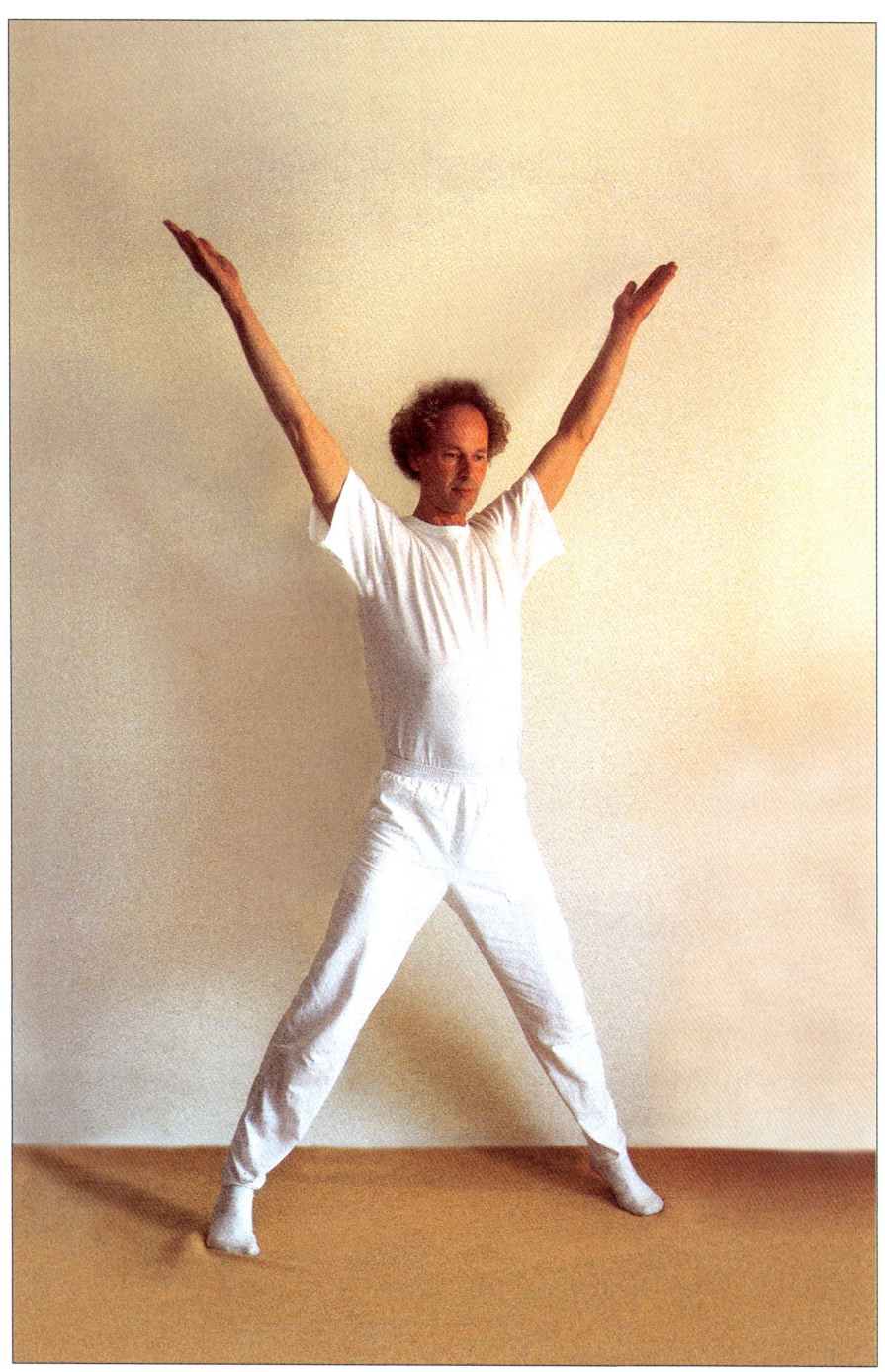

The shoulderstand
sarvāṅgāsana

The picture and the meaning of the exercise

Sarvāṅgāsana means "the pose of all parts". It is that *āsana* which has its mid-point in the heart, and from this centre it emanates centrifugally outwards into the limbs. Like a stem of corn, strong with life, the body strives dynamically against gravity into the graceful candle-like line. The image of flowing ether, flowing life-forces, out of the heart into the peripheral body is presented in a striking way in this *āsana*. The head, the shoulders and the upper arms rest on the ground during the exercise. They form the natural earthly basis for the centrifugally sprouting growth of the generative life-forces.

In this pose, less emphasis is on the strict, specified linear form, but more on the natural growing in energetic lightness out of the centre of the heart. This growth is an aesthetic gesture of the feminine element of the personality. Not the forces of the will, the outer, forceful impulses, but the invigorating ether forces with their unobtrusive, pure and joyful force of levitation give this exercise its expression. Not tension, but pictorial thinking, a relaxed dynamic, resulting in a force of growth, lead to the feminine, graceful expression of this exercise. What typifies the shoulderstand is the purity of the regenerative ether forces that meet in the heart. In the final stage the body is calmly experienced, from outside looking in, as a picture.

To practise

To do the exercise it makes sense if a few preparatory, warming exercises have already been carried out. A very good example is the plough, *halāsana*, in order to work through the whole spine and facilitate the force for uprightness in the thoracic spine. However, another preparatory exercise will also be described, which contributes to a first feeling of inwardness and perfusion through the heart centre. This preparatory exercise should be done directly before the shoulderstand.

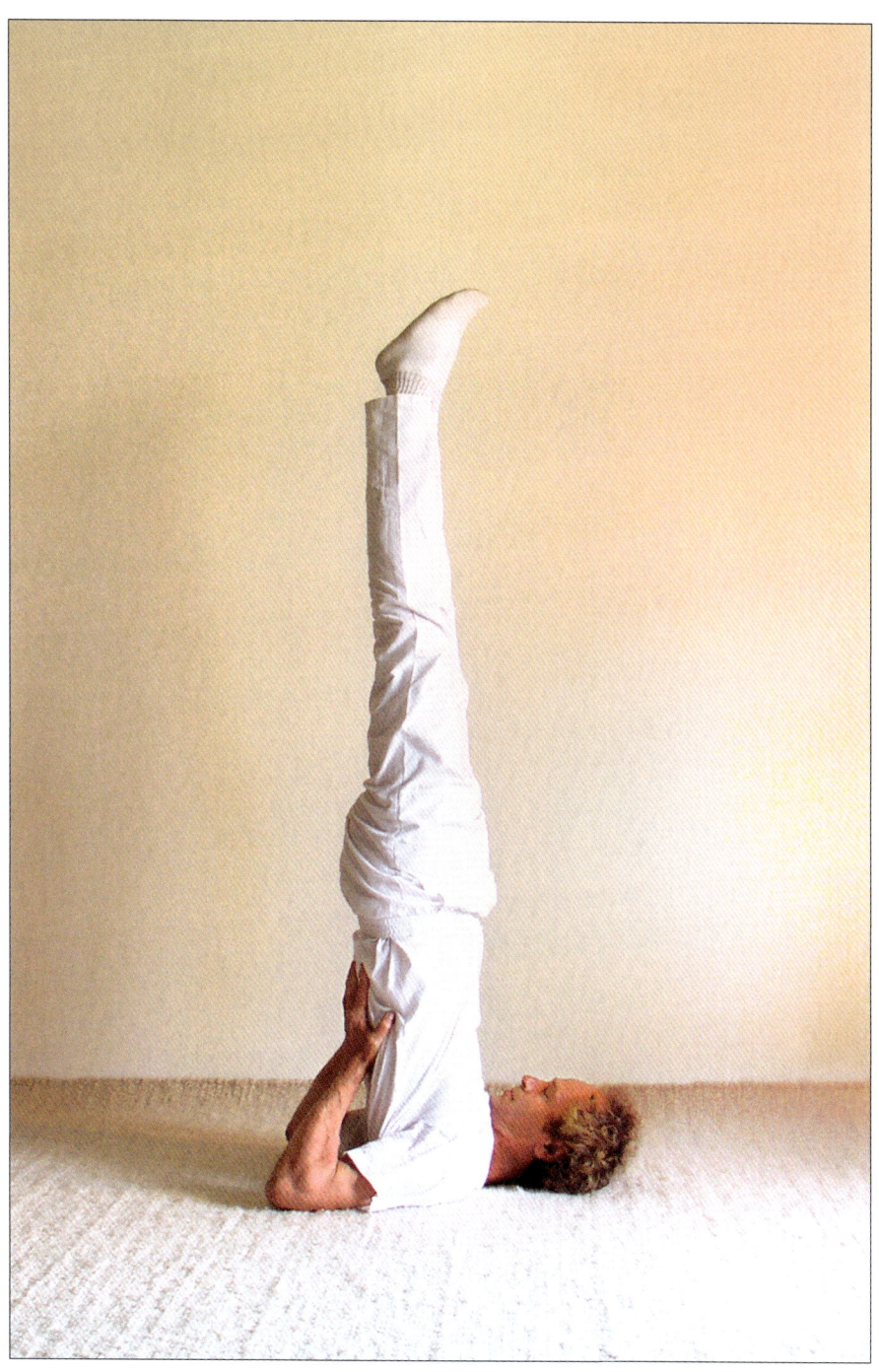

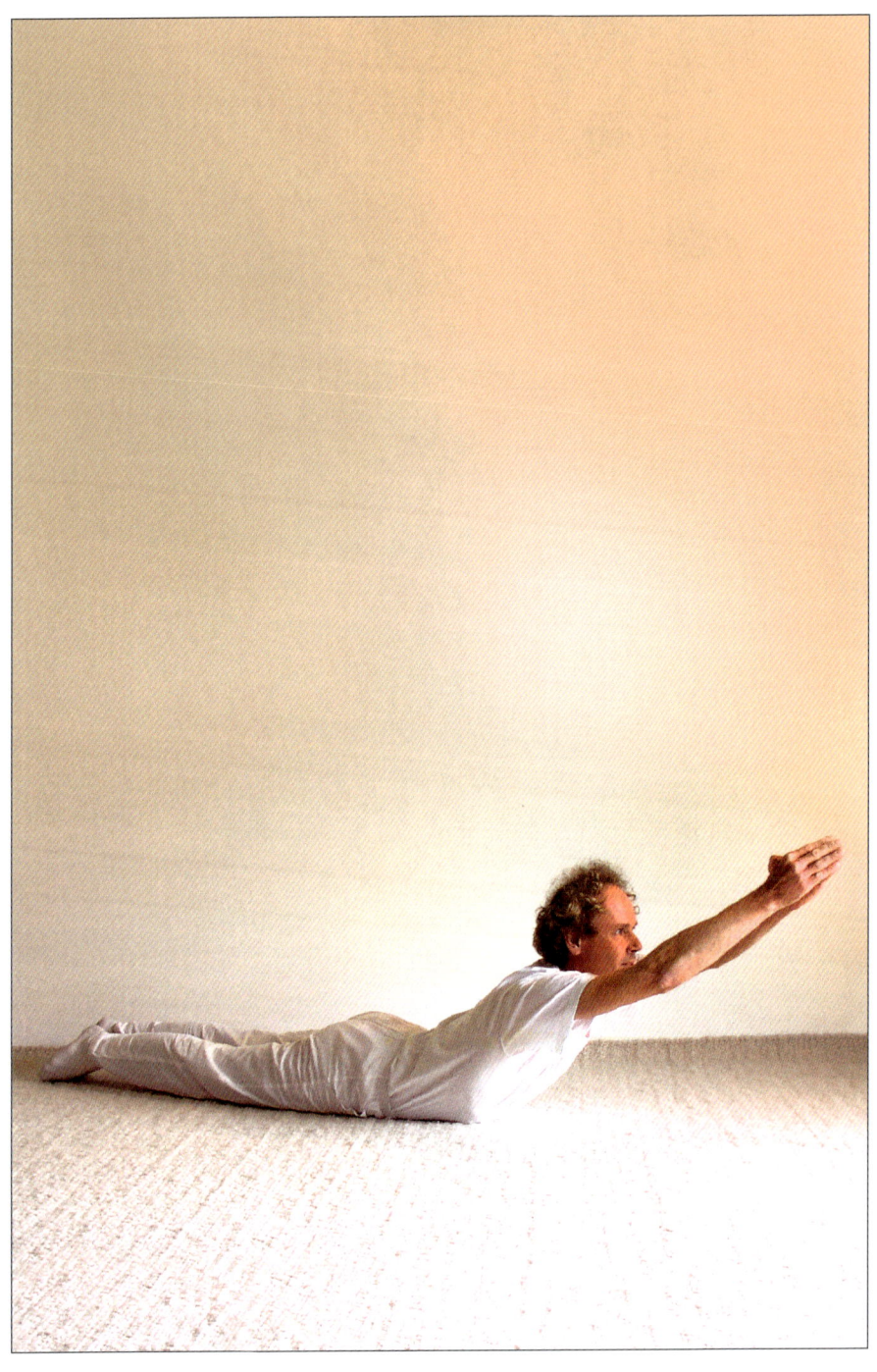

This exercise is called *utthita bhuja mukhāsana*. It is characterised by a conscious contraction of the thoracic spine, while the head and arms are lifted up off the ground against gravity. In spite of the exertion required by this position, the body should be pictorially and calmly experienced. This pictorial experiencing gives rise to a subtle process of release, and for moments practitioners usually manage to lift their upper body and arms still further. With this exercise it can become clear that the focused pictorial observation and calm brings about an ether force.

Then practitioners lie on their backs to practise *sarvāṅgāsana*. With closed legs, they lift their torso and back up off the ground and then support the kidney region with their hands. The head is aligned, the eyes usually remain open. The breath flows perfectly freely throughout the exercise and the attention is directed into the centre in the chest, the *anāhata*-centre. Without forcing the body prematurely into the vertical line, practitioners straighten up according to the ideas and picture for the exercise, and finally, depending on their flexibility, they gradually bring the body into a more perfect uprightness. The legs remain closed during the exercise. The head and neck rest relaxed on the ground.

They are alive etheric forces that do not achieve uprightness through direct vital use of the will; they are forces that emanate into the dynamic out of the relaxation and inwardness. Thinking of the body pictorially also gives rise to ether forces. Like an ear of corn, flawless on its swaying stem, effortlessly sounding in the golden shimmer of the sunlight, the inverted body is lifted into the surrounding space, a more suffused space, which practitioners who listen precisely to the subtle-feelings can experience like a bluish, atmospheric glow.

Several minutes are usually needed to do this exercise. It can be held for up to five minutes. Then return out of the position in the same way and end the cycle. It is a cycle that harmonises and activates the etheric body.

Exercises to prepare for the shoulderstand follow.

By rolling into the inversion with a skilful swing, keeping the legs high and starting with the arms above the head, the neck region is protected. Keeping the breath light and free also prevents the neck from being blocked. In this way the thoracic spine can first be activated the other way round. Reversing the direction of the spine's movement towards the pelvis has a very regenerating effect, particularly if it is done in a relaxed way.

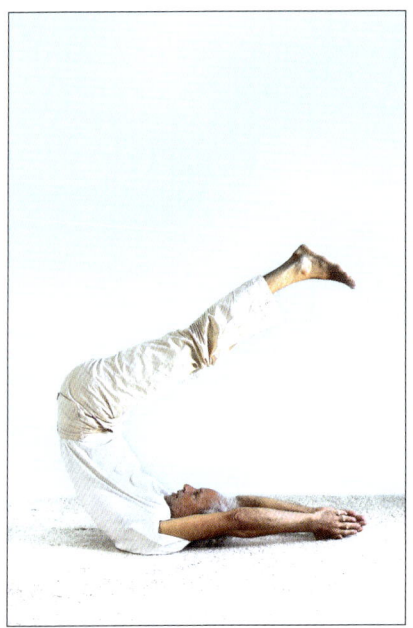

This pose is called *viparīta kāraṇī* in yoga. It represents a simplified form of the shoulderstand. The angle of the legs can vary. When first starting with the shoulderstand, or any other positions derived from it, the neck should be treated carefully. Therefore, the positions should be perfected in stages, paying attention to the relationship between the different tensions.

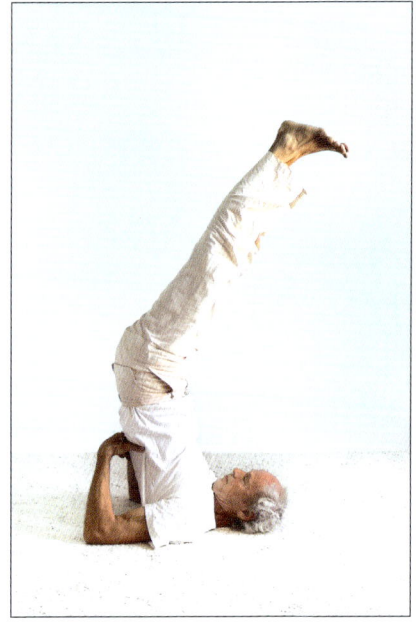

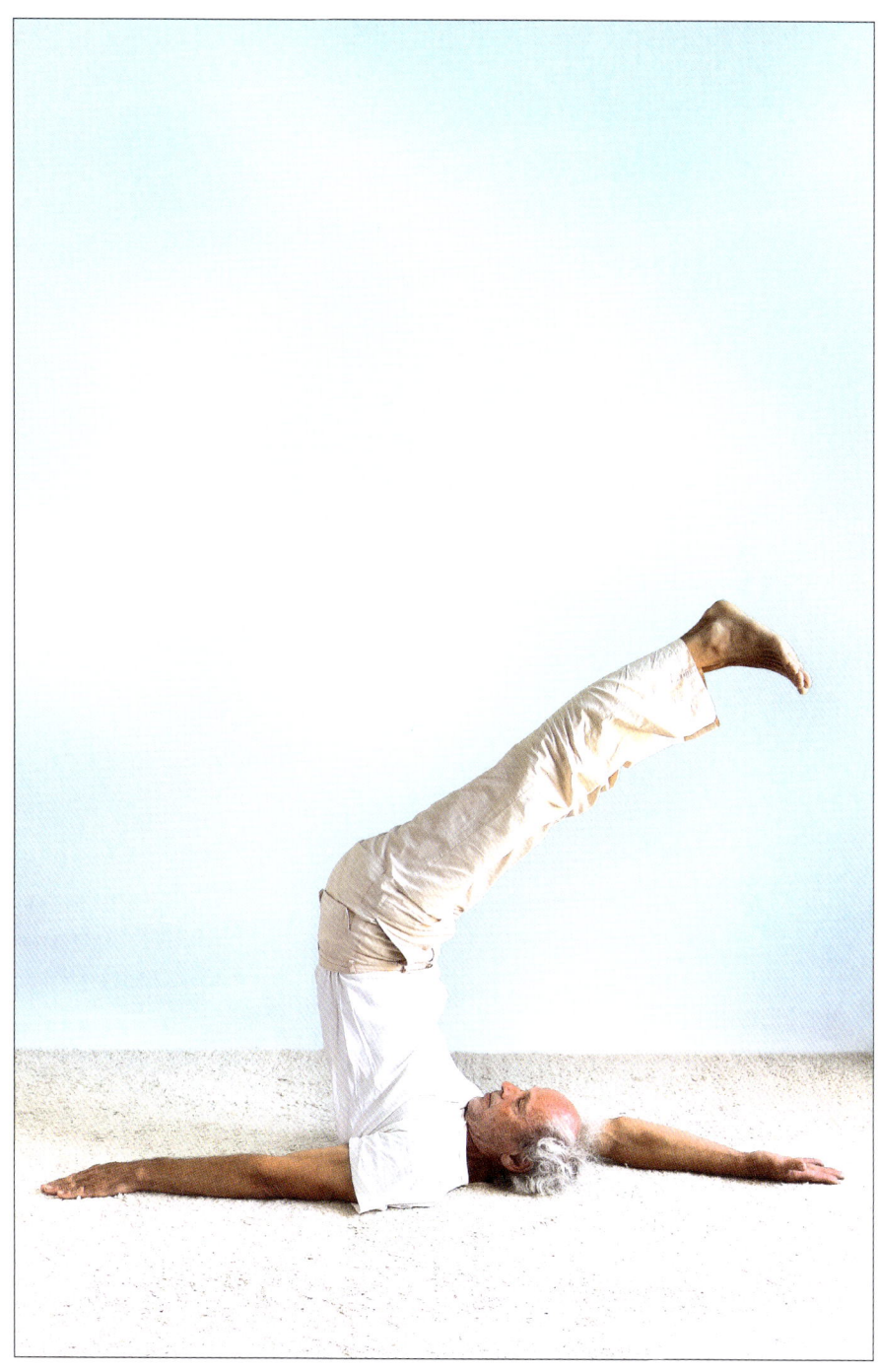

The development of expansiveness
maṇipūra-cakra

Maṇipūra-cakra is situated level with the stomach, around where the coeliac plexus is. In English it is generally called the "solar plexus", which is a small, central network of autonomic nerves. It is a centre that generates warmth because it is connected with the active metabolic organs like the pancreas, gall bladder, stomach and also, extraperitoneally, with the kidneys. This region of the abdomen is where the most important catabolism takes place.

Practitioners experience this centre through pleasant, liberating breathing in the sides of the body, which takes expression in the basic subtle-feeling of expansiveness. This subtle-feeling of expansiveness displays a clear connection to the skeletal muscles throughout the whole body, as these muscles can be relaxed, natural and elastic in their interaction, or they can be tense, over-acidic, and tend towards cramps and painful contractions. Ultimately this centre, situated above the kidney region, is essential for the build-up processes that regenerate the spine. If this centre is well developed, the dynamic strength of the spine is also freely available, and both stability and flexibility are kept in harmonious balance. The strengthening of the solar plexus is therefore of decisive importance for all spinal therapies and for the body's natural capacity to regenerate.

Central to learning is to develop an orientation towards aims, and from this a free way of relating to the outside world. From one's aims, a natural dynamic strength, and thus an enlivened and interested participation in the outside world develops. The centre at the solar plexus therefore bestows a first, natural form of love for life and for matter, by opening up a congenial expansiveness with gracefulness and joy, with dynamic strength and with inner participation in life. From interest, from inner participation and from natural empathy, finally the great character-traits of reverence, and of respect for human freedom awaken.

In the exercises practitioners learn this natural expansiveness through the free breath; they learn a dynamic strength directed towards an aim and held by the consciousness, and they learn to take up a relationship aimed towards the basic symbols of exercises. Each individual exercise, through the action of its hidden forces, encourages experiential qualities, and by means of the newly attuned and deepened soul-forces of thinking, feeling and willing, the attributes of reverence and respect for human freedom attain a greater space to unfold.

It should also be noted that the *maṇipūra-cakra* represents the reservoir of strength and will for the astral body. In a sense, it is the cosmos, with its internalised abundance of light, in the human being. For those people undergoing an intensive spiritual training, however, beyond this with each day the astral body, or the consciousness, must become ordered afresh and directed towards precise aims. When a practice is first taken up, it does not require the rhythmic discipline of constantly creating order, controlling the thinking and feeling and overcoming egoistic behaviour patterns. Initially, a certain egoistic way of life can be tolerated as practitioners are not yet equipped with the discernment as to which of the soul's tendencies are to be abolished and which ways of behaving should be developed. With increasing experience on the path of spiritual training, however, the inevitable demand arises to order the astral body through one's own efforts, one's own decisions and by properly controlling the emotions.

The basic principle that leads to order of the consciousness (astral body) can be summarised as follows: "Do not think and feel starting from your internal view, but start to think and feel as a result of having looked, as a result of perceiving others, an object or an objective phenomenon. Start to develop your thinking and feeling from the broad, real surroundings through independent consciousness and never forget the aim of a high realisation of the spirit."

With the realisation of this basic principle, advanced students can order their astral body and at the same time develop a balance between self-orientation and self-surrender, between relationship and their own standpoint, between realising aims and reverence.

A basic exercise for expansiveness
vihāyas – free space

The picture and the meaning of the exercise

It makes a big difference in social and educational situations, whether when encountering, communicating with, or teaching others, individuals open up a free space for their development or whether they constrict others through their own wilful demands or even manipulation. An open space that allows natural encounter and edifying awareness has an agreeable effect and as a result tends to appear lighter. It is actually the space, in its free openness, which can be fostered by human beings and which then contributes to a stimulating and edifying consciousness of light-filled togetherness.

Just as light has the tendency to reach out, so the human soul-life also wants to experience itself in its outreach and its expanding possibilities. Light itself reveals the spacial dimensions of this world, and the thoughts and feelings that the human consciousness creates give these already existing spaces either the feeling of antipathy and with this of constriction and darkening, or else of sympathy and thus of conscious openness, receptiveness and of luminous expansion.

The coarser element to light is air. While light corresponds most intimately with the thought-life and thus with the spirit, air possesses a certain bodily inclined, palpable reality. For example, anyone who moves their arms in space experiences how they cut through, encircle or form the air space. The meaning of this preliminary exercise lies in this conscious act of experiencing the space and its potential dimension of light through the thought-life, which wants to open up vivid subtle-feelings of expansiveness and inscribes these into the air space.

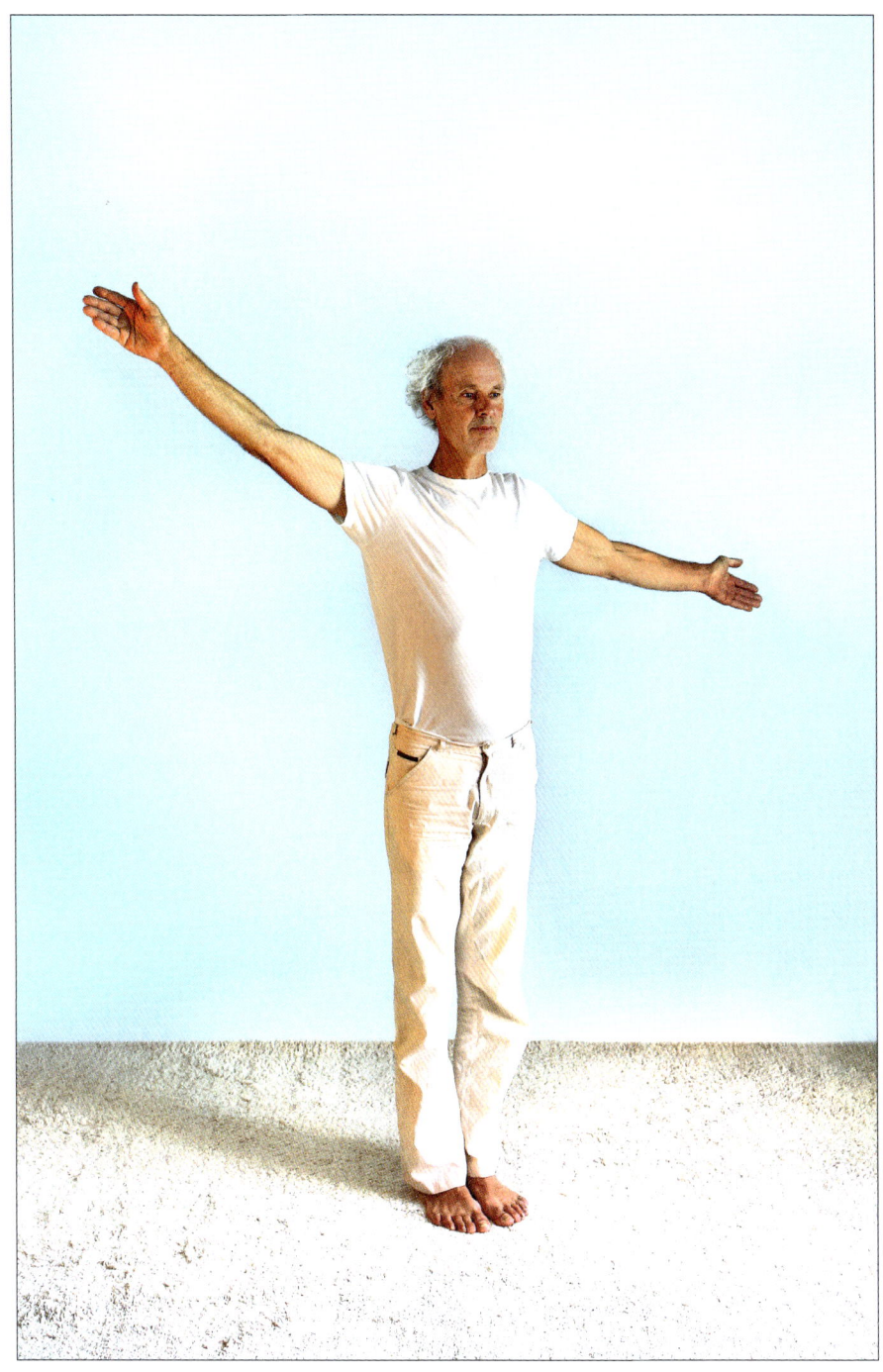

To practise

Remain preferably in a standing position and become aware of the space around you as air space, and then also become aware of your own body as an individual space in its own right. Then move the arms in a gesture of opening expansiveness taking care that this gesticulation is expressed in awareness, as if the senses are opening up a more three dimensional space of expansiveness. The element of air fills this external space and this coats the entire individual physicality.

It also seems helpful, during these opening arm movements, to remain aware of the sides of the body. The air element in its space-expanding and natural connection is felt tangibly by practitioners when they become aware of their sides, quite particularly in the region of the lower chest and waist.

When performing this gesture, practitioners can become aware that through their mental pictures and the way they enter into a field of relationship, the way they form their communication and the way they ultimately establish an expanding and open atmosphere, they are constantly shaping geometric forms, which can actually be of a more harmonious and open nature, and which can also move in beautiful proportions. Every communication that is engaged in and every relationship that is adopted therefore possesses a spacial, creative dimension, in which sensitive bodies are brought into being, and these, particularly when they emerge out of an expansiveness, freedom and truth, ultimately have a particularly, pleasantly regenerative effect on the life of the soul. It is a felt perception of space and the sphere of air becomes a direct subtle-feeling. Those who undergo training in the knowledge of these beings, which arise through an articulated consciousness, can also use them in communication to a growing extent for a liberating and health-fortifying regeneration.

In the light-space therefore, through the human thought processes, geometric forms arise, and these are inscribed right into the air-space felt with the hands. You can therefore also create geometric forms in your imagination and draw these with your hands.

When an *āsana* or a specific gesticulation is performed, then the effect is not confined just to practitioners alone, and to their own physical and mental state, rather the effect is given out to the surroundings, to other people and also to the spacial sphere. When the exercise is practised well, the space truly assumes a kind of visage.

The rhythmic and space-creating feeling which, through its character of motion and its dynamic expansion, develops into a lively, free and open relationship-whole, therefore reveals what in a metaphysical form are actually shell-like and inviting structures, appearing similar to blossoms. The space itself attains an animated aliveness and looks towards people, almost like a visage of its own. The drawing is intended to illustrate this quality of openness, receptiveness and friendly radiance, which the space adopts in its structures and lines.

The plough
halāsana

The picture and the meaning of the exercise

The plough turns over the earth so that it can produce new fruits. The exercise depicts an inverted posture in which the head is underneath and the legs swing over the torso. At the same time the form of the body represents a very simple, old plough, in which the torso forms the blade which digs into the earth and the feet show the direction in which the plough is pulled. This symbol of a plough's functioning, and of penetrating into a special and intense process of forming, contains the spiritual image of transformation.

Practitioners begin lying on their back, swing their legs over their head and first of all remain in the preparatory stage of the inversion until they then finally lower their legs to the floor and bring the movement to rest in motionlessness. From above the legs glide slowly downwards until they finally touch solid ground behind the head. This moment of lowering the legs should be consciously experienced, because it is a moment of expectation, a subtle openness within the stretch that glides out, until finally the actual nature of the plough, which penetrates with its blade into the earth, has been achieved. It is a movement that leads rhythmically and dynamically to a close relationship with the earth.

In the inverted position, practitioners experience themselves on the one hand open, but on the other hand constricted by the movement, and out of this state of tension they seek the path to the earth. The image of transformation is expressed in the inverted position and in the whole, dynamically executed movement, in which the feeling for the ground, for the earth, and the longing for expansiveness in an intimation of the spirit are vividly intertwined.

During the practice of this exercise, the mental pictures of the expansiveness achieved from the body, and at the same time the contact created with the ground of the earth, can accompany the consciousness.

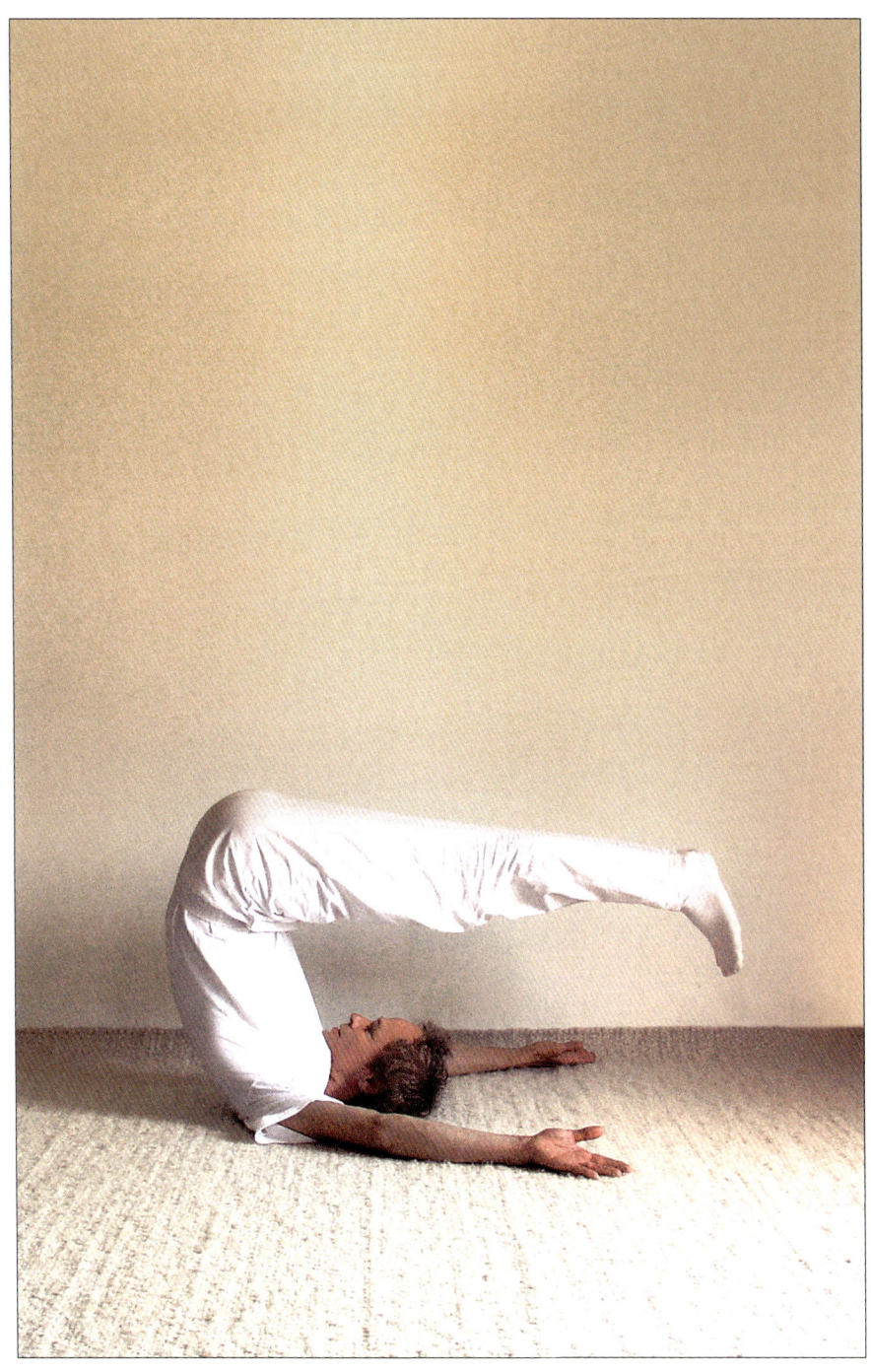

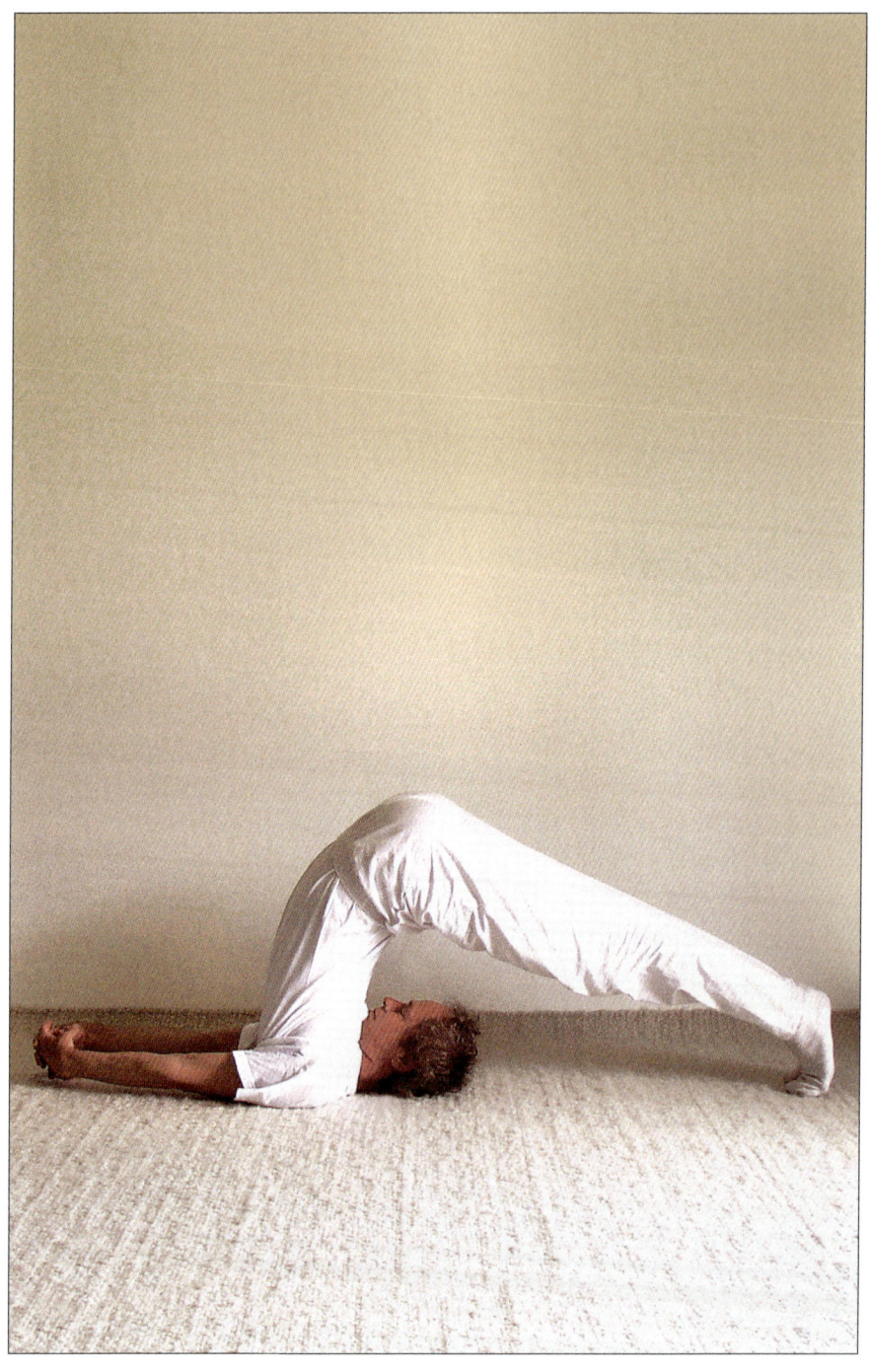

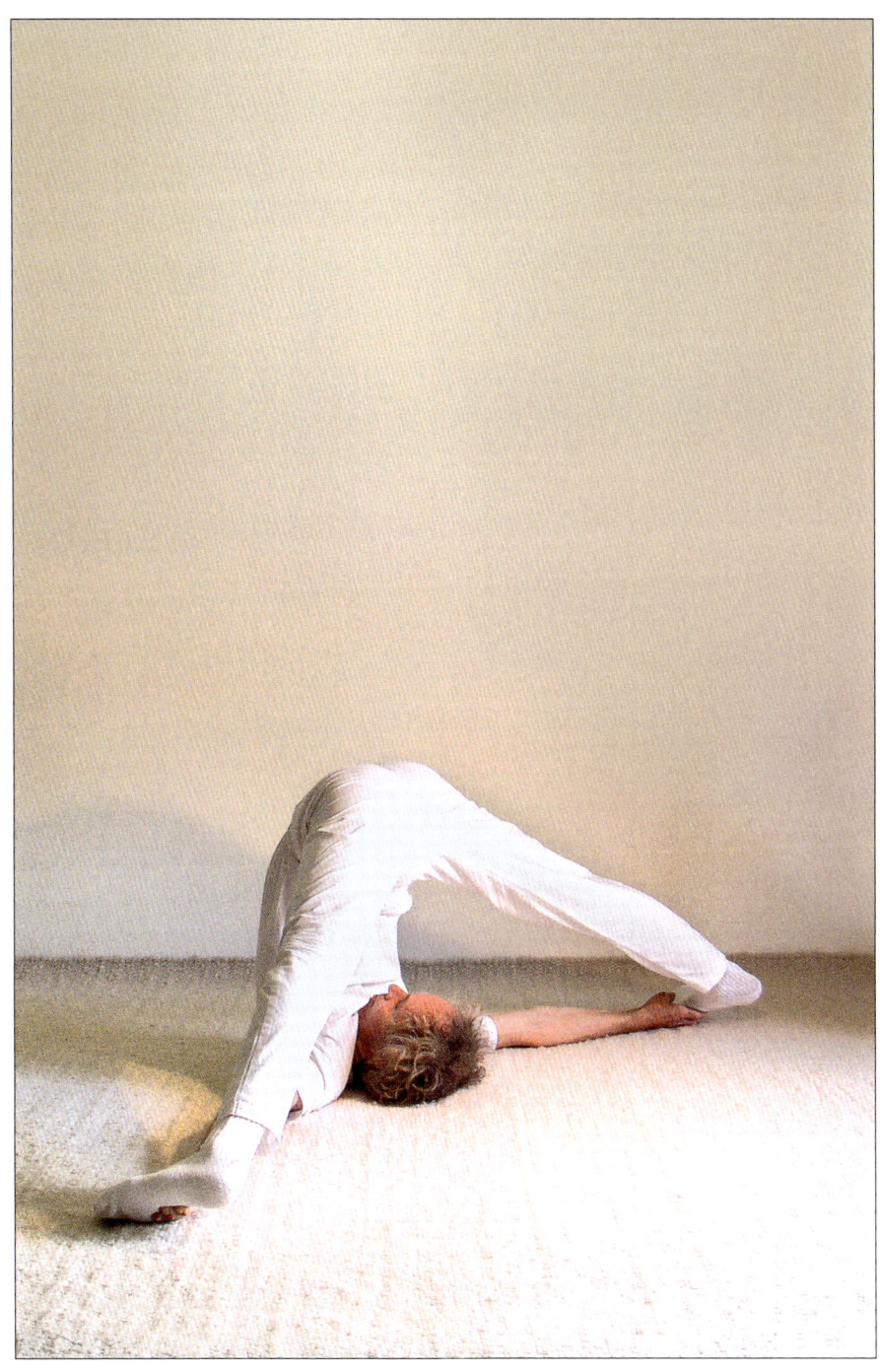

To practise

Begin lying on your back with your legs closed and your arms next to your body. In a big movement bring your legs up and continue until they are horizontally above your head. Now pause, preparing in this position and bring your arms from behind you sideways to the front, so that the moment of sensitive openness and of expansive breathing reaches conscious experience. The arms, which have been moved sideways to the front, allow the breath to flow more into the sides of the body (picture p. 149).

In this preparatory *āsana*, which can be held for up to half a minute or even a minute, the *maṇipūra-cakra* in the upper abdomen is noticeable as an energy centre. It forms the gathering point and at the same time the outwardly streaming, dynamic movement-element for this exercise. Then in a controlled way lower your legs behind your head and interlock your fingers with your arms stretched in the opposite direction. The breath always remains free both in the dynamic and in the static phase of the plough. If possible, you can heighten the dynamic strength by bringing the legs farther backwards into the stretch. However, the neck should never be overstretched by going into the exercise hastily or with wilful force (picture p. 150). Come back out of the movement rhythmically at the end.

For the plough there are a few excellent variations which are related to the experiencing of subtle openness and contact with the external space. One of the very aesthetic variations is to raise one leg into the shoulderstand (picture p. 153). In dynamic alternation, followed by short resting phases in the plough, first the left then the right leg can swing dynamically upwards into the vertical line of the shoulderstand. In this variation, a subtle openness and also a strong dynamic can be felt in the third centre. With this variation, the connection between free movement and free breathing activity can be experienced. The movement becomes all the more alive, sprouting, dynamic and free when the breath is also allowed expansively, and the act of experiencing is allowed unbound and with natural will activity. Another variation is the one with spread legs (picture p. 151). This gives rise to the feeling of expansiveness while also forming a geometric triangle.

In the plough the back extends out towards the legs. Normally, human beings straighten upwards and with the help of their arms they stretch

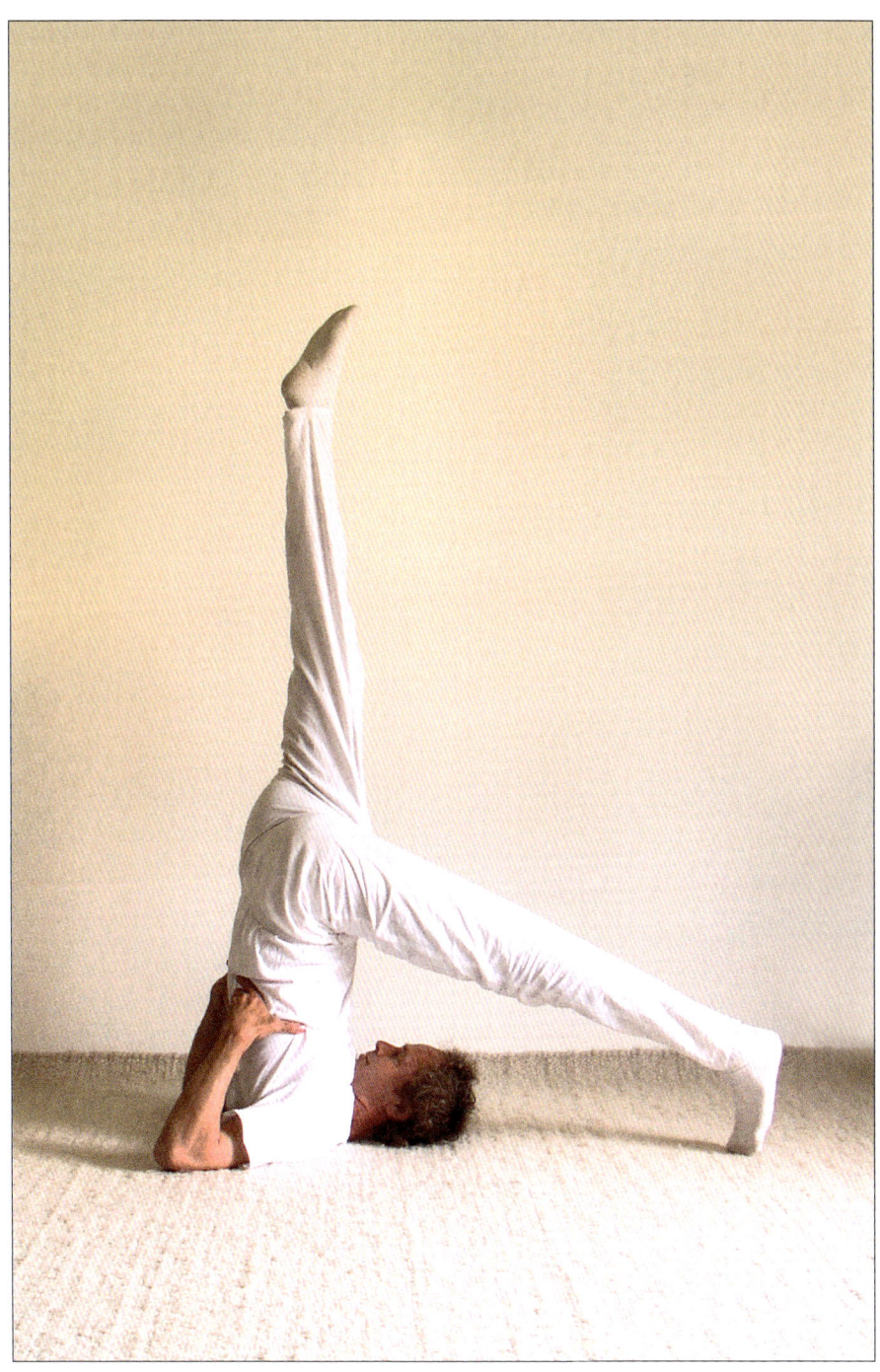

lengthways. However, during the inverted position practitioners learn a focused, lengthening stretch downwards, which they are able to continue specifically into the legs. A very good variation, which can both prepare for and follow the plough exercises, develops by straightening the back far up from the shoulder area, for one to two minutes, and bringing a dynamic movement into the legs. Spreading the legs widely out to the sides helps the movement attain its greatest possible dynamic.

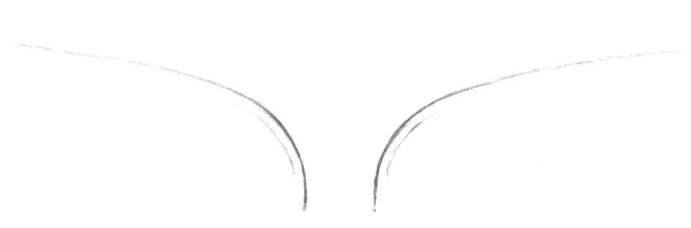

In this preparatory or follow-up position, which is a position showing a more dynamic, growing movement-element than the plough itself, alongside the inverted force straightening up the back, the sides of the body are of notable significance for the experience. Starting from the arm activity, the movement in a sense flows downwards along both sides and leads into the widening stretch of the legs. The characteristic feeling of expansiveness attains a precise form by paying attention to these roundings which arise in the sides.

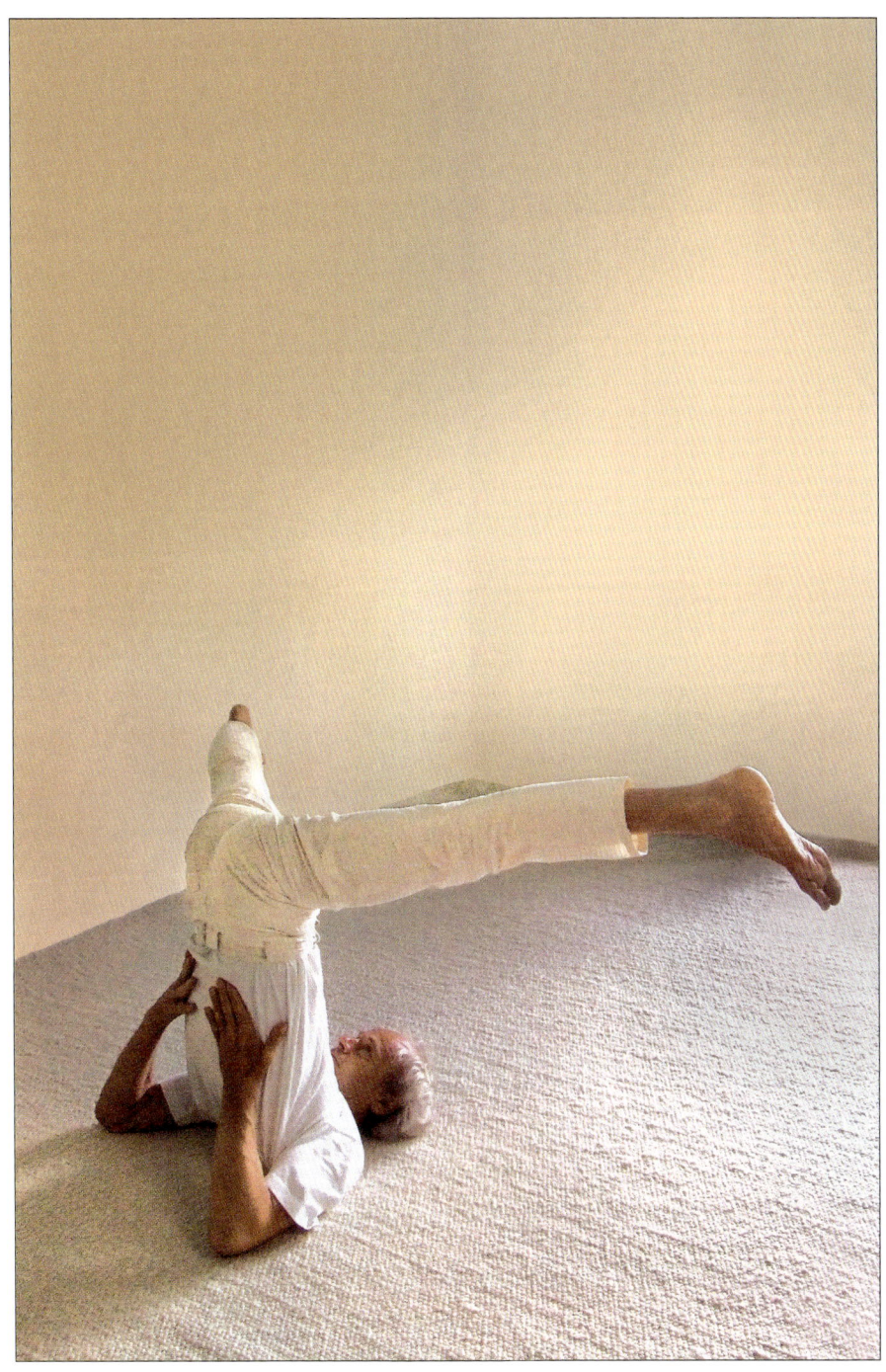

The head to knee pose
paścimottānāsana

The picture and the meaning of the exercise

This very important, central pose of *haṭha-yoga* depicts the transcending of limits, the extension of personal possibilities in the sense of wilfully performing an activity, and furthermore it indicates the inner sense of patient work and persistently "entering into relationship" with earthly matter. On the one hand expanded and stretched out, but on the other hand with depth and adeptness, practitioners devote themselves to the closed form in the movement. It is the soul picture of "going into matter", of the soul's becoming deeply touched through the form of what is earthly.

Observing the play of movement somewhat superficially, it could be thought that this far, limit-surpassing forward bend would present a gesture of humility. However, what is being addressed is less the religious gesture of humility and much more the actual active, form-giving being-turned towards matter and even the courageous entry into the tensions and uncomfortable conditions that matter offers. The pose is therefore one of the most active that yoga knows. It is connected with work, dedication and endurance. The experience of penetrating deeply into the earth, into life, into the realities with one's own creativity is the symbol of this exercise.

This is also the pose of activity which, when affirmed, expels any forcing and, through its own dynamic forming of the will, produces a joy.

To practise

Preparatory exercises like the sun prayer, *sūrya namaskāra*, the plough, *halāsana*, the shoulderstand, *sarvāṅgāsana*, or also other physical exercises make a lot of sense, as the movement, stretching beyond limits, absolutely requires a warming process. You can also do the *āsana* several times in succession and focus on building up the dynamic tension in this way. In any case, begin in the sitting position with straight legs, and with relaxed shoulders take your arms and upper body far forwards over your legs. With increasing activity coordinate your lower and middle back with the

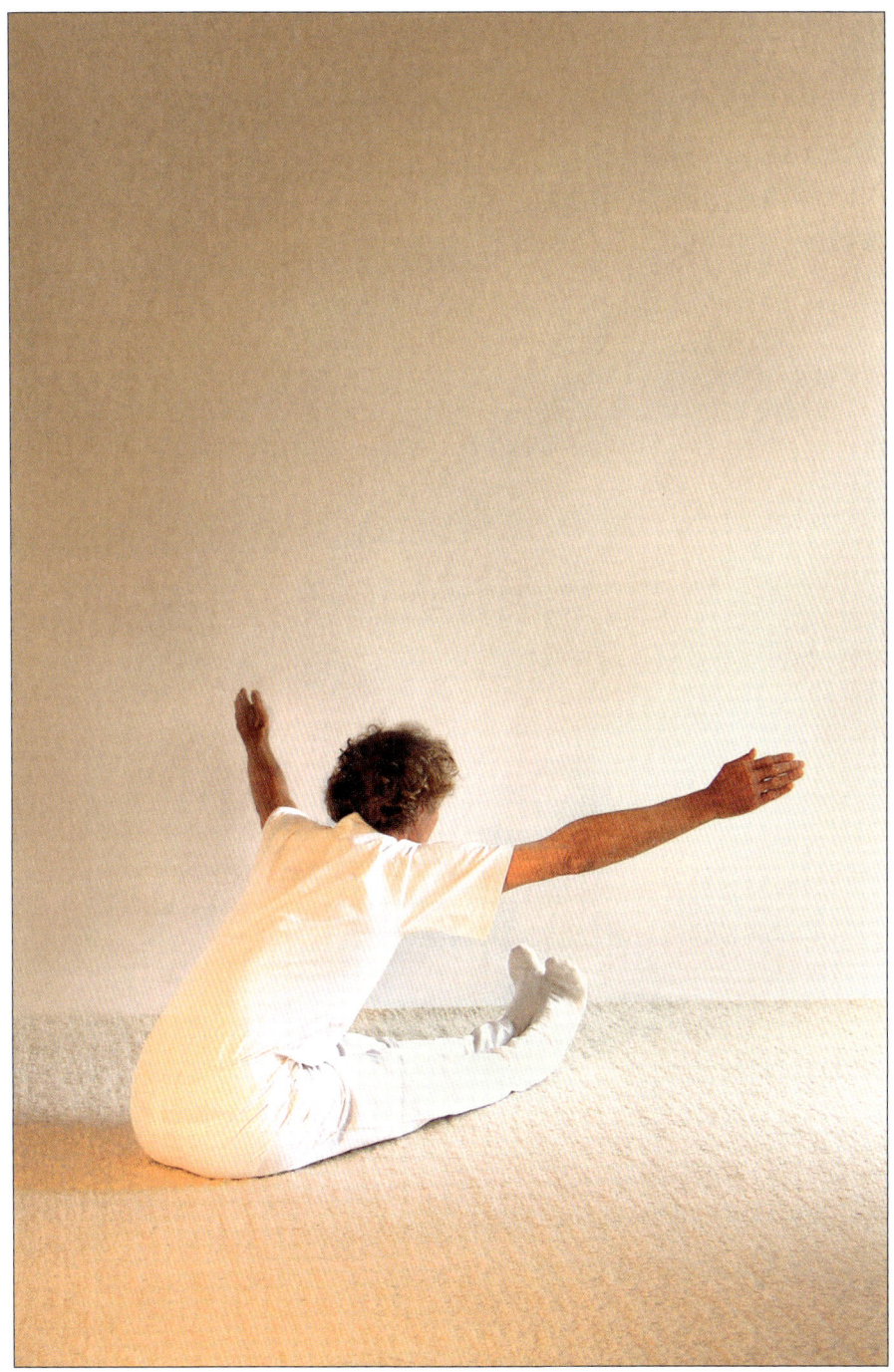

upper parts of the back, the shoulders and arms, which should be subject more and more to a relaxation. After you have led the body far into the position, it makes sense to open the arms like great wings so that the breath can be experienced once again in the sides of the body and in its liberating expansiveness (picture p. 157). Finally come into the end position by taking hold of your feet with your hands or, if possible, interlocking your fingers behind your feet. The practice itself can vary a lot in its dynamic strength. Sometimes you first have to work your way painstakingly into the forward bend and can only take hold of your feet after a long time.

The *āsana* is held in the end stage with the legs as straight as possible for at least one minute and perhaps even for as long as five minutes or more. Aim for a conscious stillness with simultaneous overseeing.

It is recommended when practising this exercise that in the whole dynamic of the movement you learn to transcend your personal limitations. This surpassing of limits is not a forceful pressing of the body into a desired form, it is much more a dynamic, highly active streaming-out of the spine into a growing stretch lengthways, which in the final stage integrates itself into an elegant and intentionally low form. Out of a great impulse originating from the solar plexus or *maṇipūra-cakra* , the movement flows into the lengthways stretch and after sufficient time seeks itself a still, closed form. The stretch with an active dynamic and lively resolve is maintained during the stationary phase. The shoulders nevertheless remain as relaxed as possible. While practising, place particular emphasis on consciously planning to surpass the limits to the stretch in the spine. After sufficient mental preparation, the movement-element should therefore be applied in a focused and very direct way. The focus is exactly in the middle of the spine, the areas of relaxation are higher up towards the shoulders and neck.

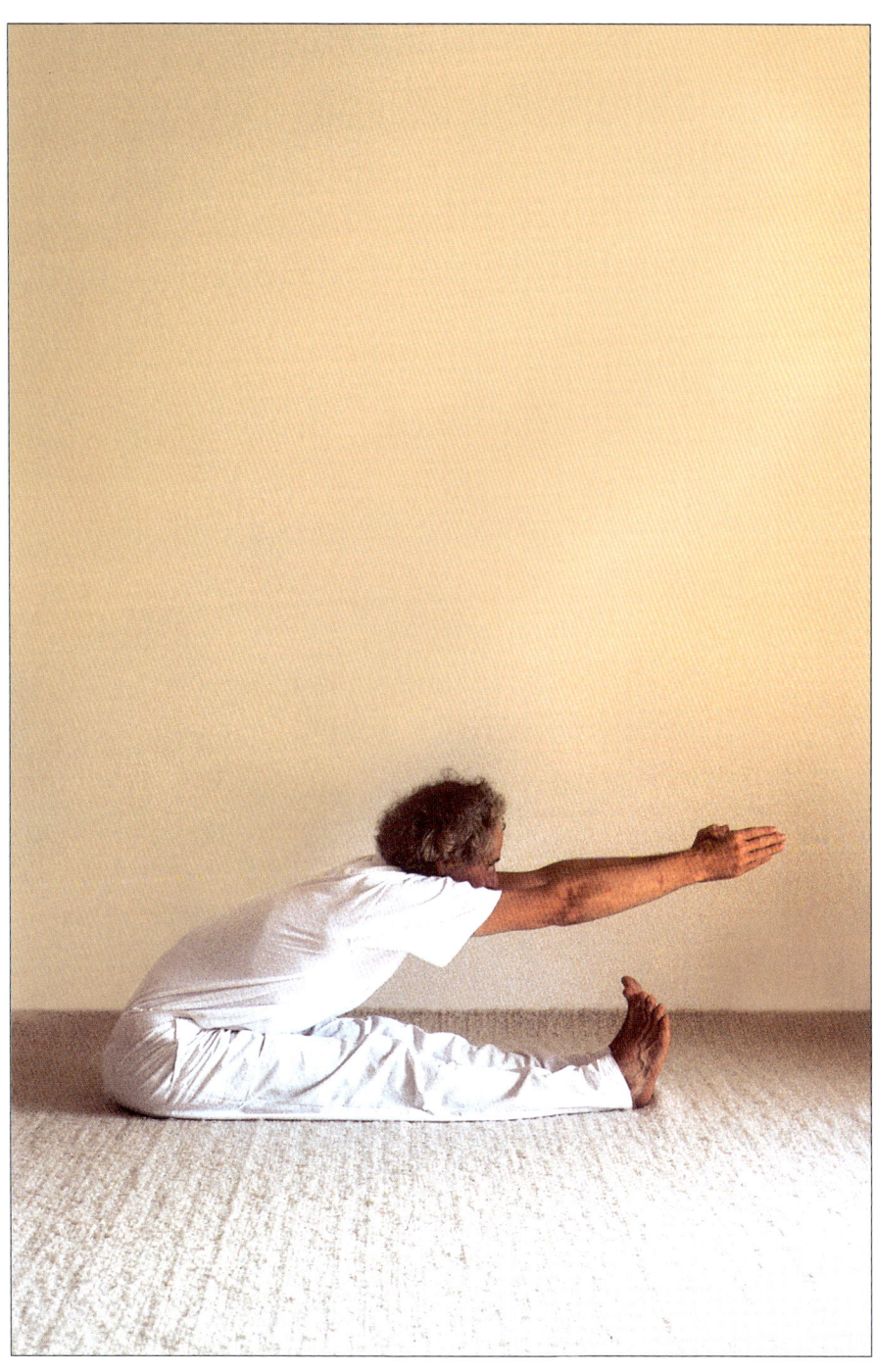

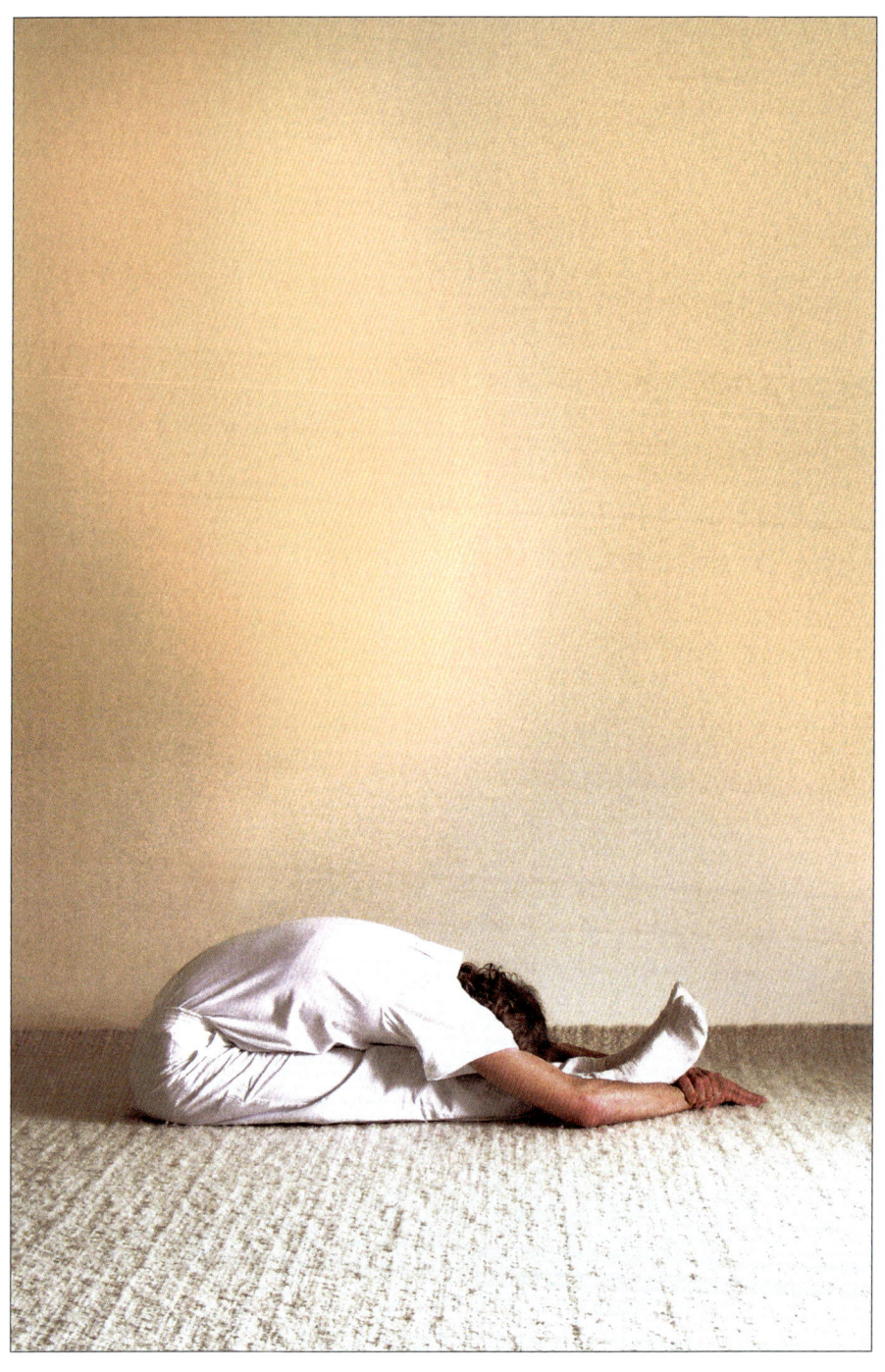

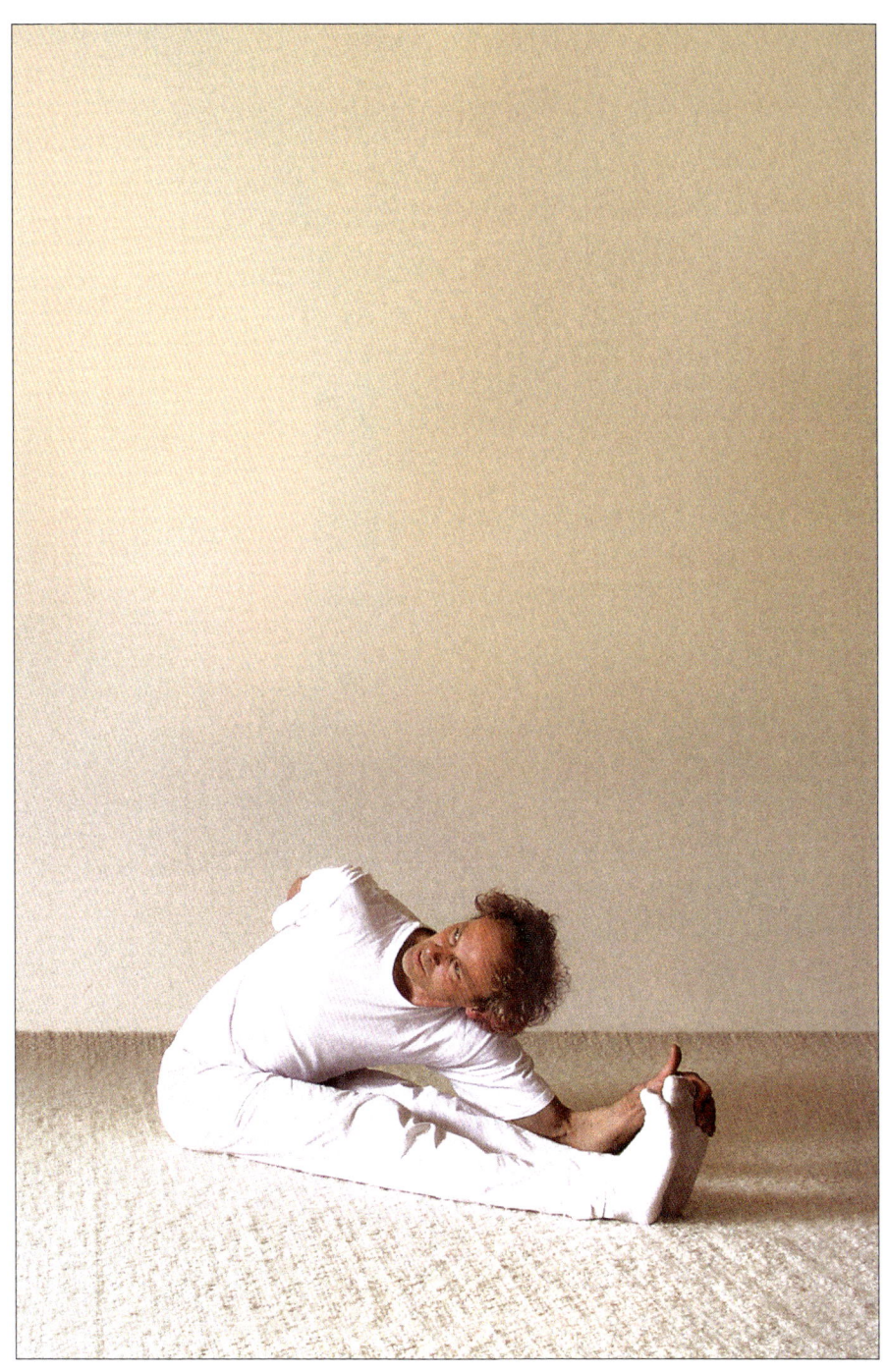

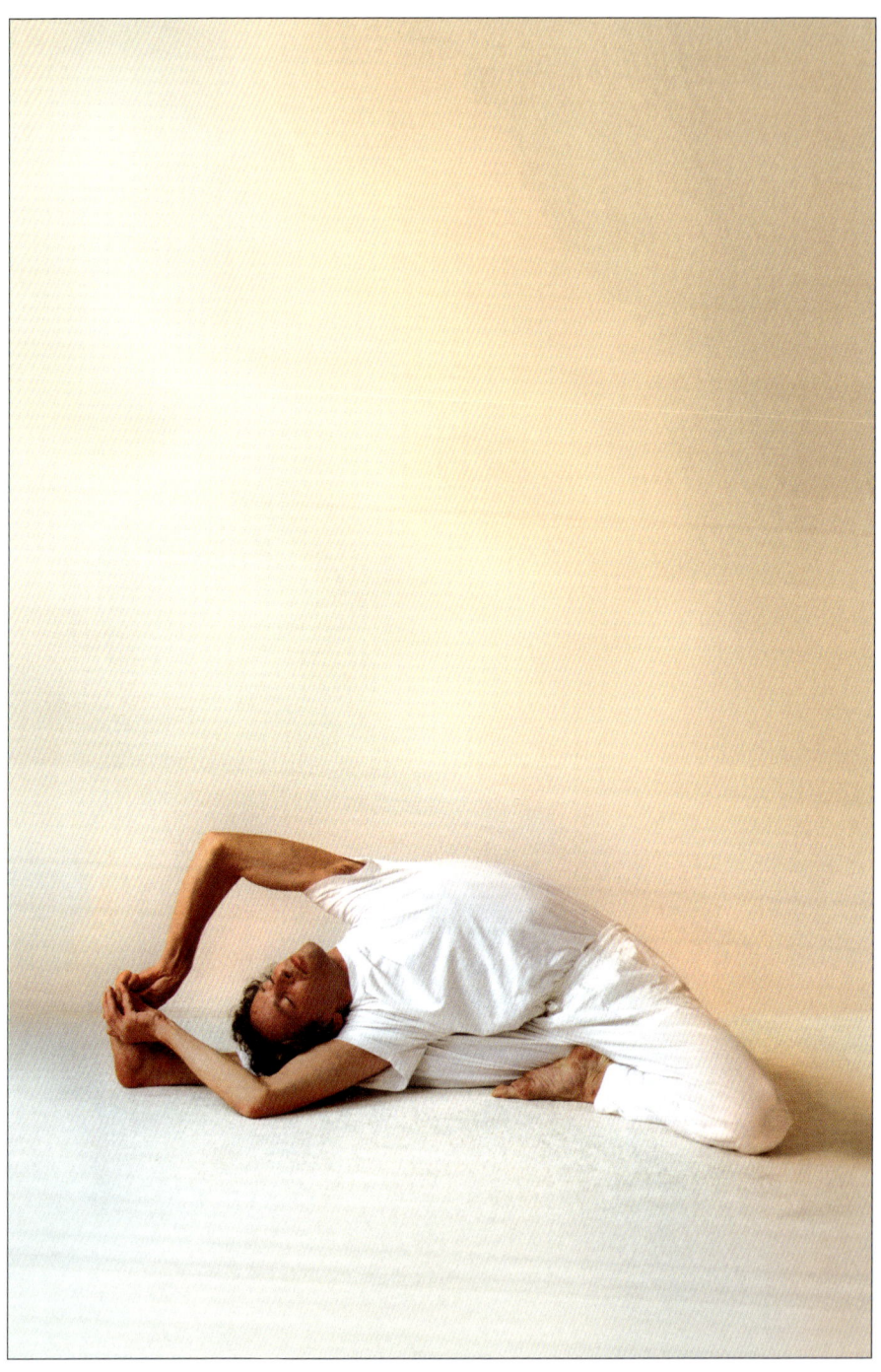

A very noble variation can ensue by adding a spinal twist, *pārśva paścimottānāsana*. When this additional twist is practised, the experiencing is refined to a greater sensibility and sensitive openness. While doing the head to knee pose, twist the body carefully and yet with a focused dynamic to the left and place your left hand behind your back on your waist to the right so that an aesthetic and graceful form results (picture p. 161). A second form arises by sitting with one leg bent in and completely twisting the whole torso and back over onto the straightened leg, *parivṛtta jānu śīrṣāsana* (picture p. 162). Both these difficult poses can be held for up to twenty seconds in the final stage.

These exercises should all be practised by articulating the will. The body is led into a twist not in one whole, unified and uniform impulse, but rather the upper body with the shoulders, neck and head are deliberately relaxed and the middle of the spine is deliberately activated. The lower back and the hips remain as a still base in the exercise. This articulated relationship between the different tensions is an important part of the exercise, and when observed will lead to an expansive experience of the surrounding space.

For the soul-life, observation is therefore to be developed. If the will is exerted in a differentiated and articulated way, and other regions of the body remain free and relaxed, new and free thought spaces open up. With undifferentiated and one-sidedly forceful impulses, and also with strong utilisation of the breath to intensify the movement, the act of subtly feeling falls back onto the physicality and the pleasant and beautiful, self-expanding space remains barred.

After or before practising the various forms of *paścimottānāsana*, a simplified, basic version of the movement-dynamic is recommended once again. Stretch your legs forwards actively and with your hands touch the ground beside and slightly behind you. The centre of the movement is formed by a dynamic stretch in the region of the third centre, which is directed openly forwards, expanding the space (picture p. 164). The upper body remains open and relaxed. This movement is intensified when you place your arms up high and work actively with the thoracic spine to bend backwards. (picture p. 165).

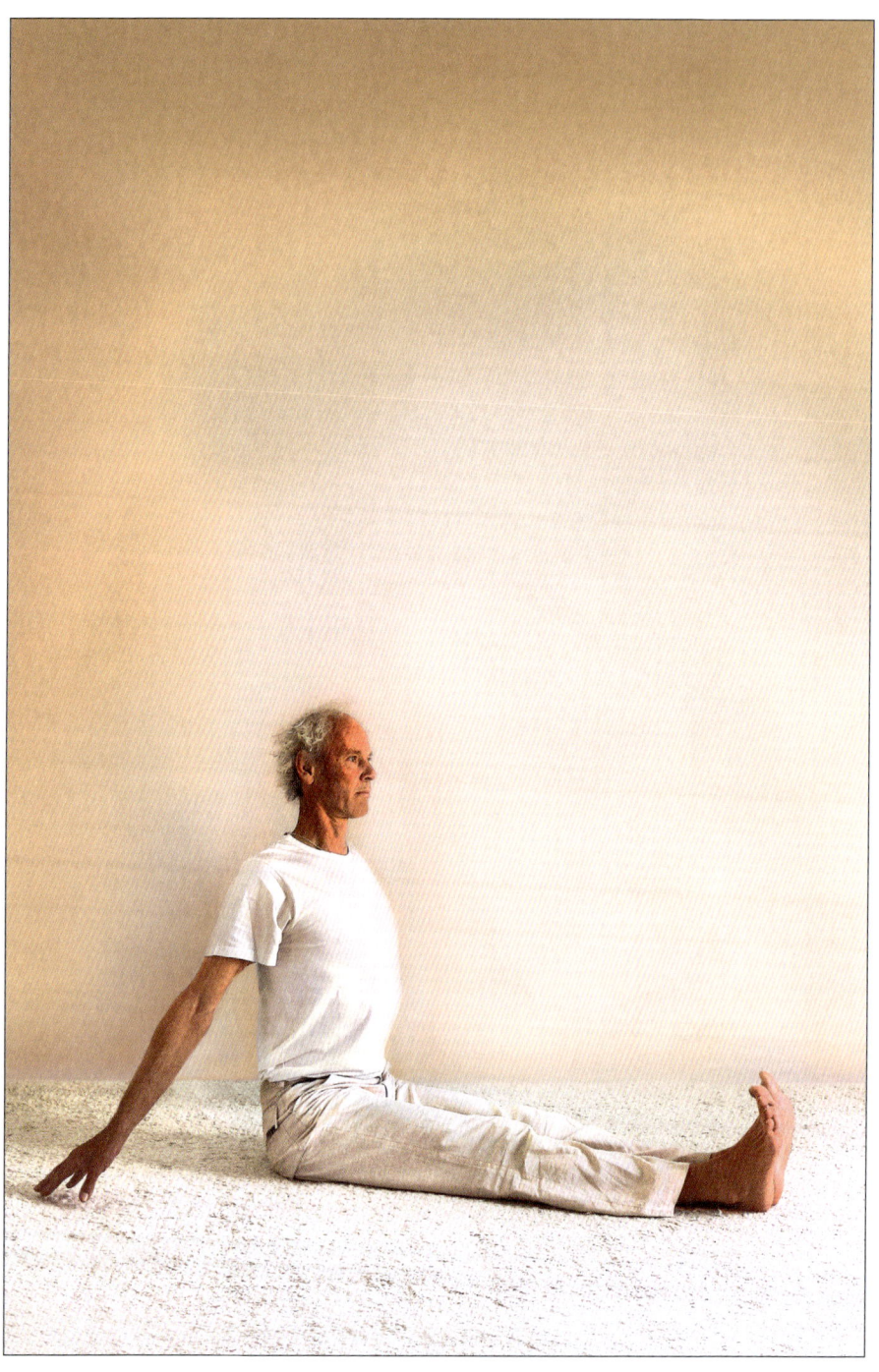

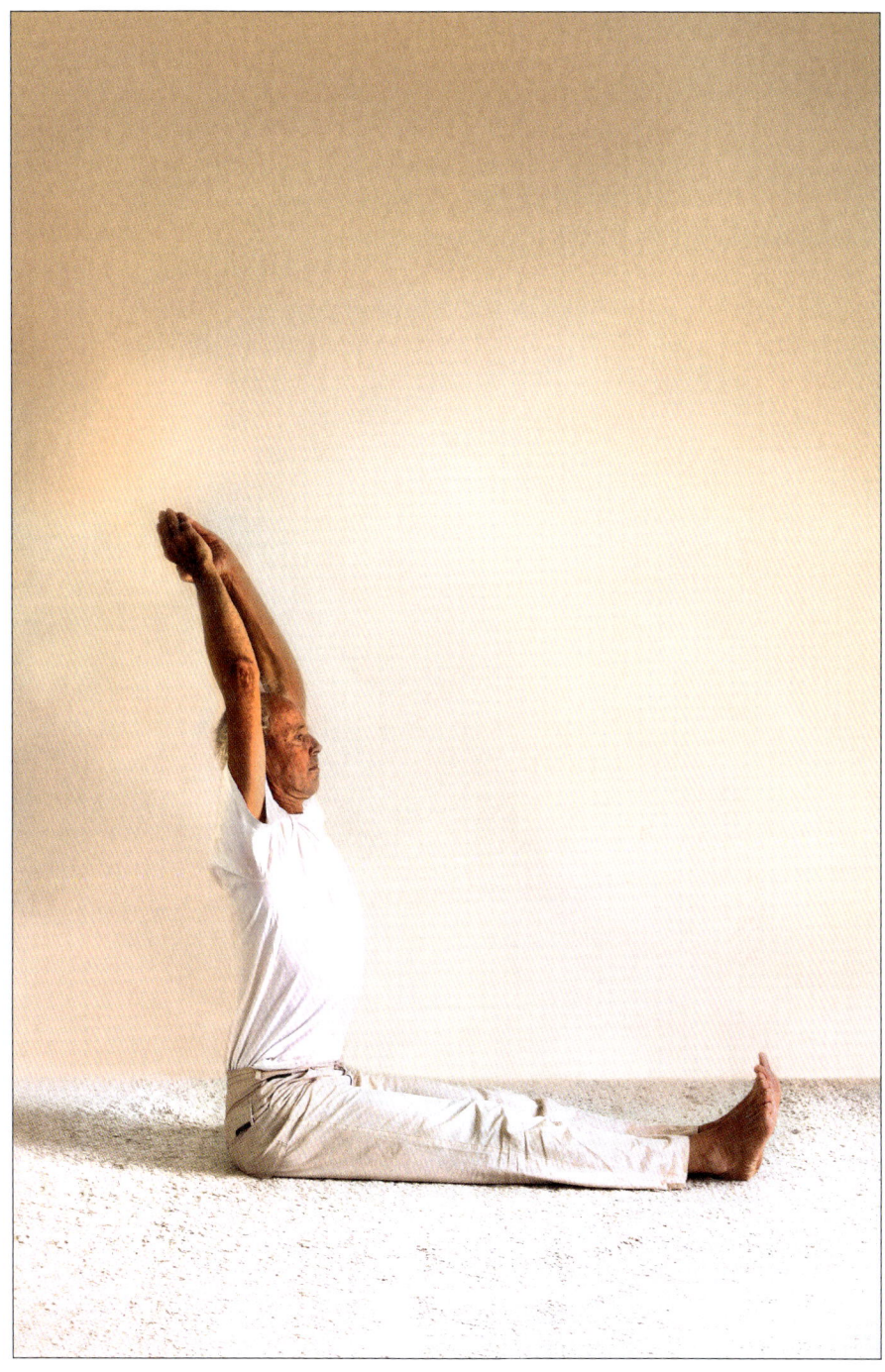

The bow
dhanurāsana

The picture and the meaning of the exercise

Just as the arrow of a strong elastic bow flies into the distance and reaches its target, so the spine should be dynamically strong and elastic so that it can set free high forces for the daily activities and people can realise their personal aims. The spine is the central axis of the personal being and through its healthy elasticity, stability and dynamic it signalises the capacity for vital, active creative-energy. Flawless, without blockages, the individual vertebrae work together to form one strong, dynamic unit. At the same time this flexibility is encompassed by soft musculature and counteracts any lability or weakness through its own dynamic strength.

The bow is a symbol for healthy dynamic strength of the nerves and the body, and represents the vital substance of concentration-capacity, which practitioners activate out of their surrounding sphere of air, and mobilise in an active response, out of themselves, through their will. In this sense, *maṇipūra-cakra* is the physical centre of concentration, which takes up the surrounding air and transforms it into a regenerative dynamic and purposefully aimed activity. The surrounding sphere and the centre within work together. In the bow this centre is designated as the mid-point of the tension. The aimed-for joyful effort of building up tension can be felt while practising, streaming vibrantly from the kidney and lumbar region, both upwards towards the head and downwards towards the legs and knees. The fullness of the vital concentration and dynamic strength is activated out of the surrounding sphere of air and out of the ability to manifest this in *maṇipūra-cakra*.

The bow is the pose of targeted activity. Just as a bow with its quivering state of tension is the instrument for realising a waiting intent, so human life is an expression for an active wanting which, taking account of the surroundings, becomes concentrated, well-coordinated and seeks a precisely defined direction.

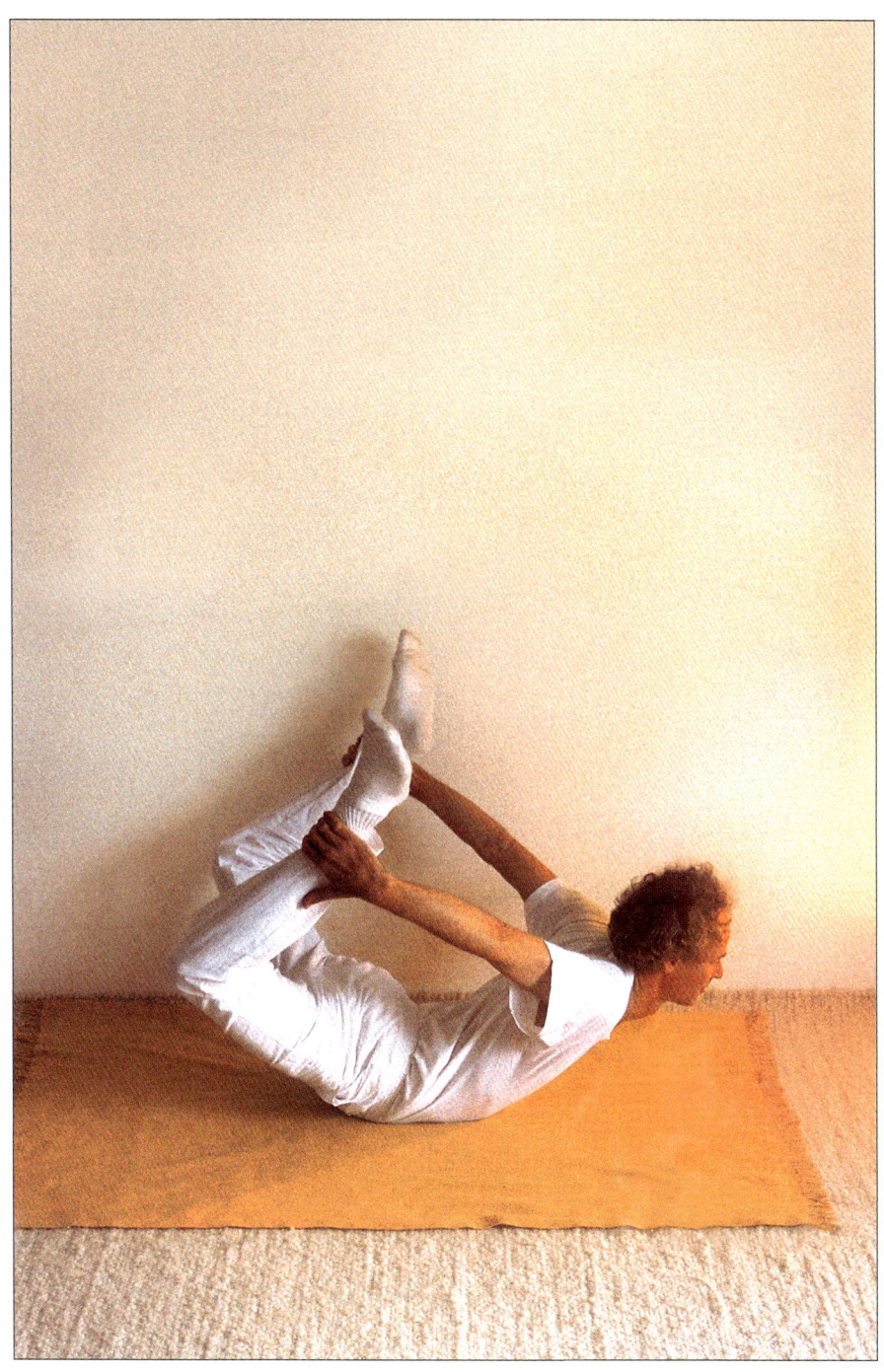

To practise

Begin the exercise lying on your front with a preparatory, aesthetic and dynamic movement. Stretch your right arm far forwards and your left arm backwards. Then lead your spine up as high as possible, both towards your legs and also towards your head, stretch the right arm up, the left arm up behind you and also the left leg up behind you. Change the directions of the arms and legs after a few breaths, several times in a flowing alternation. This exercise unites the lower and upper halves of the body through its lively play of movement. During the practice take care not to take the active movement too much from the body alone, but from the sphere of air. This movement becomes less strenuous when it takes place in the lively play of the air element like a free breath. Movement is free from the body.

Following this preparatory, dynamic exercise, you can bend up your lower legs, bring your knees apart and take hold of your ankles with your hands. With a well-coordinated, consciously planned impulse firstly lead your legs up into the tension and only secondly raise the upper body. Do not let yourself be discouraged prematurely by feelings of heaviness or discomfort in this position of heightened tension. Lead your legs persistently, in a concentrated way, out of the back as far upwards as you can and yet make sure that your neck is relaxed and your shoulders are reasonably released. The pose can be held from half a minute up to as much as two minutes. Concentration firstly on the surrounding sphere of air and then on the centre and on the focused, growing movement, is indicated in the exercise. Never sink back, but increase the dynamic. Movement is formed breath-activity.

The tension out of the centre of the spine is created all the more joyfully and easily the more the upper body and the arms remain relaxed and the more you experience the breath as a whole in the surrounding sphere. Repeated practice, connected with study of the spiritual picture of the bow, can be very beneficial for those who are frail because the metabolic forces are strengthened and the will-possibilities expand. The centrifugal movement-dynamic on the one hand unburdens the inner organs and on the other hand stimulates the cardiovascular system and imparts a pleasant regeneration afterwards.

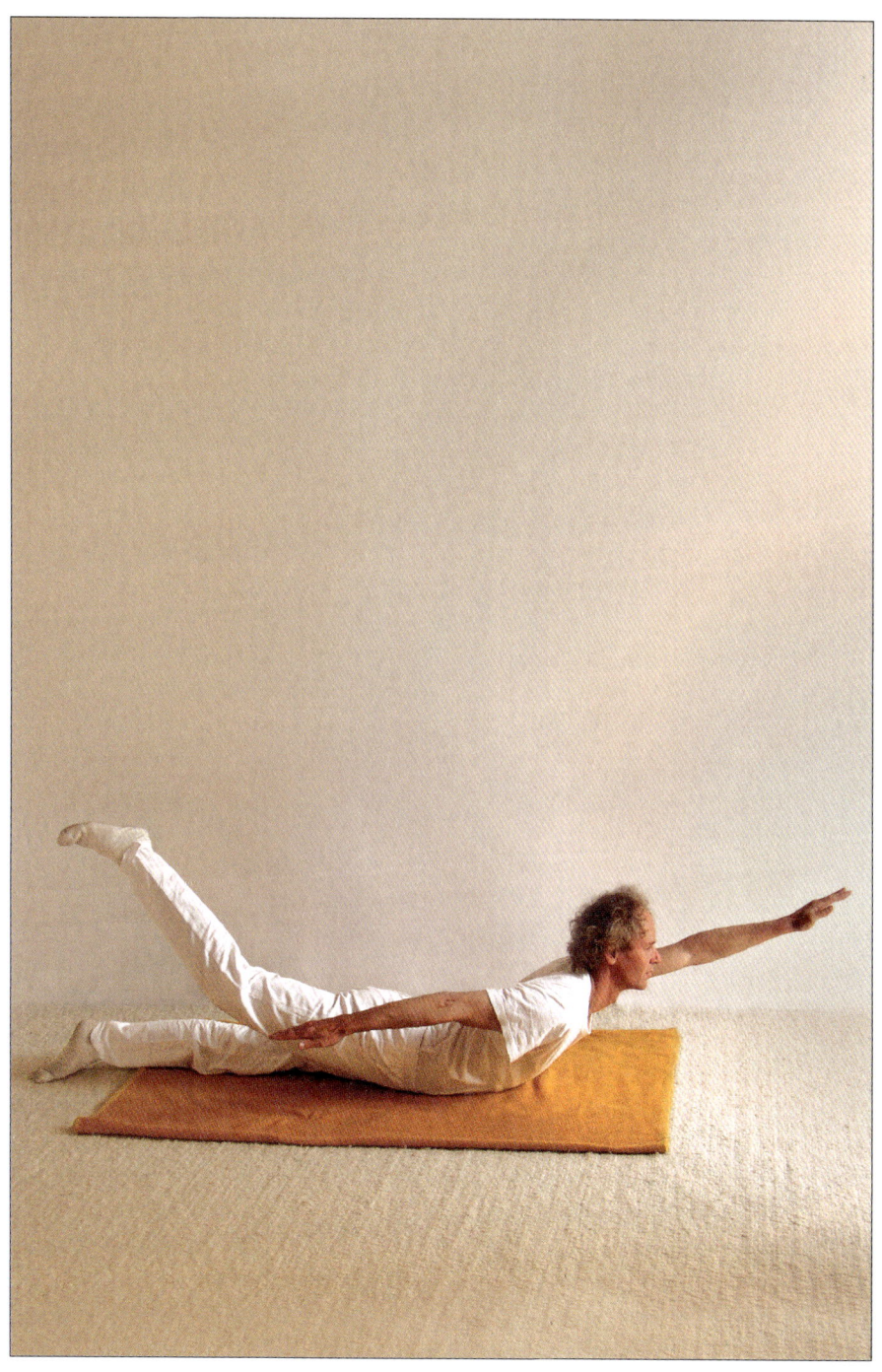

169

The camel
uṣṭrāsana

The picture and the meaning of the exercise

In this *āsana* the movement is built up and rounded into a wide open gesture of bending backwards. The lively and outwardly gliding arch backwards is supported through a big circular movement formed with the arms. Only lastly do the arms come behind and the hands touch the heels, so that the movement is given a natural order and the body a closed form. The body, however, is built up further in its dynamic strength, and the spine is rounded upwards.

This daring openness, which can be experienced in the camel, demands a stable and in all parts flexible spine, which with its enclosed nervous system possesses the coordination to combine an outer expansiveness and an inner calmness. So this camel pose describes an initial form of conscious devotion, for devotion is characterised by the capacity of developed stability and by the boldness to step away to some degree from oneself and the body. The exercise is a symbol for *kṣamā* or for the capacity to be able to bear the consciousness as a conscious instrument of awareness itself.

The spine, with its skilful capacity to extend and its dynamic fluidity, is representative for the processes of the personality's unfolding and for the conscious, wilful use of the actual human possibilities. Practitioners must nevertheless firstly permeate and build their thinking and also their feeling as well as their acting in a soulful way, in order to come into an ordered inward- as well as wide opened outward-relationship. The camel describes this capacity of the consciousness itself, which is that practitioners do not only devote themselves unprotected, but train themselves in thoughts and feelings and with this they also build the spine, which they lead up into an expansive, shaped arc. The large circle that practitioners perform with the sweeping arm movements helps to stretch the spine in a healthy way and to lead it up dynamically into the shaped arc. The better the building-up process succeeds, the freer and more released individuals feel also in their encounter with the external world. Seen this way, practitioners do not merely bend, but build up a beautiful, aesthetic and uniting structure in the way that an initial devotion requires. The life of the soul relies on a

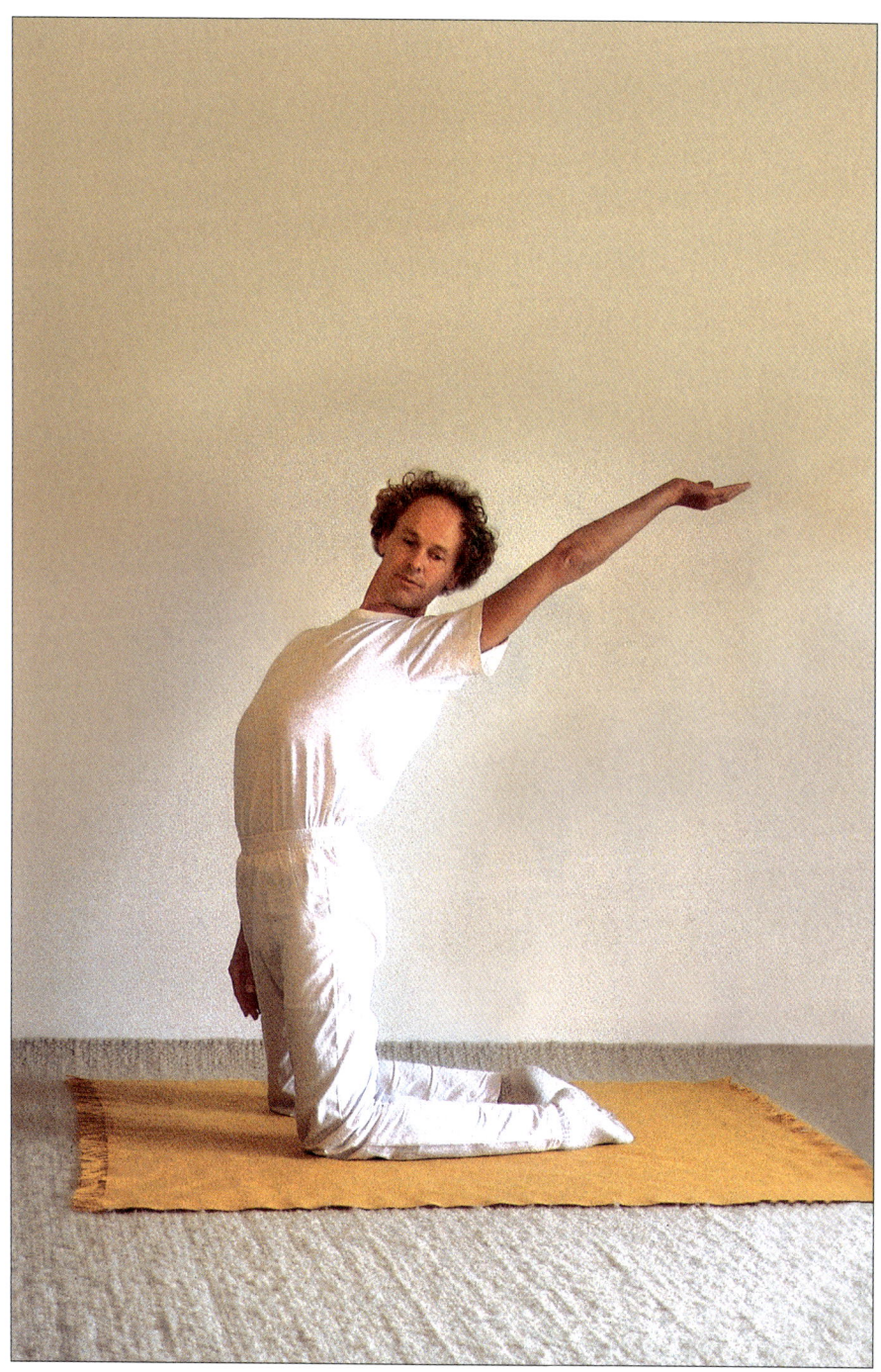

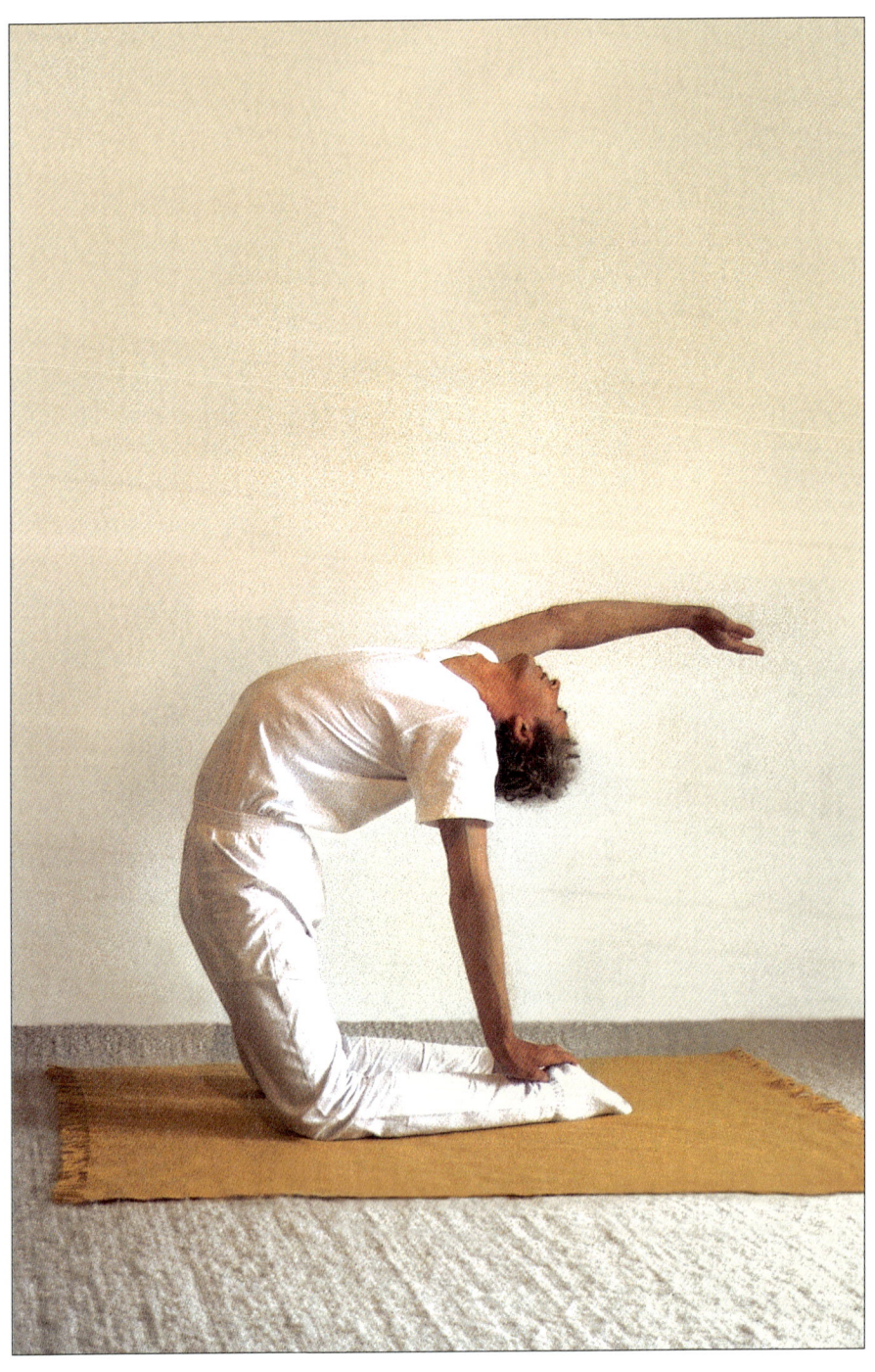

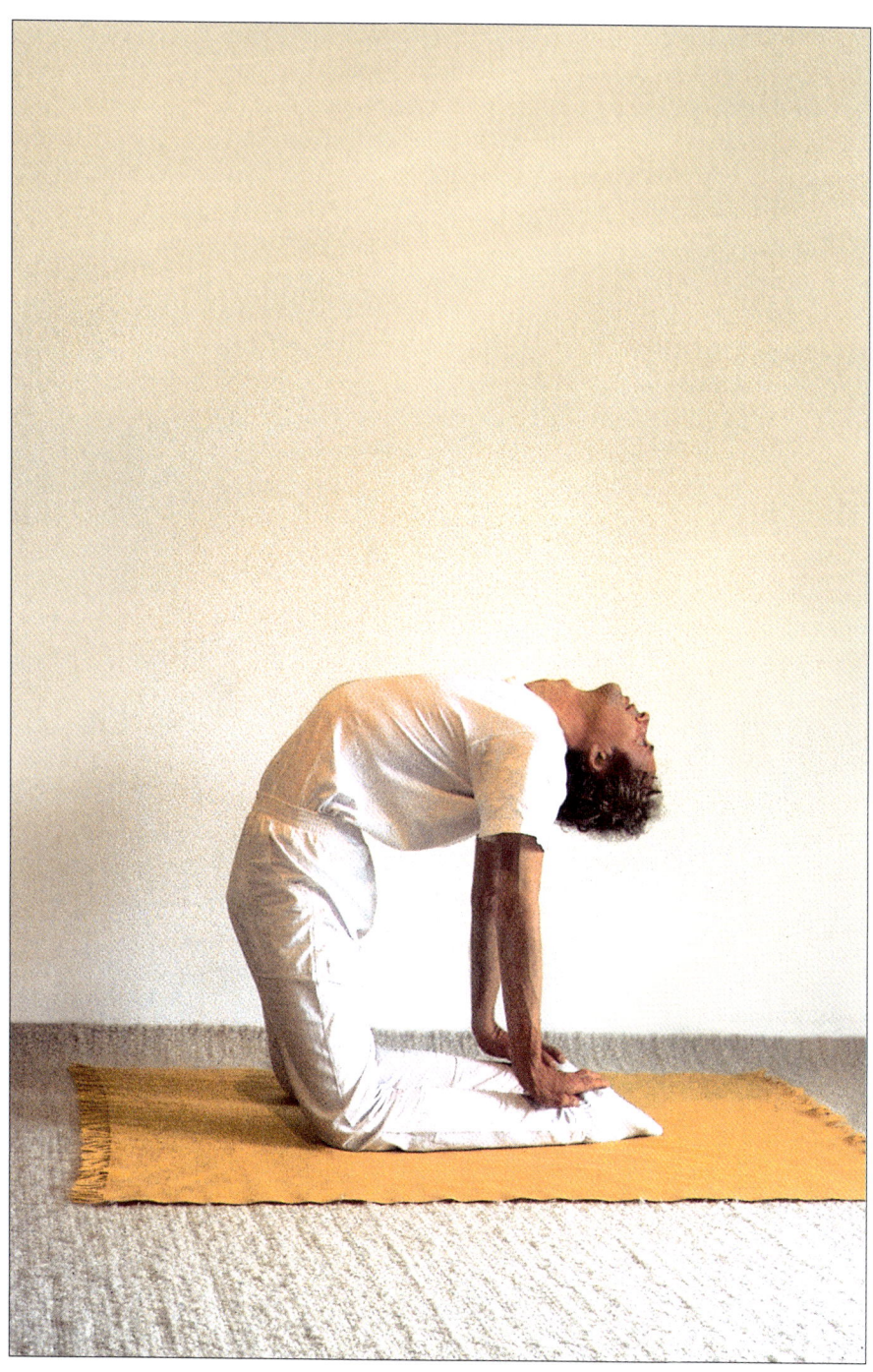

building-up process and on the capacity to shape. Thus the body recedes and practitioners give the external world space. In the reality of their self, they build a connecting, aesthetic structure, and this is expressed pictorially in the shaped arc of the spine ascending from the centre. *Kṣamā*, the capacity to carry and bear, develops with growing, higher wisdom.

To practise

First begin with what could be called an awful starting position. In Sanskrit this pose is called *adhomukha trikoṇāsana*, the downward facing triangle (picture p. 175). With your feet about a metre away from your hands, press your heels powerfully onto the floor. The dynamic is directed towards your heels. In this position your field of vision is restricted. The specifically chosen physical posture also makes you feel as if you are bound into your own physicality. The senses do not look outwards but, as if imprisoned, into one's own existing space. Hold this unpleasant position for up to a minute and then come onto your knees for the actual pose.

Begin this pose with a wide sweeping movement of the left arm upwards, forming a circle from front to back to motivate the expansive stretch outwards. Like a great circling breath, the spine is built up out of the surroundings. With this arm movement, the spine is actively stretched and arched. Also look back and lead your hand towards your heel. While acting as a base the knees are slightly opened. Then the right arm also glides in a widely extending circular movement from front to back and takes hold of the right heel. Lastly the head falls back into the neck and the spine continues to be stretched through all its parts actively upwards. Hold the position for about half a minute with free breath and return rhythmically back in the same way. A strengthening in the spine is evident.

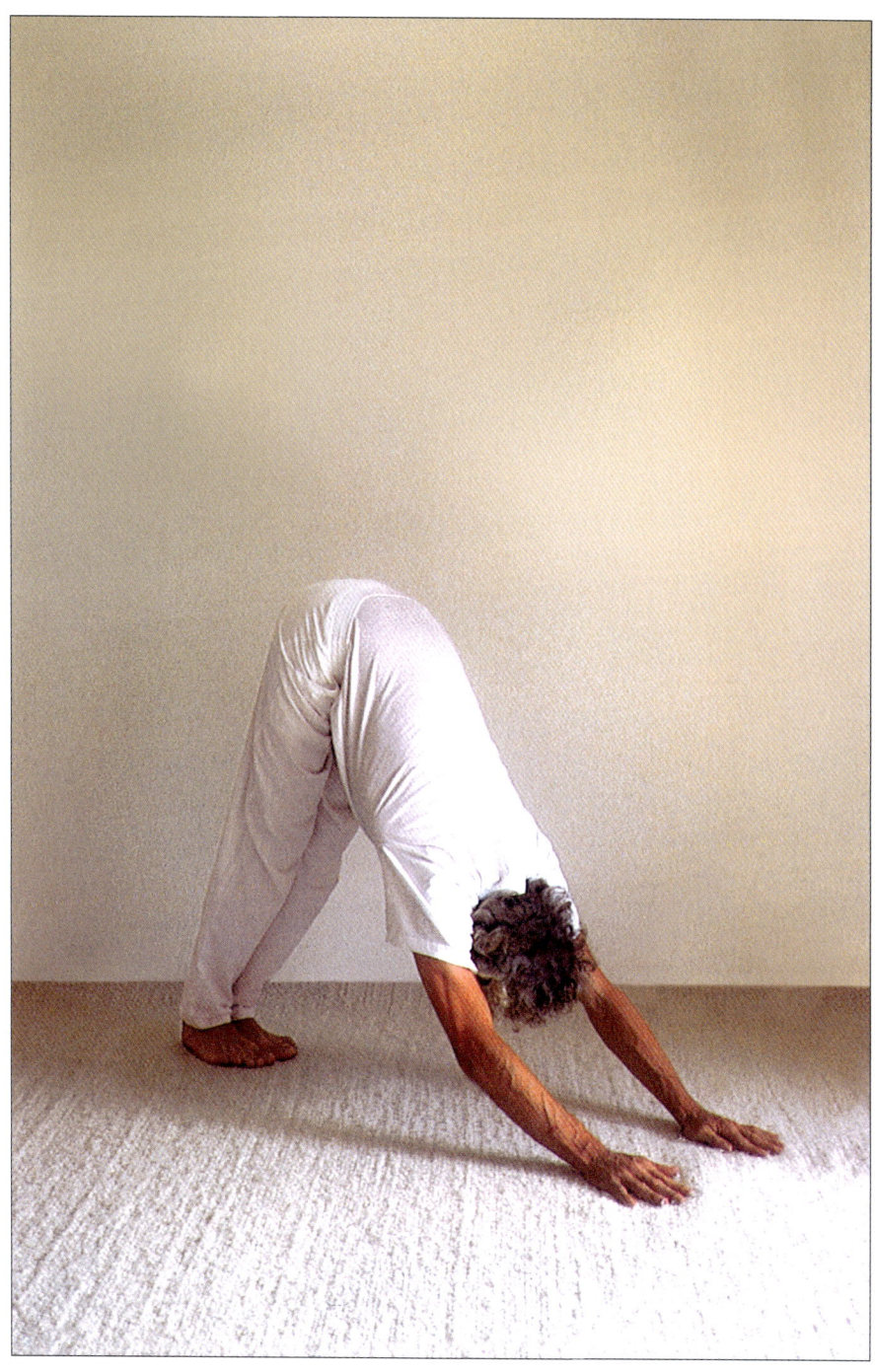

The triangle
trikoṇāsana

The picture and the meaning of the exercise

In the stable triangular base practitioners bend alternately from side to side while maintaining a free movement of breath. These precise movements sideways stretch the sides of the body and lead to an intensification of the feeling of expansiveness along the body. The simultaneous stretching and movement sideways is connected with a venturesome, joyfully courageous feeling, which is experienced almost as if in a spacial relocation. The meaning of this pose lies on the one hand in the natural activity connected with the movement, for practitioners experience themselves secure in the base, active in the middle and relaxed in the upper neck, shoulder and head region. They actually experience themselves in three parts, which is characteristic of the three soul-forces of thinking, feeling and willing. Beyond this, however, the exercise also holds a meaning through the unusual activity to be achieved. In earthly life, any physical movement initiated or any relationship formed begins as a form of courageous extension, which is still free from good and bad. Activity is given by nature, and the need to expand the will out to new possibilities is even health-giving. If a daring activity takes place while preserving the different planes in which life moves, that means preserving a free space for others and a nonetheless sensitive connection, then this activity leads to harmonious expansiveness and health as well as to ordered integration and easing of tension.

The conscious feeling of the three planes in which life moves, the right, insightful knowledge of these planes and then the active, natural development of movement, portray this pose. Expansiveness is the result of a progressive, ordered, active will-life while preserving a free space for others. This is the sense in which this very important yoga pose has its meaning. Expansiveness and an understanding of expansiveness describe, moreover, the nature of activity and the specific character of *maṇipūra-cakra*.

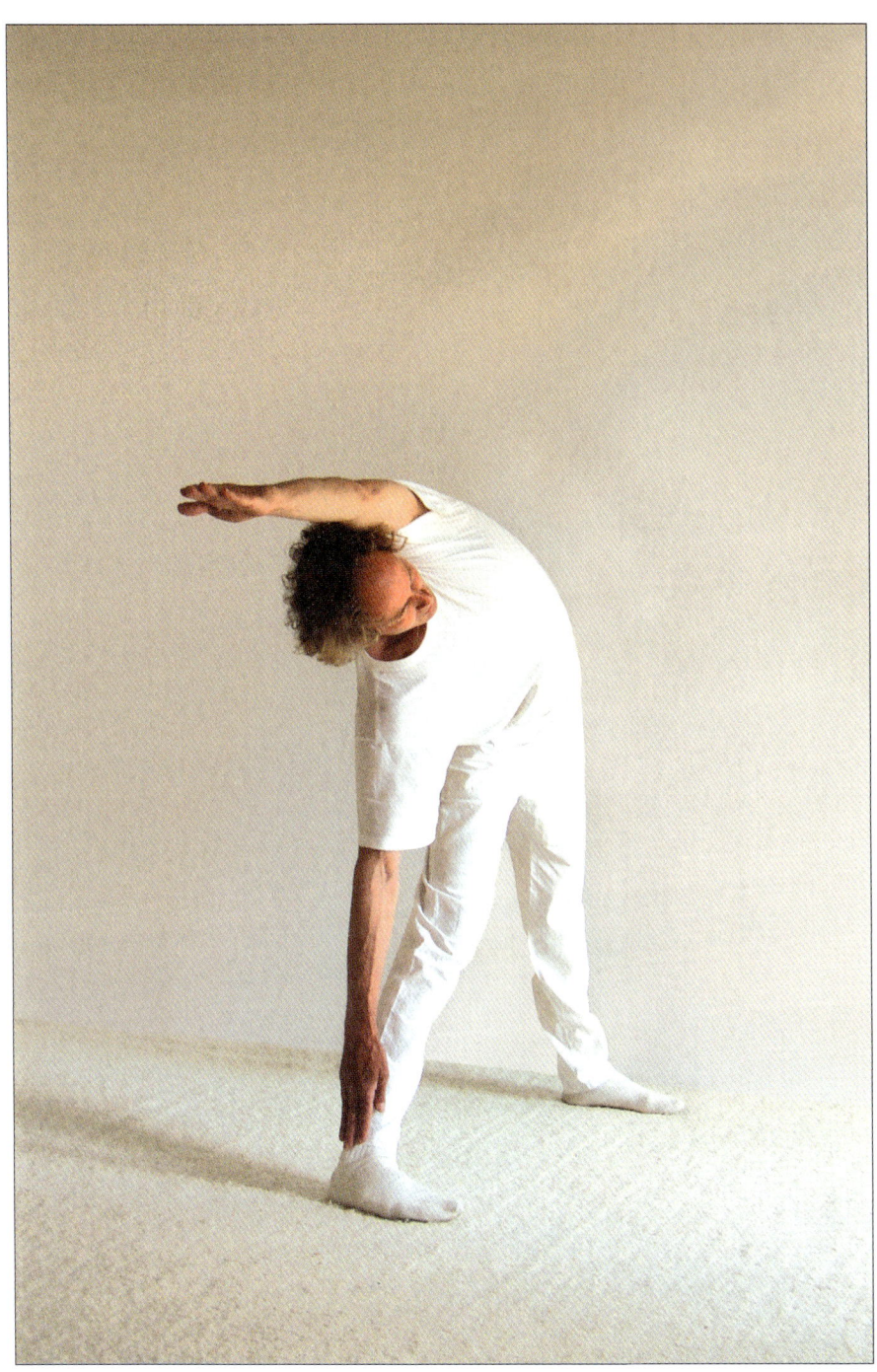

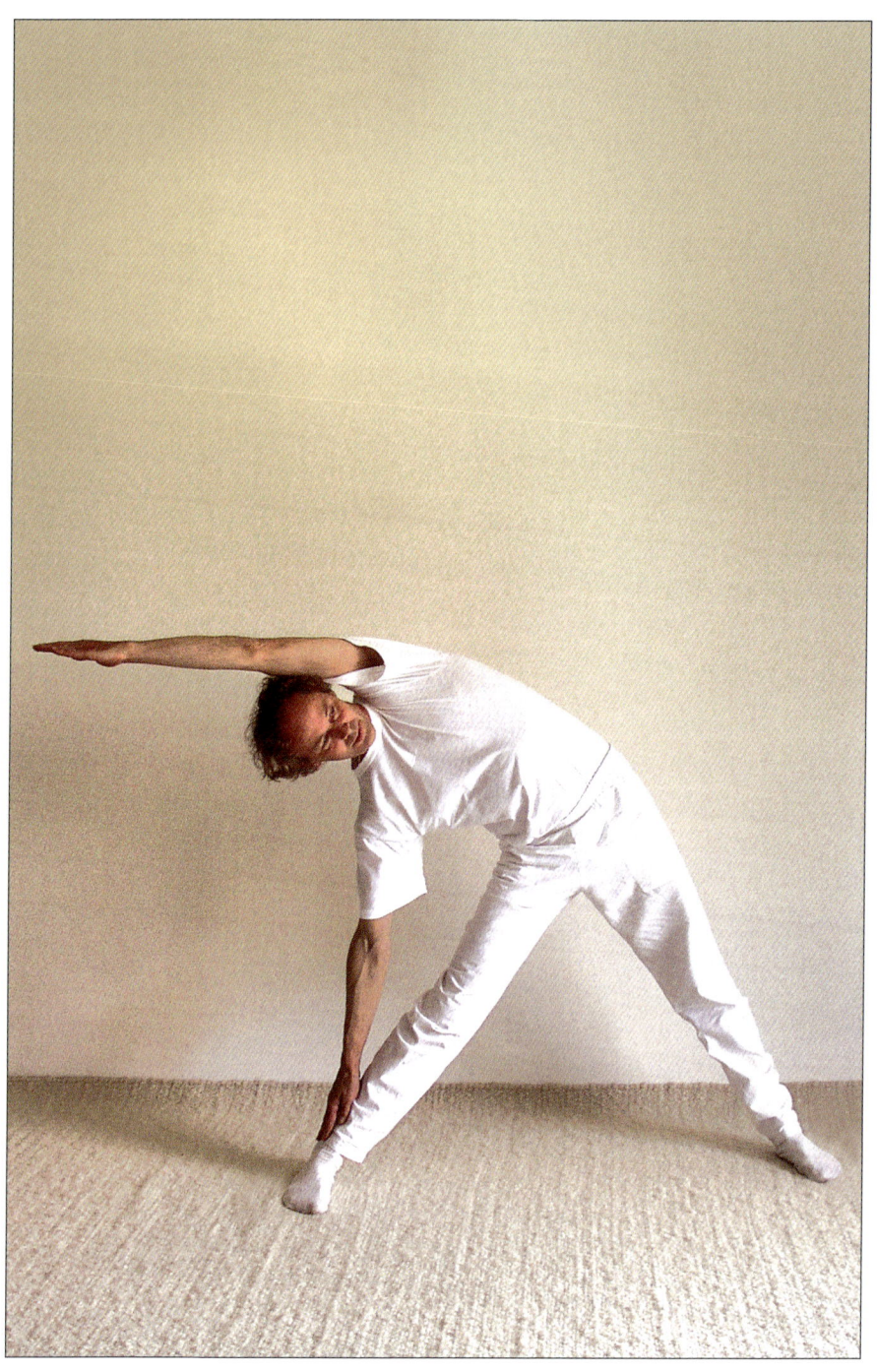

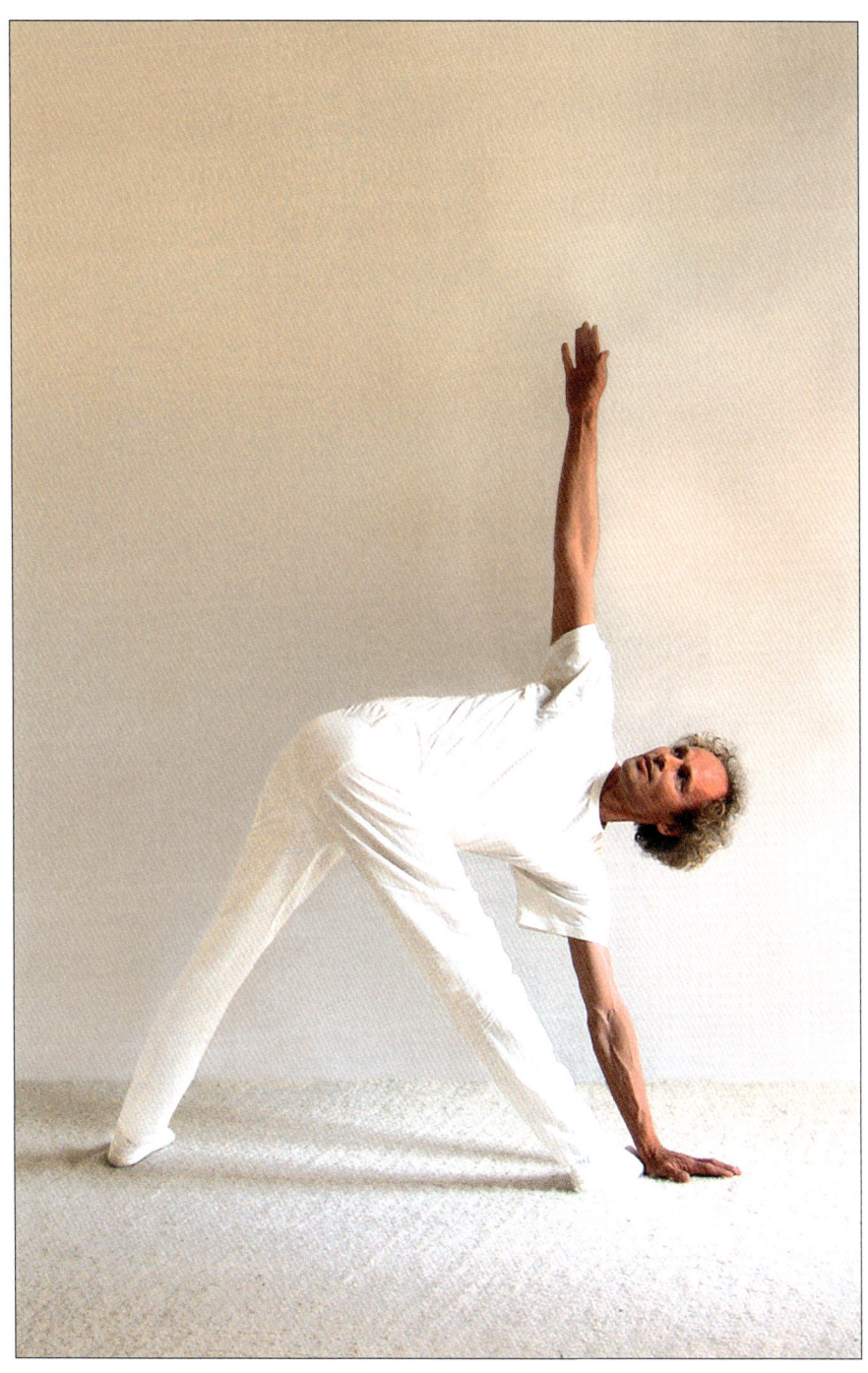

To practise

Form an equilateral, stable triangular base. Bring your left arm up alongside your head and your right arm horizontally outwards. Then bend to the right exactly in the same plane and take the left arm, straightened next to the head, with you into the movement. Throughout the standing position and the dynamic practice pay attention to the threefold articulation of the different bodily regions. The base remains stable. The dynamic is precisely in the area of the solar plexus, the shoulders and head remain as relaxed as a leaf in the breeze, the arms also merely continue in a relaxed way the movement-dynamic existing in the solar plexus centre. Return to the middle after about fifteen seconds, become aware once again of the threefold articulation in the body and then with the reverse arm position stretch to the left side.

Practise this triangle pose preferably several times for a short time on each side. Let the breath flow naturally, expansively and intensively. A rhythmic and dynamic feeling should motivate the practice.

A variation of the triangle is done with a specific twist, *parivṛtta trikoṇāsana*. Once again, the active centre of the movement is the solar plexus. Right from the start this variation should be done with an expansive, free feeling of the body. From the triangular base, lead the right hand to the floor next to your left foot and the left arm vertically upwards. The head follows your gaze towards the upwardly directed hand. The body is twisted about its own axis yet the centre in the solar plexus is felt and held as stable.

In this position, one triangle is formed by the legs and also an additional smaller triangle is placed next to this big one through the arm variation. One hand touches the ground of the earth and the other projects dynamically up into the free region of space. In this way, the upper body is stretched out between earth and free atmosphere. Nevertheless, in the middle of the solar plexus, the stability of the dynamic is maintained, and the triangle that was formed at the beginning with the legs rests evenly in its base. The twisted triangle, *parivṛtta trikoṇāsana*, describes on the one hand activity, on the other hand the shoulder region positioned between earth and free space symbolises the wisdom of the spirit. From the vital activities that life demands, an expansion of the personality occurs into the spacial regions of earthly existence. An expansion of these conditions, ordered in wisdom, coupled with experiences of consciousness, leads to the synthesis of life. Wisdom, the ability to form and earthly activity should eventually come to unite in life to form a harmonious centre. The image of *parivṛtta trikoṇāsana* expresses not only active stretching into the expanse, but symbolises a first synthesis between celestial forces and earthly forces and thus describes a first ideal of the ordered relationships of will in human existence. The twisted triangle is therefore a symbol for wisdom together with the capacity to act.

Another highly recommended triangle variation which, however, has an energetic effect on the second *cakra*, and brings to light the experience of dynamically unified and flowing movement, is *pārśva trikoṇāsana*, the triangle of the sides. This pose is somewhat more challenging than the others, nevertheless it can be practised by beginners.

Practitioners develop a very intensive will-dynamic into the leg pushed up sideways during the exercise. Through this effect of the will, the energies flow from the third centre downwards into the second and first centres. In the process of gathering, however, the *svādhiṣṭhāna-cakra* is experienced, as the movement displays a flowing and coordinating character, and the upper body is experienced as differentiated from the lower body or legs, yet integrally connected with them. The upper body remains relaxed, in the hips and waist a powerful dynamic develops, flowing out into the periphery of both legs. With this the hand is led from above downwards and lightly touches the ground without supporting. The strength is applied from the legs.

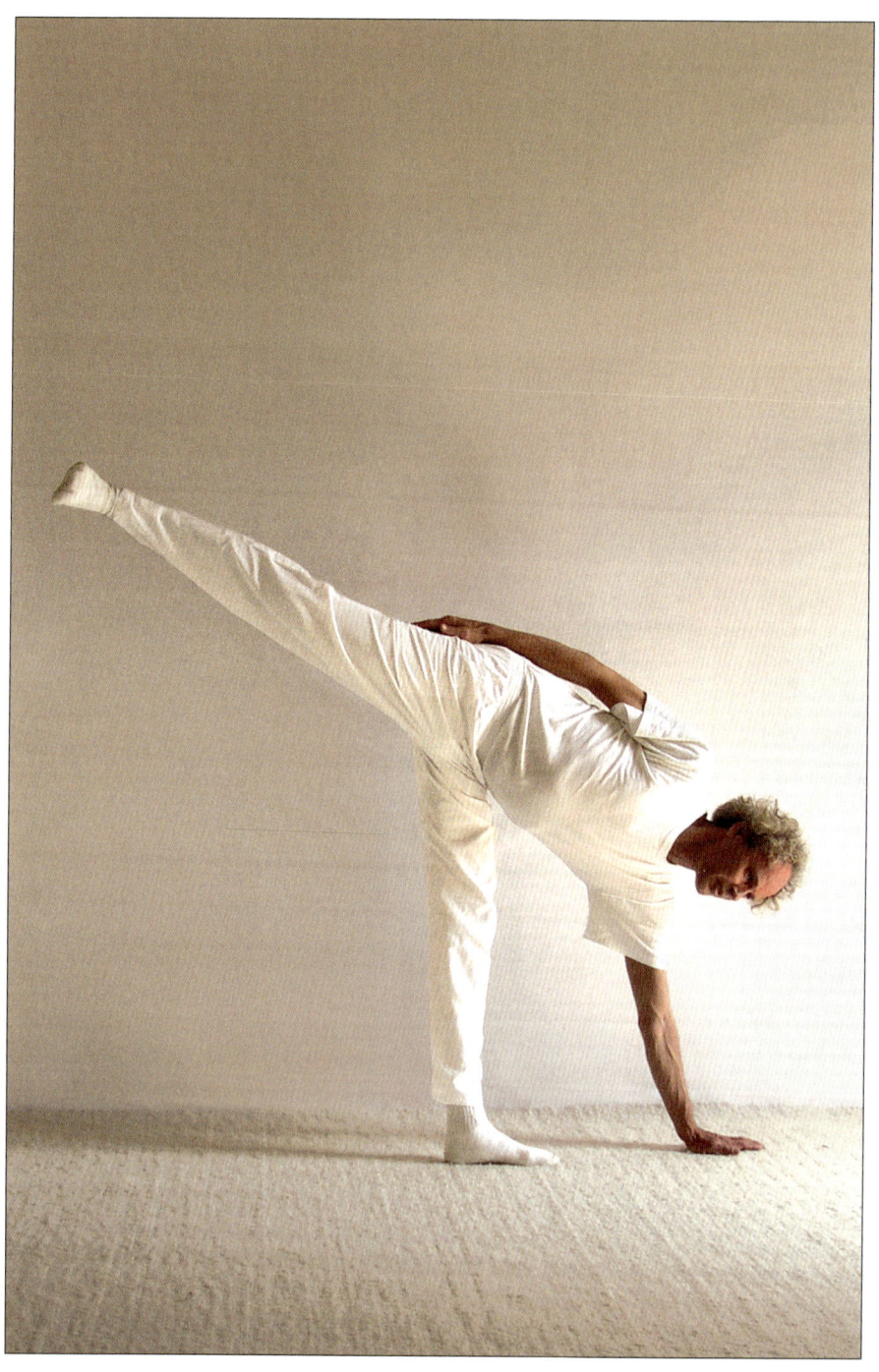

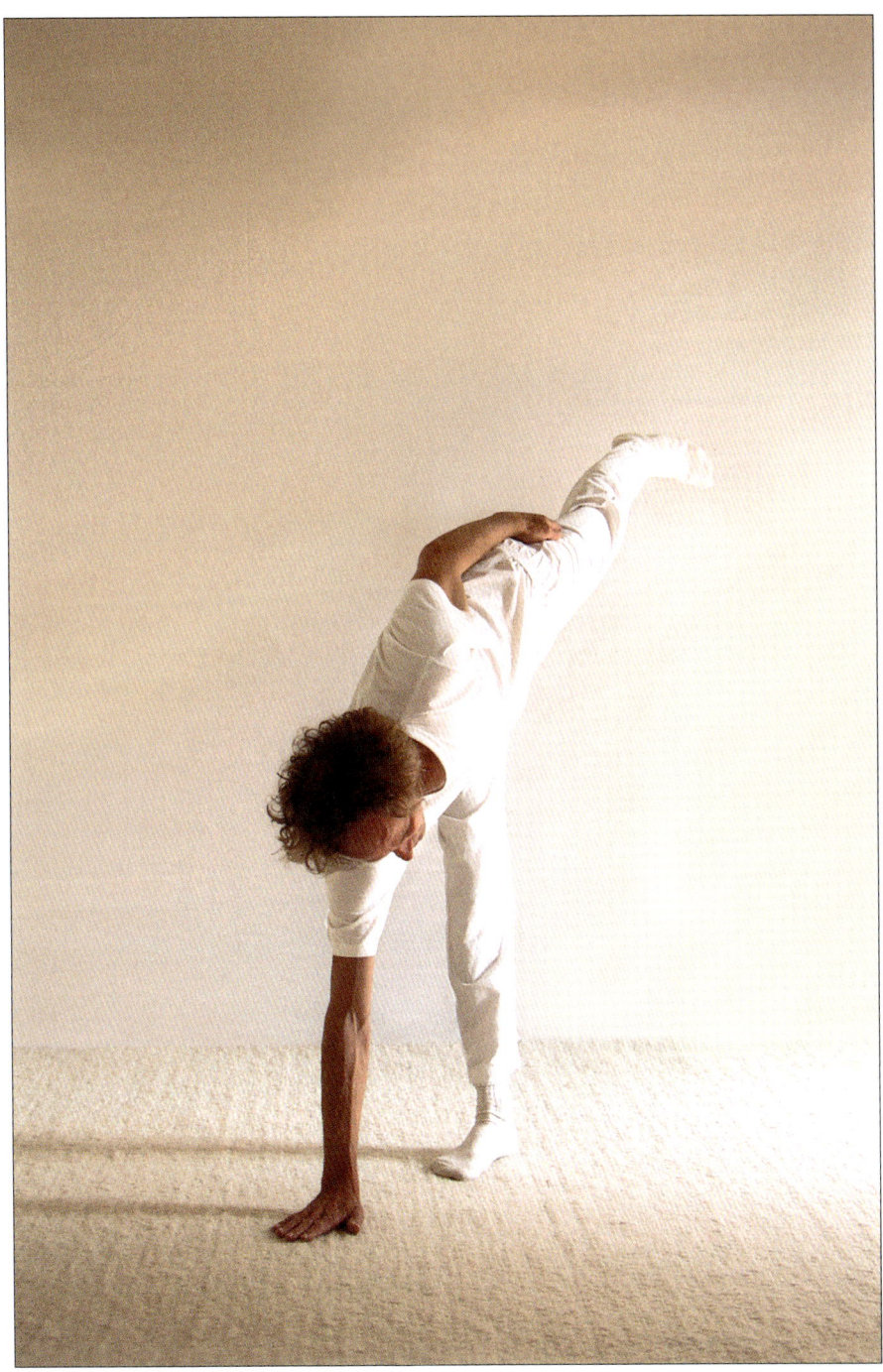

The lying triangle
anantāsana

The picture and the meaning of the exercise

All exercises of the third centre are concerned with the question of how the space can be experienced as a subtle-feeling. The space itself is three dimensional, with height, breadth and depth. The human soul-life, if we venture to draw a comparison, possesses three dimensions, or in other words three different forces. These are the thought-life, the feeling-life and the will-life.

In all exercises, and in particular in this triangle form lying on the ground, practitioners develop a careful articulation into three different sections. They identify the will centre in the limbs, with an out-streaming and mobilising dynamic, they experience the relaxed parts of the body in the free and contemplative light of the thought, and finally they sense the midpoint of the feelings as if in a connecting and coalescing centre. The three regions that work together in an exercise are experienced in an articulated way.

This experience of articulation of the body results in a natural, sensitive consciousness of space, as if space opens up as a universal and protecting dimension with its height, breadth and depth. It acquires a true, sensitively open form, becomes expansive and tangible. Space is a characteristic of earthly reality, but now it begins to live and to gesture to the sensitive soul with joy and expansion. In this experiencing of space, through articulating the human soul-life, there emerges an accommodating openness and freedom for others.

To practise

Lie on your side and stretch your arm along your head so that your body makes the longest possible line. Then bring the top leg up high and with the top arm take hold of your toes or the outside of your foot. The dynamic flows purposefully out of the legs in both directions. The foot can remain flexed so that the balance can be held more easily.

The centre of experience in the exercise lies in the regions of the *maṇipūra* centre. The head, the neck and the shoulders remain relaxed, while in a really flowing dynamic the legs give the body a support rising up from underneath, preventing it from tipping backwards at the sacral region. Dynamic and relaxation therefore meet in the middle of the body and encourage the ability to subtly feel a connection between above and below. This connection is characteristic for the experience of harmony in the threefold articulation and denotes the third centre.

In the various forms of movement, which are created by actively implementing a previously pictured idea, certain specific forms of experience develop. The exercises of the third centre, and particularly the different triangle poses, further human subtle-feeling to become an articulated capacity for perception. The will is centred at specific areas of the body required for the dynamic. Independently from this, however, practitioners consciously decide to remain relaxed in the upper parts of the body. The result of this articulated and experiential activity is the experience of form and space, which is directed to the earthly world, and depicts a soul experience of the gentle yet fluid will.

A noticeable effect of these exercises is a subtle receding of the body, as the will is concentrated in precisely chosen regions. Once the body has receded, the subtle-feelings and thoughts can then enter more freely into what is for them a pleasant and tangible space. They will always contribute to peace and sociability. An exercise which particularly emphasises the threefold articulation encourages the involvement of those inviting beings of subtle-feeling, which allow a space to manifest softly, expansively and non-violently and which ultimately contribute to a natural connection and participation in the external world. Those beings or spiritual substantialities are created that give human beings freedom from fear, and a feeling of being received.

An easier variation of *anantāsana* can be developed by raising only your knee and placing your foot on the lower part of the thigh of the horizontal leg. The lengthways stretch of the position should quite consciously feature as an experience. Finally, the hand is placed on the knee. At the mid-point of this position is *maṇipūra-cakra*. A light dynamic that develops from the middle of the back in both directions, both upwards towards the chest as well as towards the straightened leg downwards, emphasises the subtle-feeling in this centre. The position resembles a first, simple triangle shape.

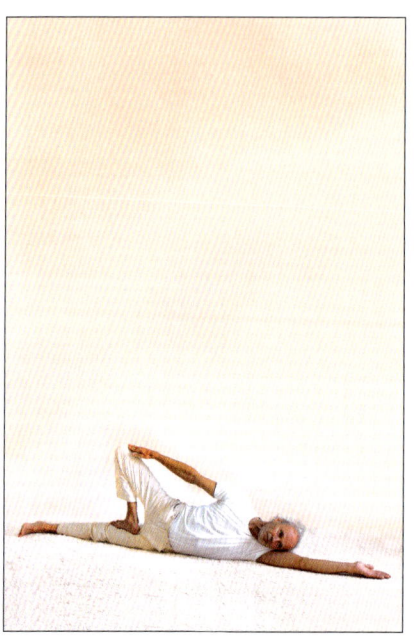

The practice of the final pose enjoys an active leg-dynamic, which can most easily be developed in relation to the relaxed upper body. The experience of the third centre happens predominantly when you keep the arm straightened and yet at the same time relaxed. Falling backwards can be prevented by actively stretching the leg lying on the floor. Between the shoulder-blades the breath space expands, its centre being formed by the sides, precisely at the diaphragm.

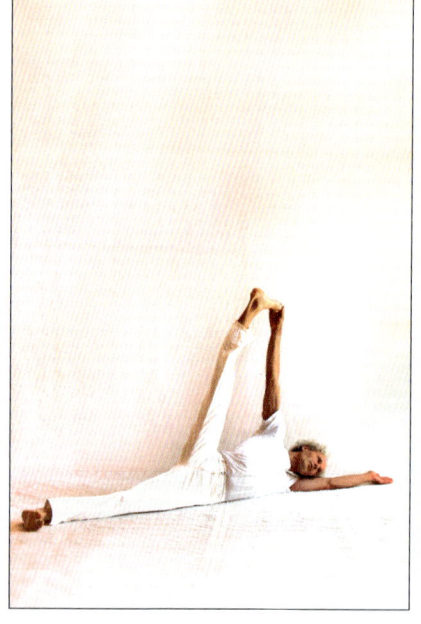

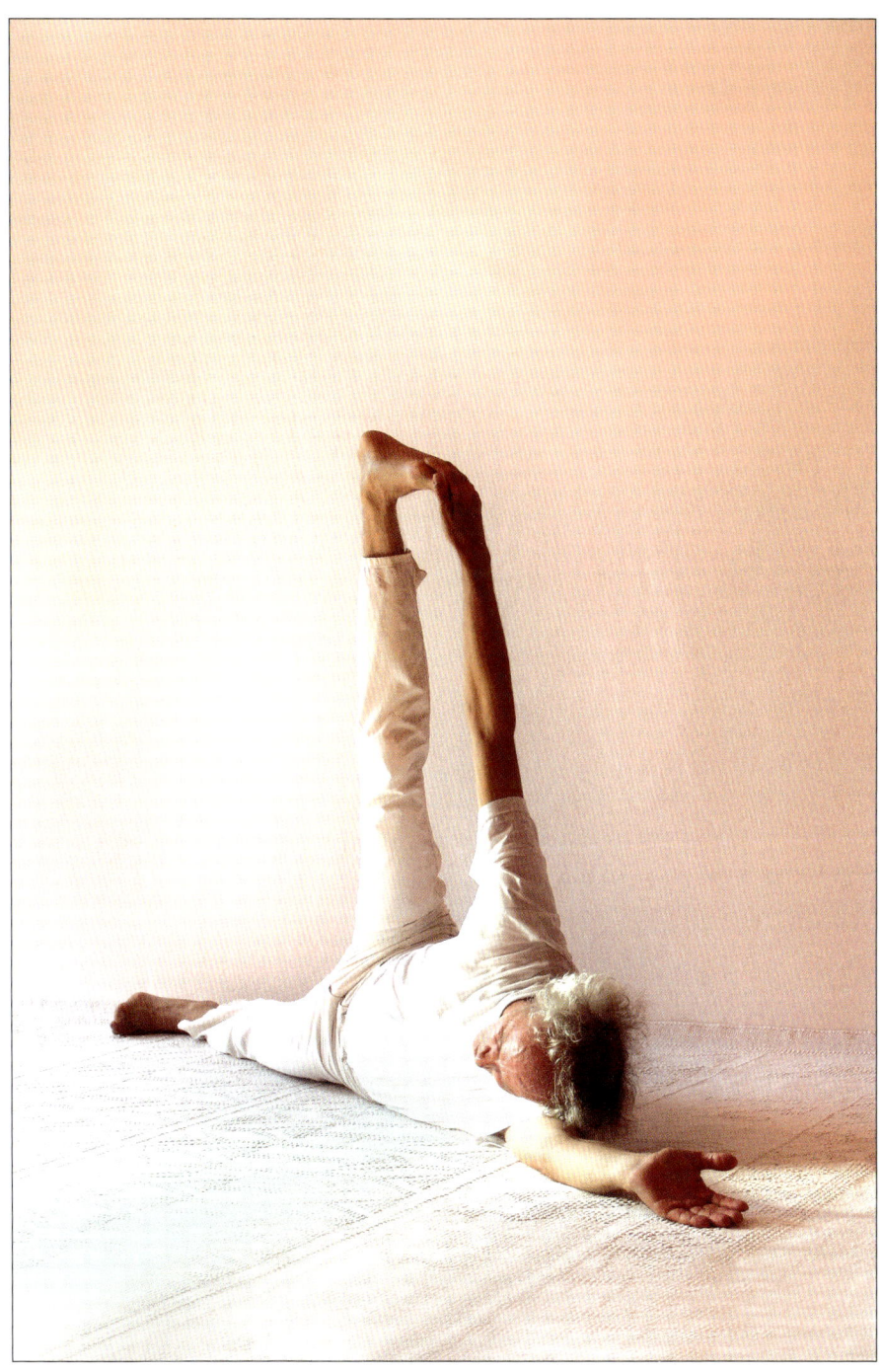

Openness through developing mental pictures, releasing the old and beginning anew – *viśuddha-cakra*

Just as the cosmos, in its constellation of stars, never produces an exact repetition, so too is the consciousness, which in reality never exactly replicates a former situation. Although each day begins with similar temporal rhythms and similar moods, which may remind us of previous days, on closer inspection the days are different from each other and the subjective moods of the consciousness likewise are never the same as the previous ones. A real replication does not exist in the rhythmically interacting activity of the consciousness. Something similar yet becomes something subtly different, and what appears identical is born again anew in its immanent uniqueness. In all the repeating rhythms of time, there is revealed an infinite, transforming and proliferating creative force of the eternal, autonomously active spirit. Consciousness is the activity in which something eternally new, unique and – in the truest sense of the word – incomparable is created.

With the development of *viśuddha-cakra*, the centre at the thyroid gland, students get to know the sensitive openness of the consciousness in the sense of continuously creating mental pictures out of new sources. For example, they practise an exercise which they may have already performed several times before. Through this repeated practice, certain learning steps, such as the practical technique, can become natural and automatic. Yet in their consciousness students release themselves to some degree from previous experiences and impressions, so as to witness the exercise in an entirely new way and to pause in the sensitive moment of the present experience. Through this releasing of old experiences that occupy the consciousness and bind it to the past, a learning requirement emerges, which demands growing alertness, sensitivity and calmness of consciousness. Only in calmness and in observation can the old experiences succeed in receding and give space to the new impressions coming. Here at this stage, practitioners get to know the alert and free calmness of the consciousness. In the sensitive openness, free working forces of active picturing breathe, lighting up the periphery of the body.

Normally we think with a certain exertion, wilfully, using the capacity we have been given. We think less using our capacity for observation or our actively created mental pictures. The breath is therefore very subtly connected to the soul-forces of thinking, feeling and willing, and so its flow is intrinsically bound. But when the sensitive openness, alertness and power of observation comes to unfold out of the consciousness itself, practitioners can then allow their breath to flow more freely and they can recognise the living process of picturing as a first activity of consciousness belonging to the spiritual dimension of existence. We think neither using our will nor through certain superimposed feelings, but in reality we think by observing, and by forming real mental pictures. The more the flow of breath becomes free, and the more it is possible for the body to move freely, the more, ultimately, the free potential is opened up for activity of the consciousness. This activity of the consciousness, meaning an activity of building mental pictures independent of the body, should be recognised and trained at this stage of the path.

A further learning step consists in developing discernment about the expression that can be perceived in the exercises. The exercises should ideally show a freer, lighter, purer consciousness of the fixed bodily tensions. Whether the exercises are harder or easier, they should describe in the expression of the limbs, in the movement of straightening up the spine, and in the form that is pictured, a clear light of freedom and differentiation. With some training on this path, practitioners get to know whether their own practice is more bound and fixed or whether their approach is differentiated, and eventually on this basis they learn to really bring the various pictures belonging to the exercises into their practice. To some degree, naturally only after some training, they then see the more subtle underlying quality of the exercise. They gradually acquire first impressions of the radiance created by the consciousness, and learn to appreciate the value of differentiating observation.

The wings
pakṣati

The picture and the meaning of the exercise

Consciously developed thinking, that is built up into mental pictures, can give people a natural protection for their lives. The way in which we think creates forms, which at first are only visible in a spiritual way. A consciously constructed mental picture is not merely imagined, but exists like a companion to people and so they are not alone. And now, when they are no longer alone, but in luminous company, they feel calmed within themselves and through their accompanying mental picture they experience a natural protection towards the outside. Mental pictures give human beings a protective, luminous sheath. So all thought processes which the human consciousness carries out have the effect of creating forms, and if these are carried out with best efforts they can in turn order and illuminate the space and make it seem accessible in its differentiatedness. Thinking is a forming and spiritual activity.

Someone who has consciously learnt to think, builds with this thinking forms of light, which appear arched or like wings, slightly curved, running from top to bottom. These forms gently touch the periphery of the human body giving a very luminous and congenial coating. However, this coating does not close off contact, it opens the person's whole being to the outside and yet still gives the calmness of a natural protection and the feeling of being ordered within.

To practise

Practitioners can directly imitate a form close to this experience using bodily gestures. To do this, come into the standing position and then bend your body as far forwards as possible. This movement is also the third position of *sūrya namaskāra*. After about half a minute come back up to the starting position.

Now start afresh by raising the arms, bringing the hands together at a point high above your head. Then glide down with your arms, creating a smooth arc, in a wider movement, and finally lower your upper body too into the forward bend, until you finally touch the ground, with your hands out sideways to the left and right of your feet. The hands are as far apart as possible, the body depicts a triangle.

Return again in a natural way, this time without describing the arch from the bottom up. The exercise should specifically be done only from above to below. Afterwards you will notice that the practice conveys to the subtle-feeling a kind of calm and at the same time a pleasing form. It is good if you consciously remember once again the shaping of this arch, which is somewhat bigger than your own body and so in a way encloses the body.

When this exercise is practised, the consciousness is never experienced as entering too far inwards, into the physicality. It sooner experiences itself active in the external surroundings and in formulating the gesture. For the fifth centre, the *viśuddha-cakra*, it is extremely important to see the activity of mental picturing in a radius of action that always takes place at the periphery of the body and not inside the body. The forms which are developed through making mental pictures actually shape the peripheral surrounds of the body, but they do not sink into the body. This relationship is extremely important. Therefore, with the activity of mental picturing, the natural surroundings light up, and individuals experience how they can move and reside with their thought-life in a space free from the body.

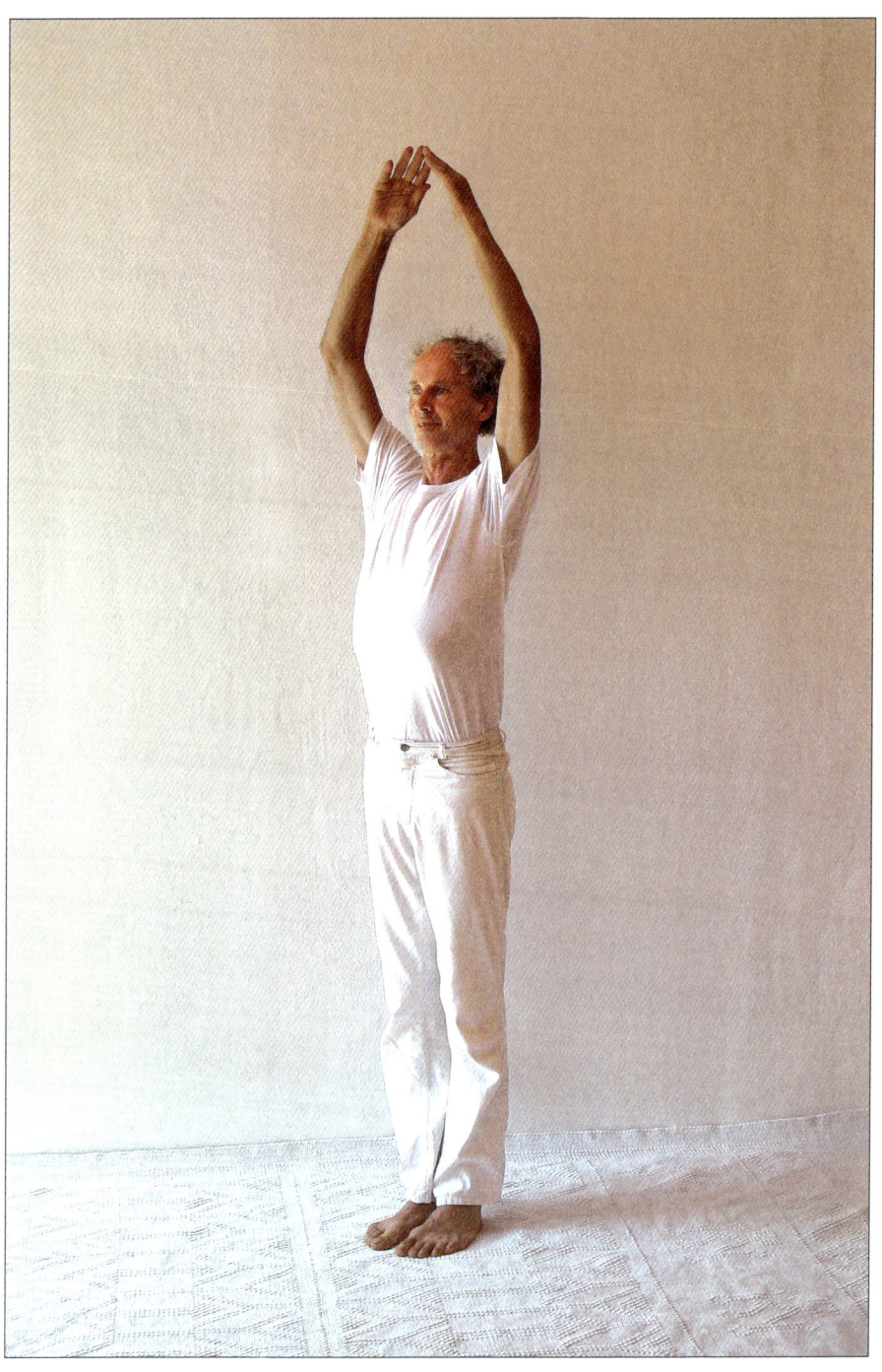

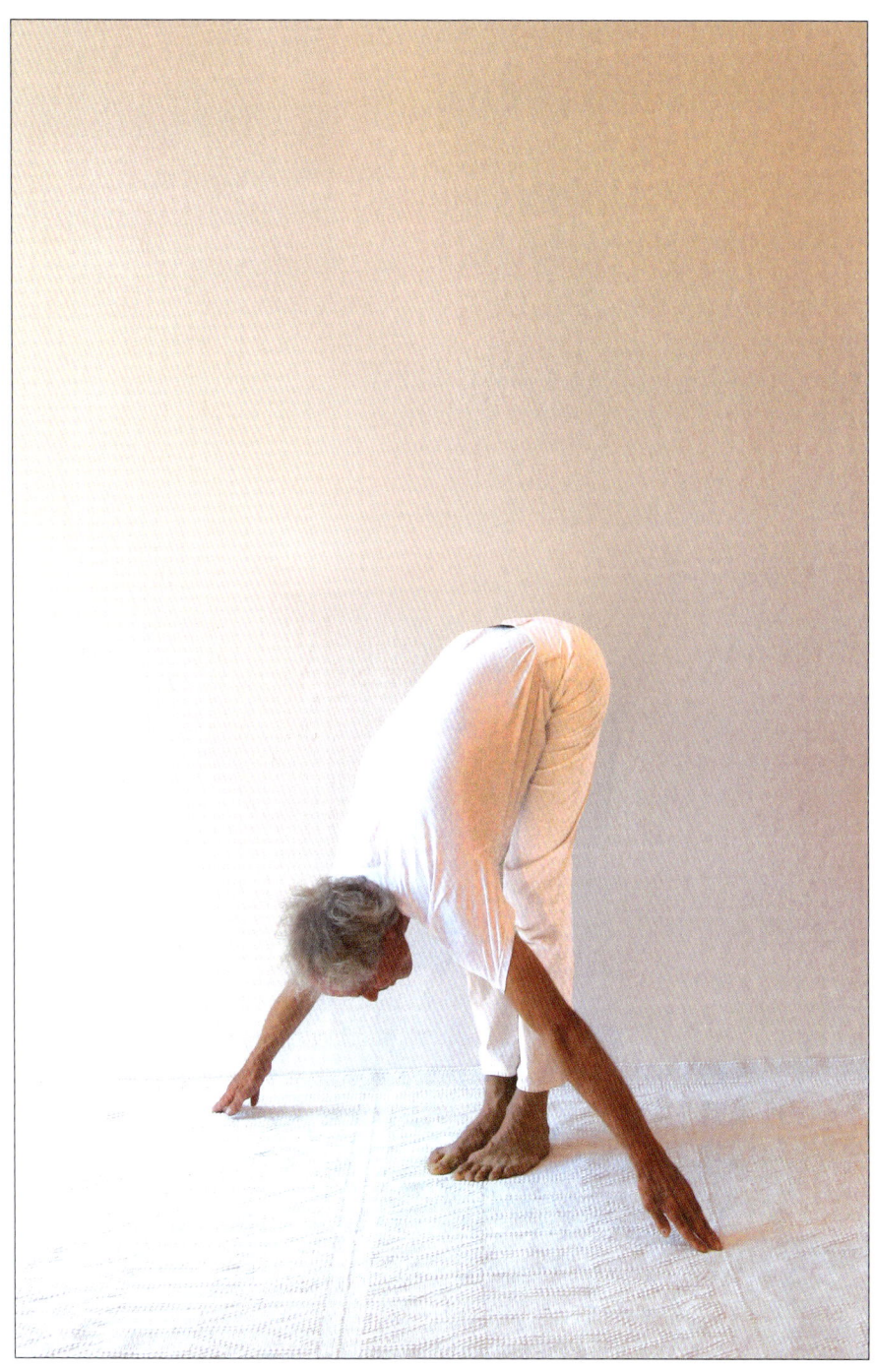

The yoga gesture
yoga mudrā

The picture and the meaning of the exercise

This exercise, which is reminiscent of bowing down in devotion, should illustrate the true nature of self-surrender. What is true self-surrender, and the devotion connected with it? Is it a form of subservience, of skilfully being able to subordinate oneself, of the ability to painfully endure, or of passive abandonment? Or is it not more an inner, dignified attitude based on the wisdom that only the body is offered up, but the consciousness establishes itself in a greater alertness? Do practitioners give up their entire consciousness on the path and allow themselves to fall into a seeming meditative feeling? No, with every form of dedication to another they preserve a conscious state of discernment, and with every act of devotion they develop a greater consciousness in the sense of overcoming lower character traits. But what is true discernment and the exemplary art of a chosen devotion?

Yoga mudrā is a gesture of actively devoting oneself while preserving honour, and is opposite from a passive, dreamy giving-up and a passive letting-be without understanding. The consciousness is directed to an actual ideal, to a greater aspirational theme of life, and in doing so gives up all dependencies, leanings and attachments bound to the body. The consciousness is therefore highly active and is never surrendered, while all the other forces bound to the body are released and subordinated to the greater feeling. With this distinction, *yoga mudrā* helps bring about a first discerning experience of the principle of consciousness, which is a principle of inner alertness. *Yoga mudrā* depicts a process of physical release and of a delicate, sensitive new founding in the active state of the consciousness forces. The meaning of this exercise lies in this discernment between a body that is offered up, and a consciousness that becomes delicately awakened to a world of attachment and to freely available activity.

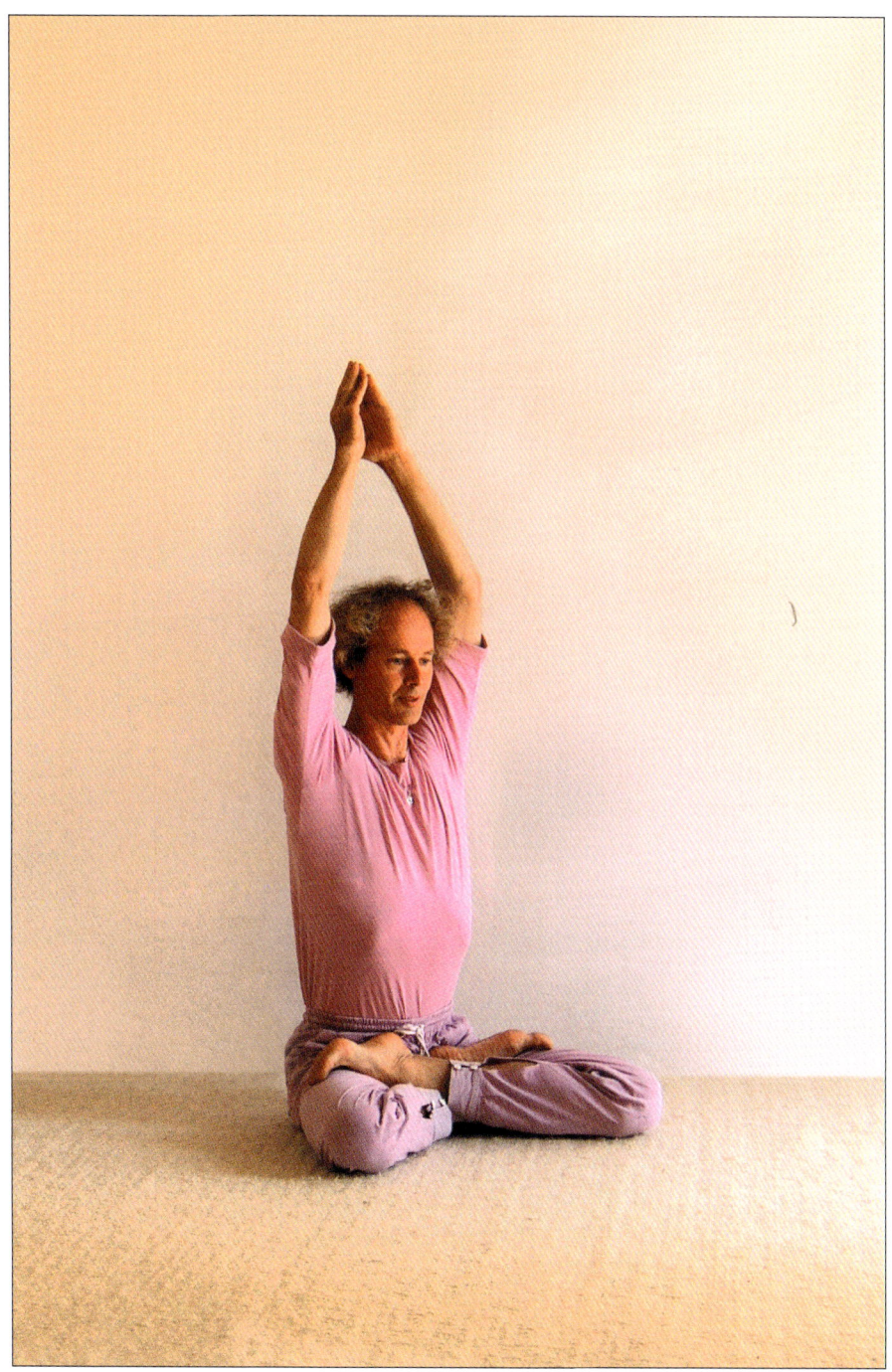

To practise

With the gesture of *yoga mudrā* you take the body into a most intensive, closed bowing form, which is reminiscent of completely letting go of the will, as if the body is reconciled with the earth, motionless, timeless, untouchable, as if dead. The exercise comes into being like an arrival at the gate of death, where the body remains behind and the consciousness can from now on expand freely, victoriously over the earth.

Take a position with your legs crossed or in half lotus, or if possible in full lotus. Stretch your arms above your head with the palms together. Pause, become absolutely calm and let the breath flow freely. Become conscious of yourself in this position with the body upright.

Tilt the body forwards, without much strain or exertion, until the head and arms touch the ground, relaxed and stretched out. The whole upper body, arms and head should rest bowed down, as released as possible. Only the breath remains freely flowing. Contemplation should increase in this exercise, until a subtle-feeling of release comes about, which can be described as if the body were dead. The consciousness nevertheless remains sensitive, watchful, overseeing.

After about twenty seconds straighten the body up into the sitting position again and remain conscious of yourself in the present. Repeat the exercise a few times.

In contrast to the head to knee pose with its very active tension, in which the aim is to stretch beyond one's limits, in *yoga mudrā*, the bowing gesture, the emphasis is more on the sensitive alertness of the consciousness, which gives the effect of contemplatively looking upon the body, and in doing so allows the body to sink into a complete, released relaxation.

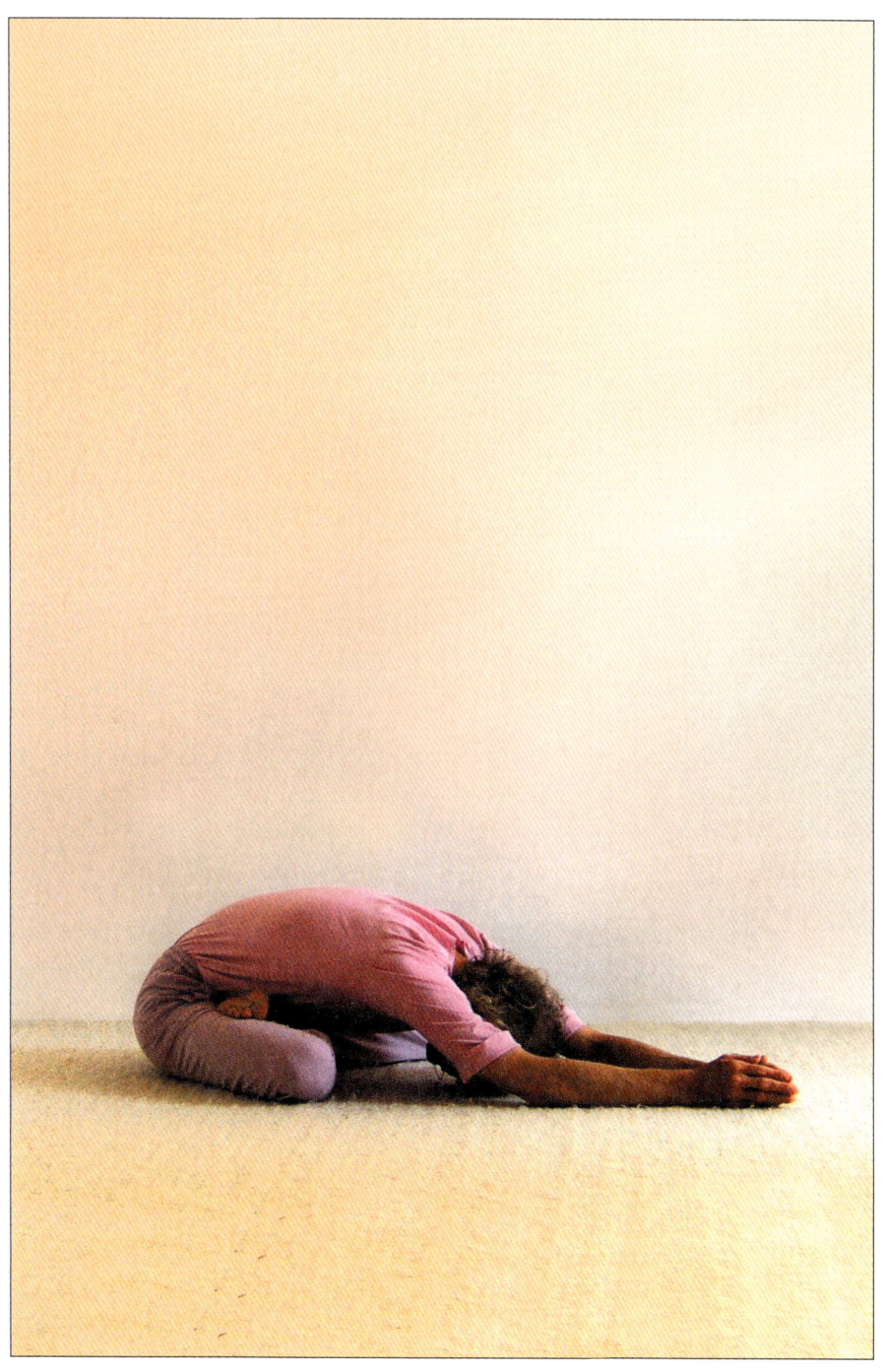

The fish
matsyāsana

The picture and the meaning of the exercise

This very important, central pose in yoga, which can be done at any age, develops its inner sense through the particular and carefully guided distribution of tension into which the bodily position is integrated. The head falls back, the thoracic spine is lifted into the farthest and most thorough stretch, and the hips and legs rest on the ground. The thoracic spine is the middle section or link between the lower, metabolically active regions and the upper nerve-sense regions of the body. With the lifting of the thoracic spine, the lungs are also lifted up. They are, so to speak, lifted out of the natural line of the body. When the lungs are sunk too deeply into the body, and this is a kind of psychological state in a lot of people today, melancholy and sadness, a kind of hopelessness arises. However, if the feelings are freed from their constriction and the lungs are lifted up, life becomes what it actually represents in the sense of possibilities and tasks: Hope, confidence and joy with an interest in others.

The consciousness can be likened to an arched gateway, erected by individuals themselves. When the consciousness itself becomes capable of creating order in its own inner space and can assign the past to the past and the future to the future, and the consciousness itself can be experienced as active consciousness, then with each day, that sensitive, spiritually-seen arched gateway of life and of hope in life can be subtly felt. Inwardly, human beings are constantly erecting this gateway by achieving new perceptions, learning steps and courageous actions. In this sense, similarly to the spiritual gateway, the fish depicts the hope of an ordered life of the consciousness, that can always experience itself in the present. Individuals do not rush into the future too quickly, meaning that they do not race through the existing spiritual gateway, but they remain for long enough in the forming of suitable mental pictures, and only act these out after a reasonable time period.

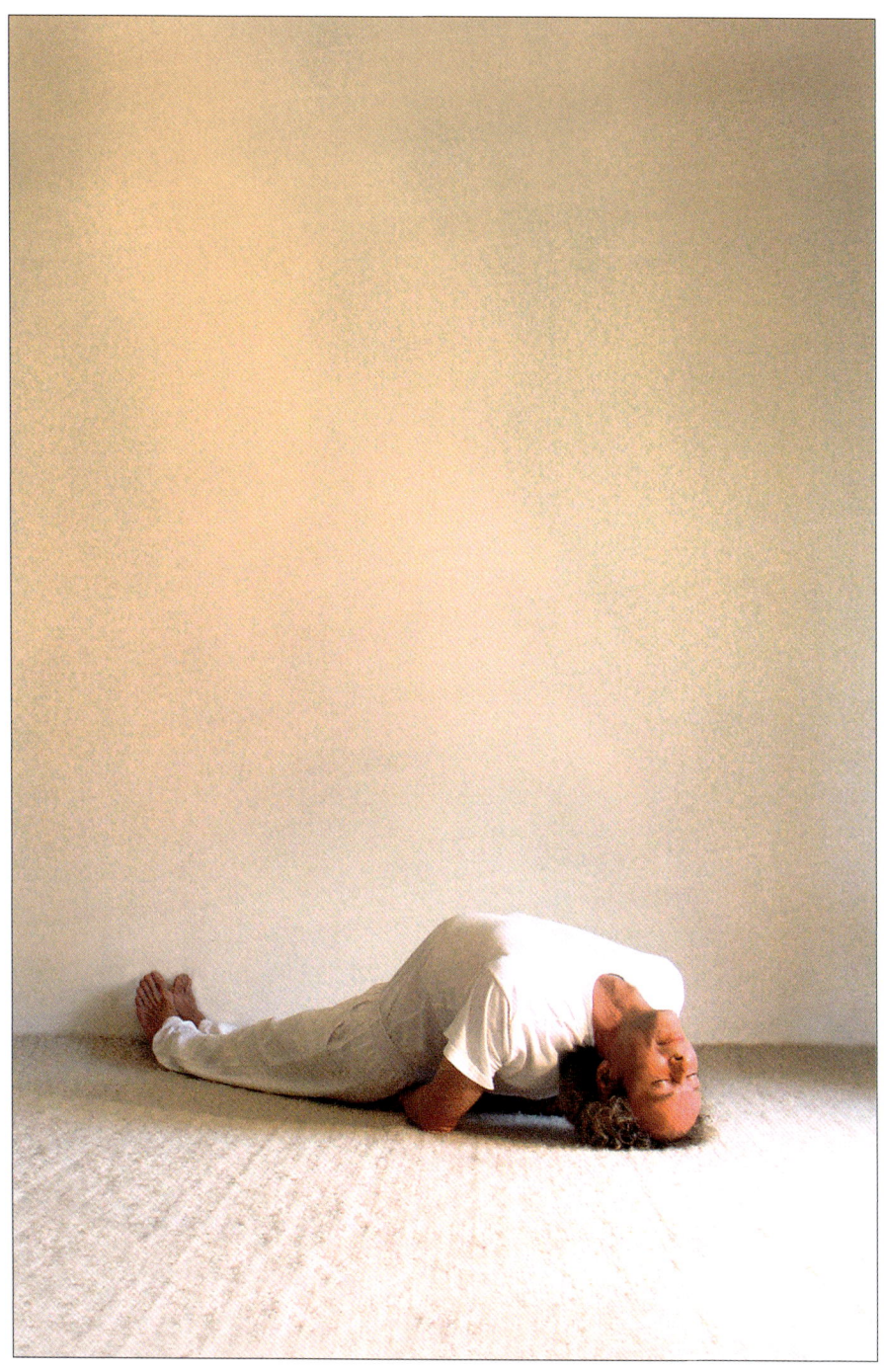

Neither a physiological withdrawal nor nervous haste identify the harmoniously, actively chosen movements of the consciousness. The fish describes an ordered and sensitive state of awareness, a kind of exact, well-tuned, forward-looking consciousness-activity of rational and also hope-filled thought-activity.

To practise

With the practice of *matsyāsana* you enter into an attitude of consciousness of the precise distribution of tension and concurrent sensitive openness for the light of the still unknown future that lies ahead. Lie on your back and bring your arms under your body, the palms are placed on the floor under your buttocks. Support yourself on your elbows as you come up and direct your thoracic spine upwards as far as possible. The head then gently drops back at the neck and the crown touches the floor with the weight of the head. The collar bones are extended right up. The breath flows into the chest and remains free, light and sensitive.

Hold the position with precise distribution of tension for close to a minute, remaining aware of the body in all its parts. You can vividly experience the sections of the legs, abdomen, chest and finally the head in their analogy and meaning, and allow a feeling that in the light of the cosmos the future awaits. In the fish you experience the body with all its parts ordered and differentiated, while a very centred dynamic lifts the lungs up against gravity.

An advanced variation, in which the position is experienced as being more unified and centred, is the fish in lotus. In this classical *āsana* the emphasis is even more on stretching through the thoracic spine and lifting up, even lifting out the chest, as the body does not tail off into the space beyond as much with the limbs, but dynamically hones in on a central point. The exertion in stretching through the length of the thoracic spine shows pictorially and tangibly how effort is demanded in order not to fall into one's old mindset or habits, but to orient the thinking towards new perspectives. The fish is the health-promoting, progressive pose.

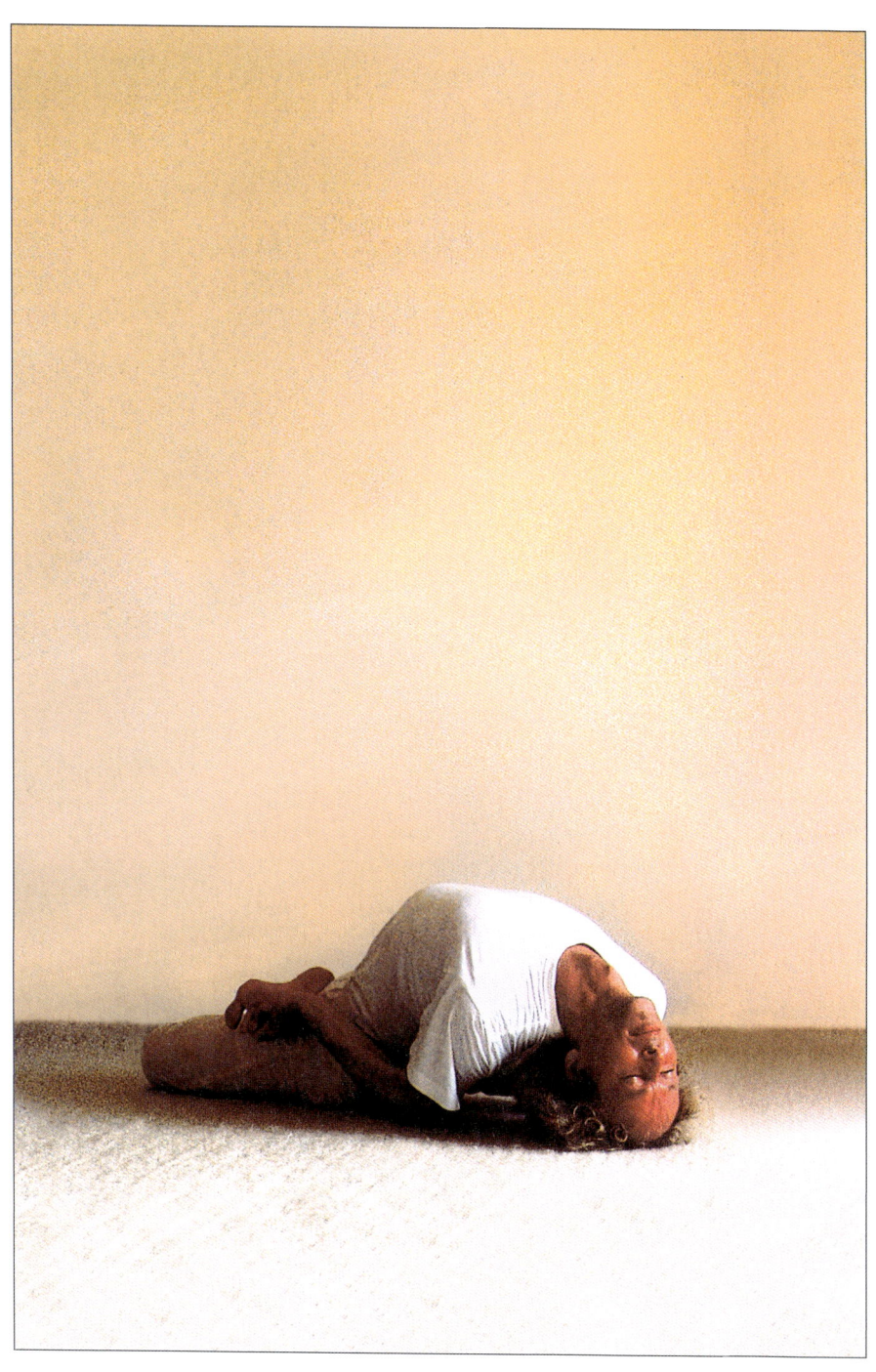

The half moon
āñjaneyāsana

The picture and the meaning of the exercise

The half moon is the symbol for the consciousness, which is woven out of light and active in the light. Practitioners actually notice during practice how through their attention it becomes imperceptibly brighter around them.

This superb pose depicts the two directions of movement that the consciousness, or to use the technical term the "astral body", takes. These two movements are on the one hand towards expansiveness and openness into the world and into cosmic space, and on the other hand towards the earth and integration into the earth. These two directions of movement are expressed in the exercise. The astral body constantly seeks to expand, it is like the light of the cosmos, which is always active, shining out both to the earth and to the spaces of the worlds, longing for sensitive contact.

Practitioners sink forwards in the leg position, gently and far, so that the hips come down as near to the ground as possible. This is the first form of movement, representing the sensitive nearing of human nature to the ground of this earth. The other movement is formed with the back and with the rising arms, which move into the half moon, *ardha candra*. That is the cosmic activity of gliding out.

Practitioners feel the connection between relaxation, sinking into the base close to the earth, and the possible stretch through the spine into the openness, towards the cosmos. The directions of movement are actually interdependent, the way to the earth and the way into the light of the cosmos. The farther one can manage to sink into the base, the more easily one can stretch through the thoracic spine and lead it into the openness. In the insightful knowledge of these two directions of movement and in developing an experience of being devoted to the inner, hidden, profound aims that the consciousness wants to find, lies the sense of this very important *āsana*.

To practise:

Dedication, close proximity, like the noble, knightly court gesture, and a fine round dynamic streaming into the ether, are combined in this exercise to form a unified picture. Bring your right leg forwards and your left leg far back. Transfer your weight onto the front leg but keep the heel on the ground. Relax your shoulders and arms and sink down farther and farther into the base. You should feel yourself to be like a bowl that receptively opens upwards in this starting position. Only after at least half a minute of preparation in this base position can the hands be brought together and the arms glide up over the head. With this movement the thoracic spine extends back into the half moon.

The stretch through the spine should not be felt in the lower back during practice; the activity of stretching flows into the various sections of the thoracic spine, which is released vertebra by vertebra. This happens all the more easily if the upper body remains entirely relaxed during the exercise.

With increasing practice, you can take the thoracic spine into a farther stretch. The breathing should nevertheless remain free and the position should not tense up. Hold this position for up to half a minute and then come back out of the position in the same careful steps by moving systematically until you reach the first position of initial concentration again. Then change to the other side.

When doing the exercise, also pay attention to the connection between the third and fifth energy centres. In a pleasant way these two centres connect with each other through the precise, well-coordinated and sensitively perceptible dedication. The half moon is a sensitive movement, which comes about less through strength, but through an articulated, careful, contemplative and relaxed differentiation in the way the active tension is built up.

The following pictures depict a short sequence, leading from the initial concentration (picture p. 204) via the normal, basic pose (picture p. 205) to an intensive development of active tension in a very advanced version of the half moon (picture p. 206).

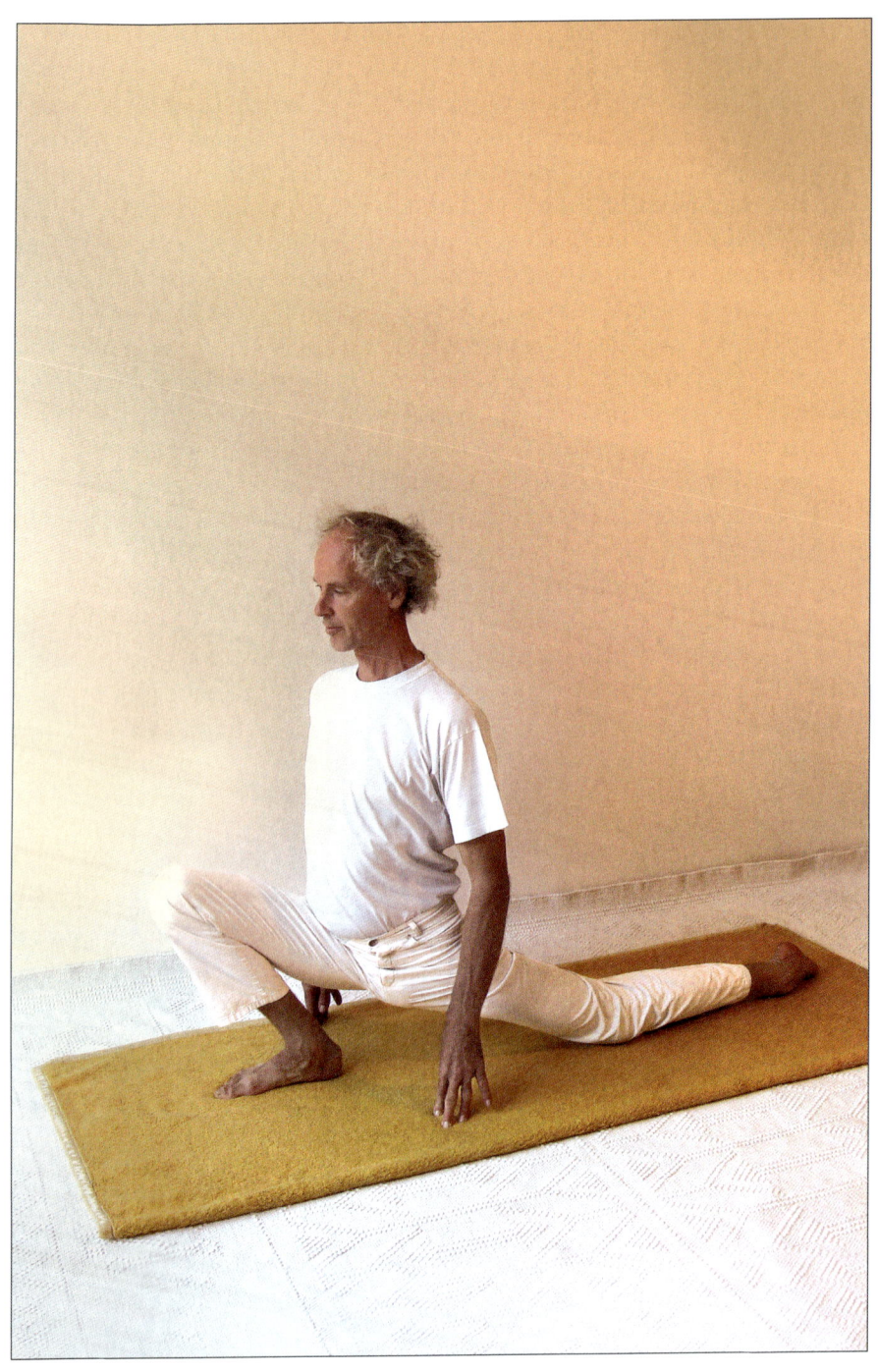

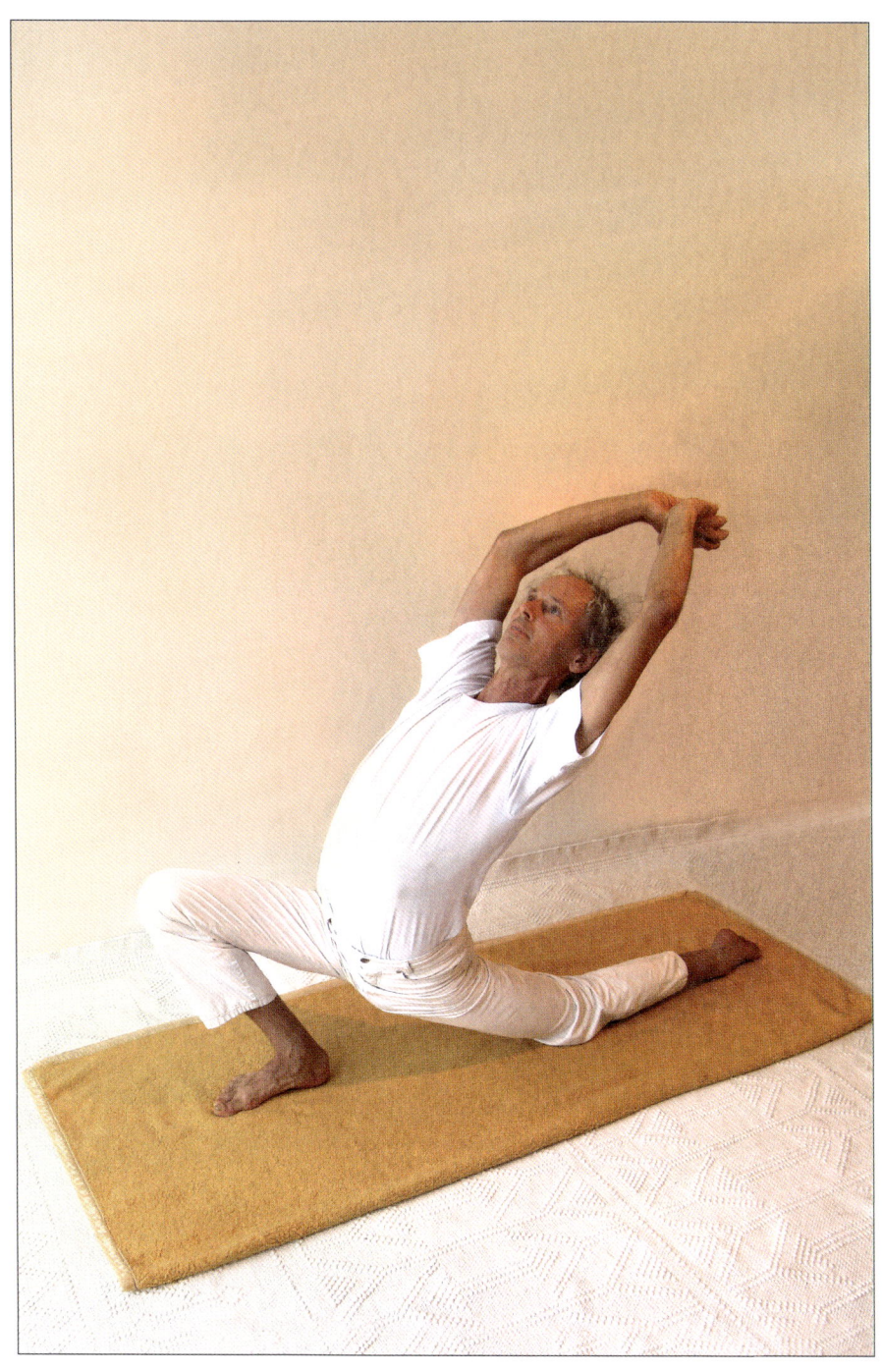

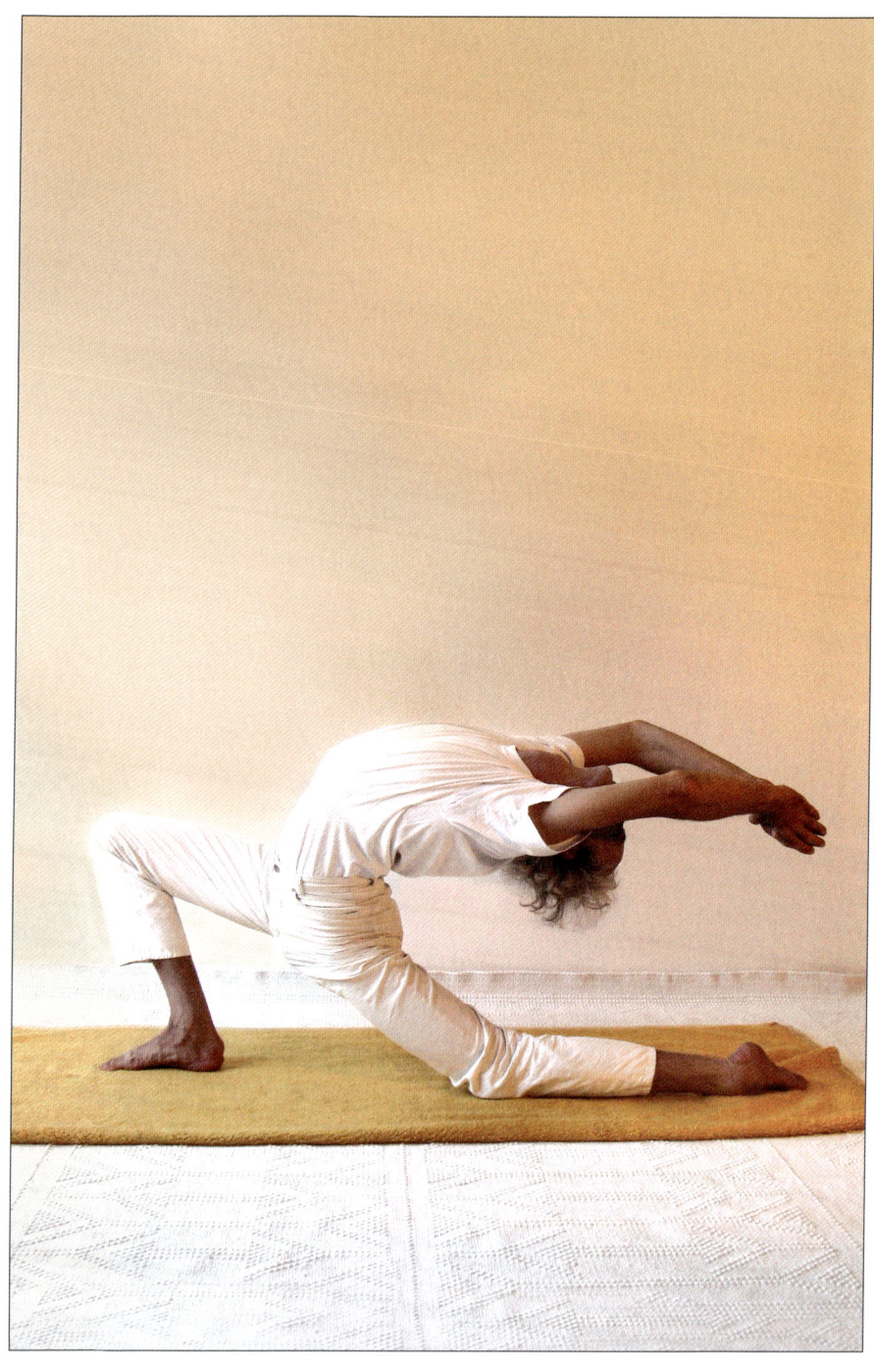

The following simple sketch shows two directions of movement; a bowl and an arch, which pictorially outline the experience in *āñjaneyāsana*. In every phase of the exercise, the body is experienced as if in a calm picture.

To integrate and apply these two directions of movement in a social sense, the sinking into the base can be transformed into, and equated with, a capacity to perceive earthly life and other people. From this capacity for perception, combined with a path of spiritual training and aims for greater ideals, the light and free ether force of newer and nobler thoughts then awakens, symbolised in the exercise by the rising half moon. Sinking into the base is a female gesture, while the thought-forming or ascending process represents a male gesture. However, both gestures together complement each other and create an ideal.

The head to knee pose in half lotus
eka pāda padma paścimottānāsana

The picture and the meaning of the exercise

Adults are only able to develop and progress towards spirituality in a truly satisfactory way if independence, free decisions, active focus and conscious self-motivation underpin their learning steps and experiences. An independent focus and activity of consciousness, however, usually first need to be learned, as human beings are shaped by many unconscious, body-instinctive energy structures, psychological patterns and learned, passively acquired beliefs.

If a human being succeeds in replacing instinctive ways of behaviour, motivated by the body, with clear, pictured, newly oriented objectives and with perceptions that are realistic and true, then these are consciousness-steps of a new beginning. They have an extremely beneficial effect on the immune system and even during the exercise they appear as a star-like glow in the area of the fifth energy centre, *viśuddha-cakra*. This exercise is directed predominantly by this centre, while the head to knee pose, in its classical practice, is motivated more by the third centre with its driving-force and its dynamic that transcends limits. With this exercise, practitioners now experience the difference between the fifth and the third centres. To develop a free will to form mental pictures, with appropriate care, control and mental concentration towards the body, are the learning steps of this exercise. First the consciousness attains an ordering overview and mental picture, in order subsequently to attain a differentiated will-activity. The exercise places the subtle-feeling acquired out of present-moment perception above unconscious will-activity anchored in the body.

Were practitioners to enter into this exercise with only impulsive, almost instinctive will-power, they would not get to know the exercise and they would not need to consider their motives in order to find a new beginning. But by going into the exercise carefully, with an alert, sensitive overview and clear control of the thoughts, they notice how the consciousness, with its guidance, gradually develops a new kind of subtle-feeling for the body and in doing so remains at the periphery. Order, with its guided activity of thought and deliberate care, takes precedence over emotional,

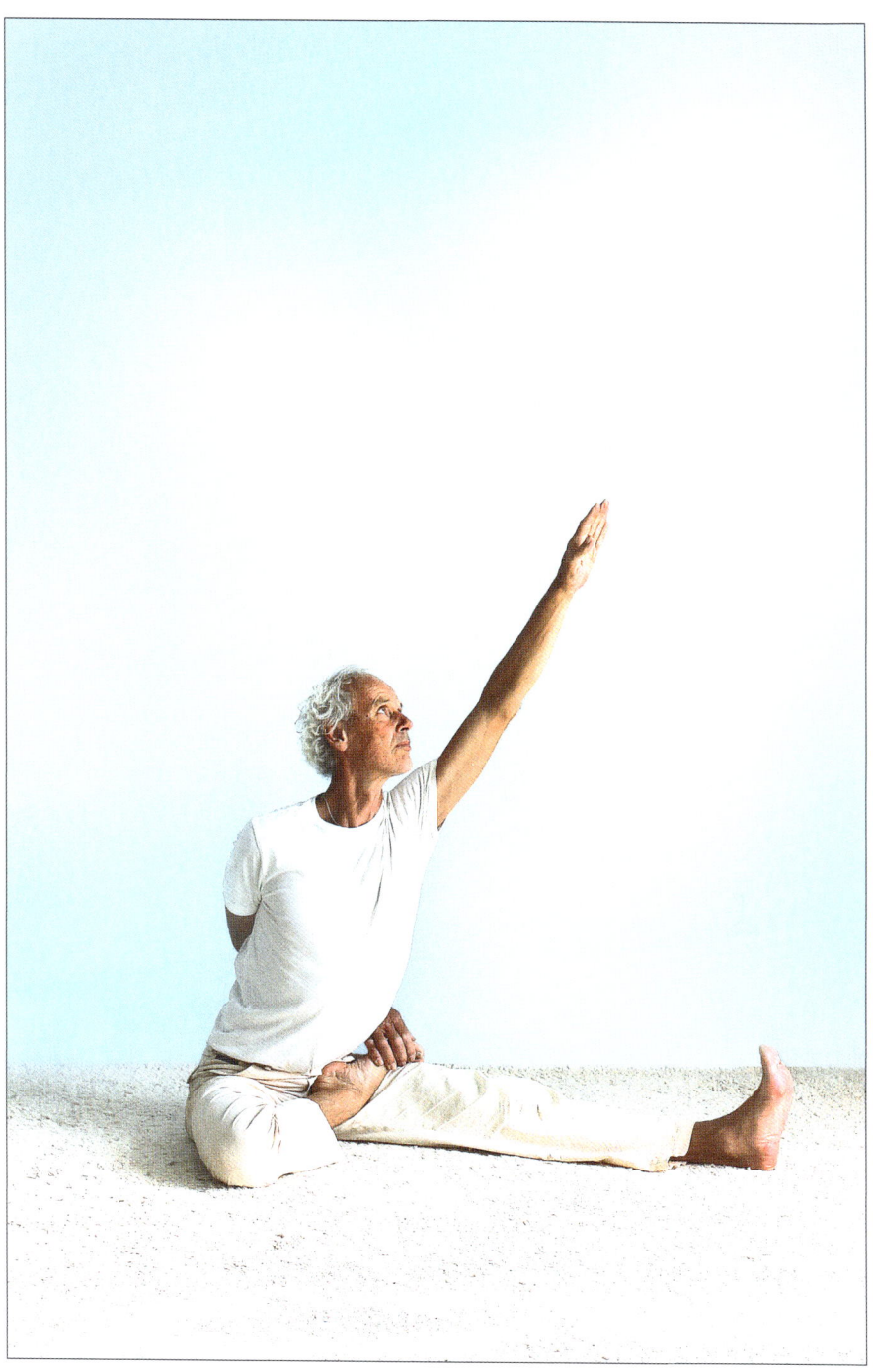

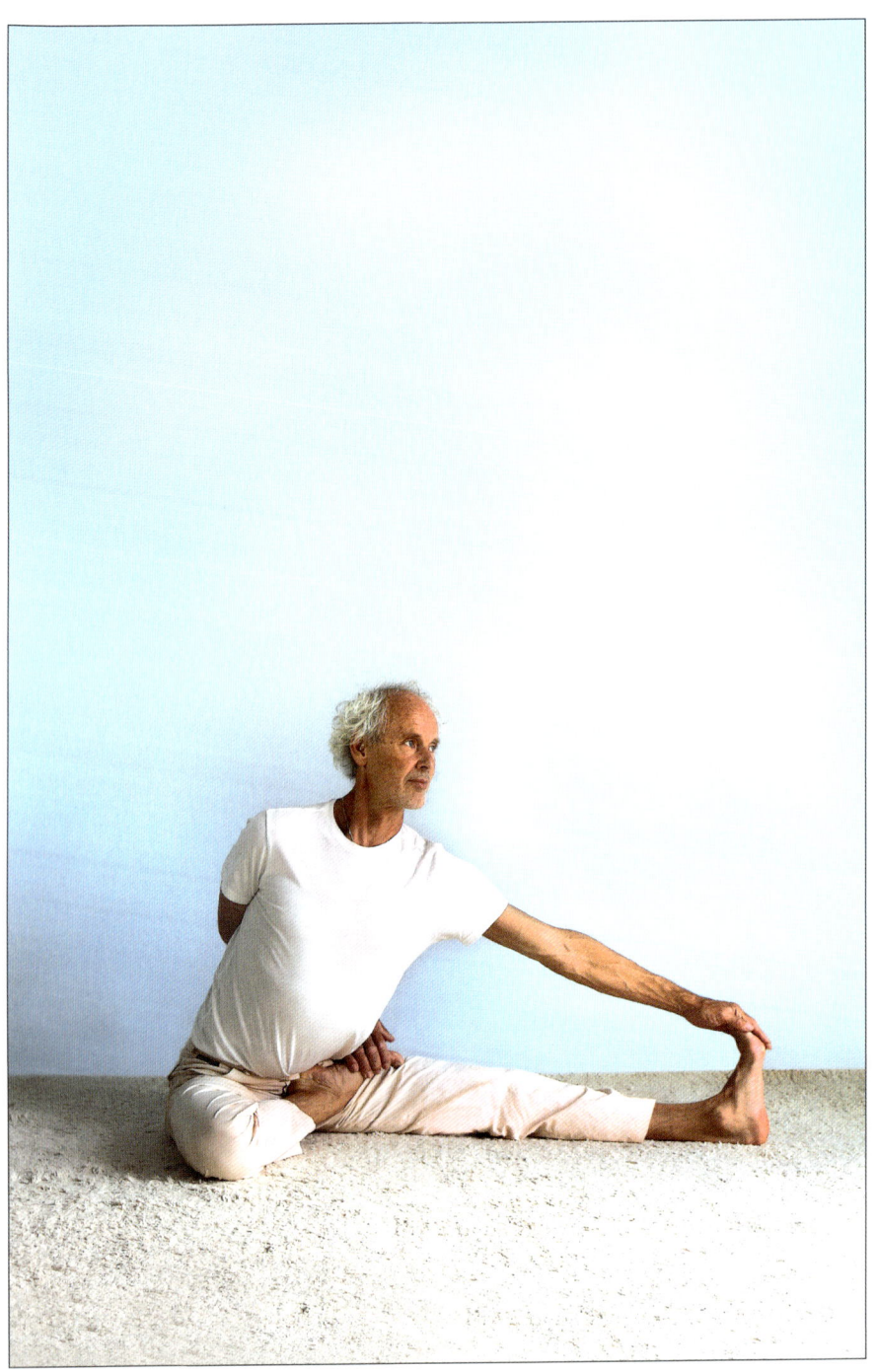

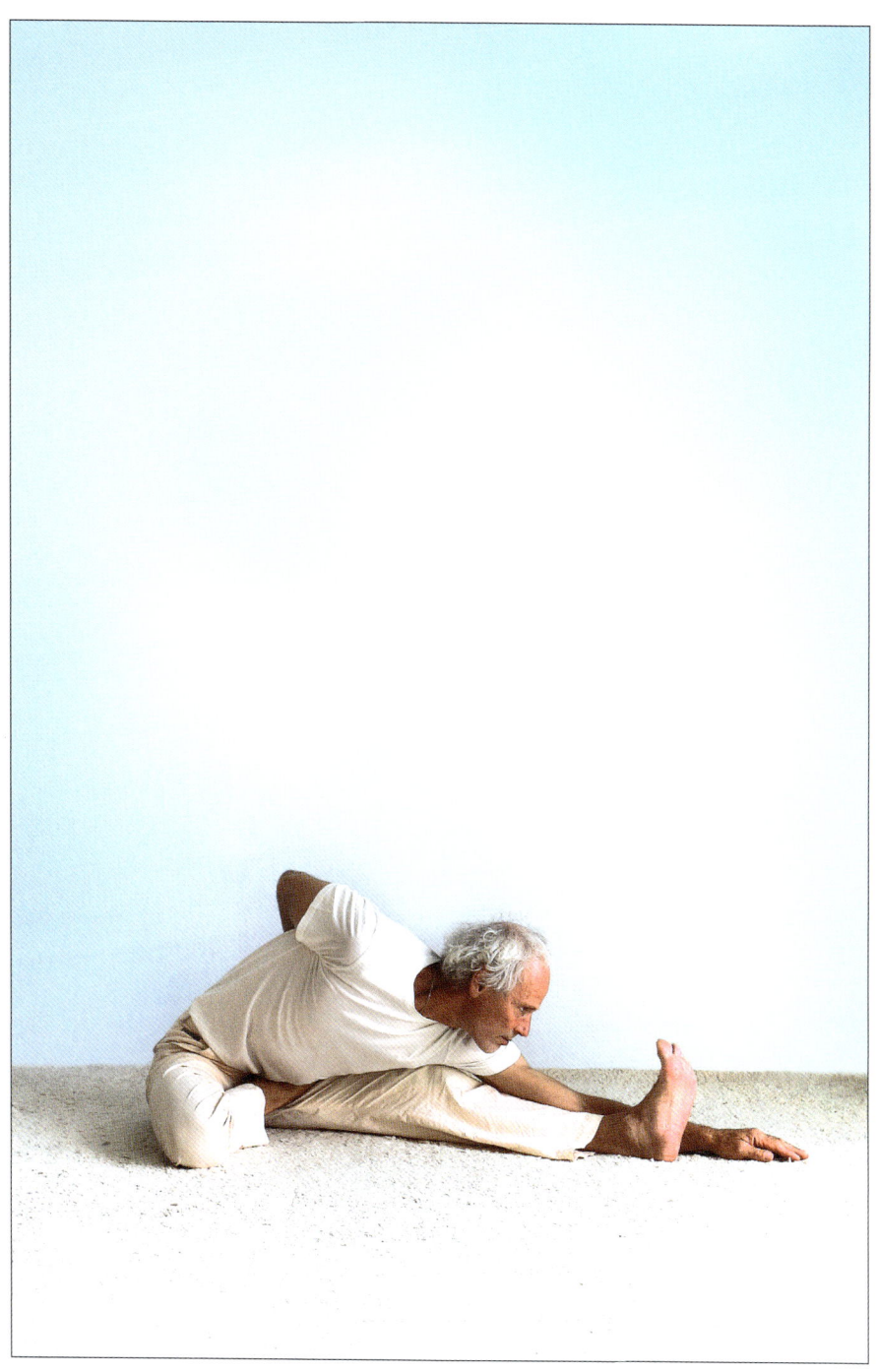

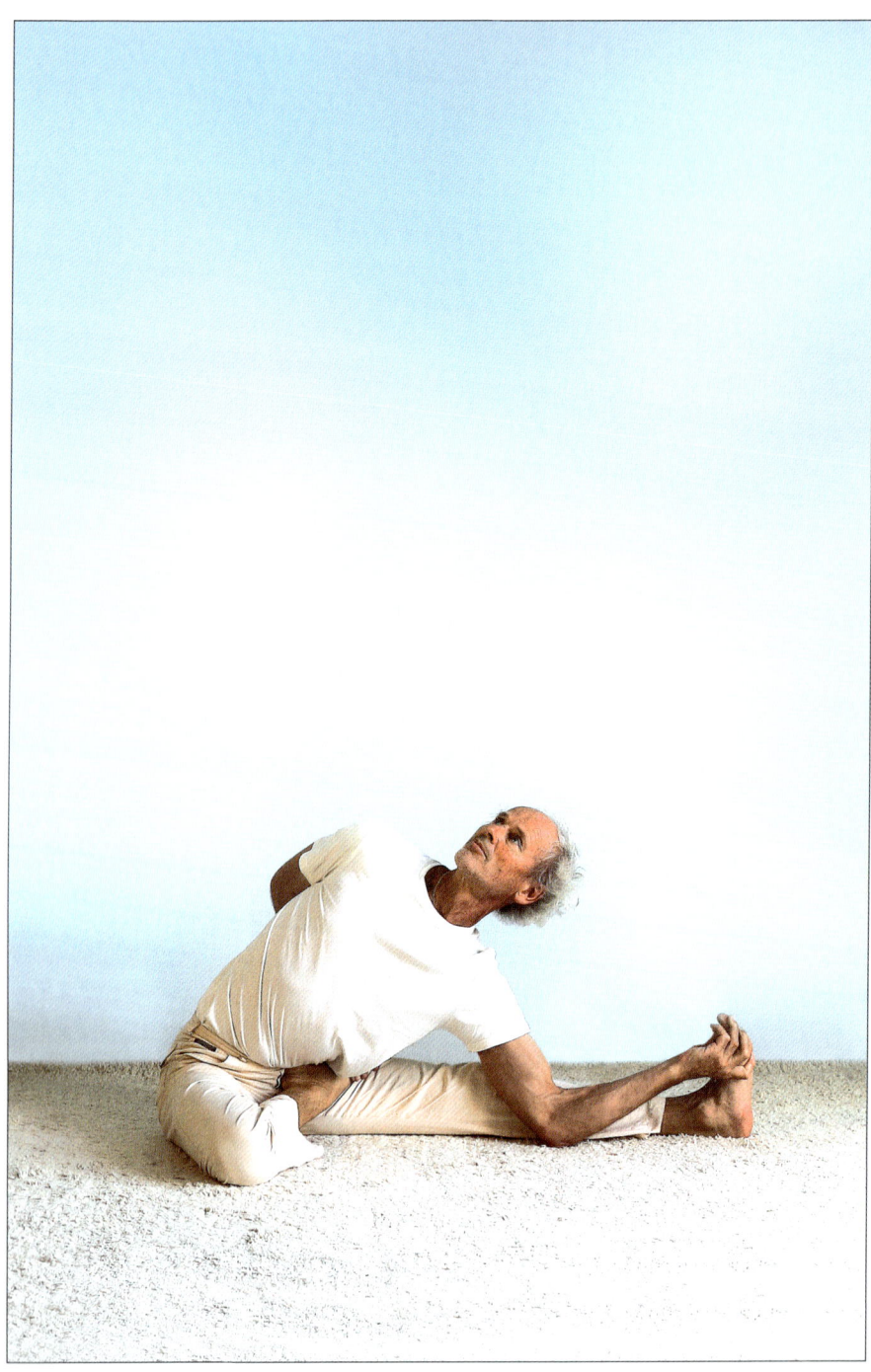

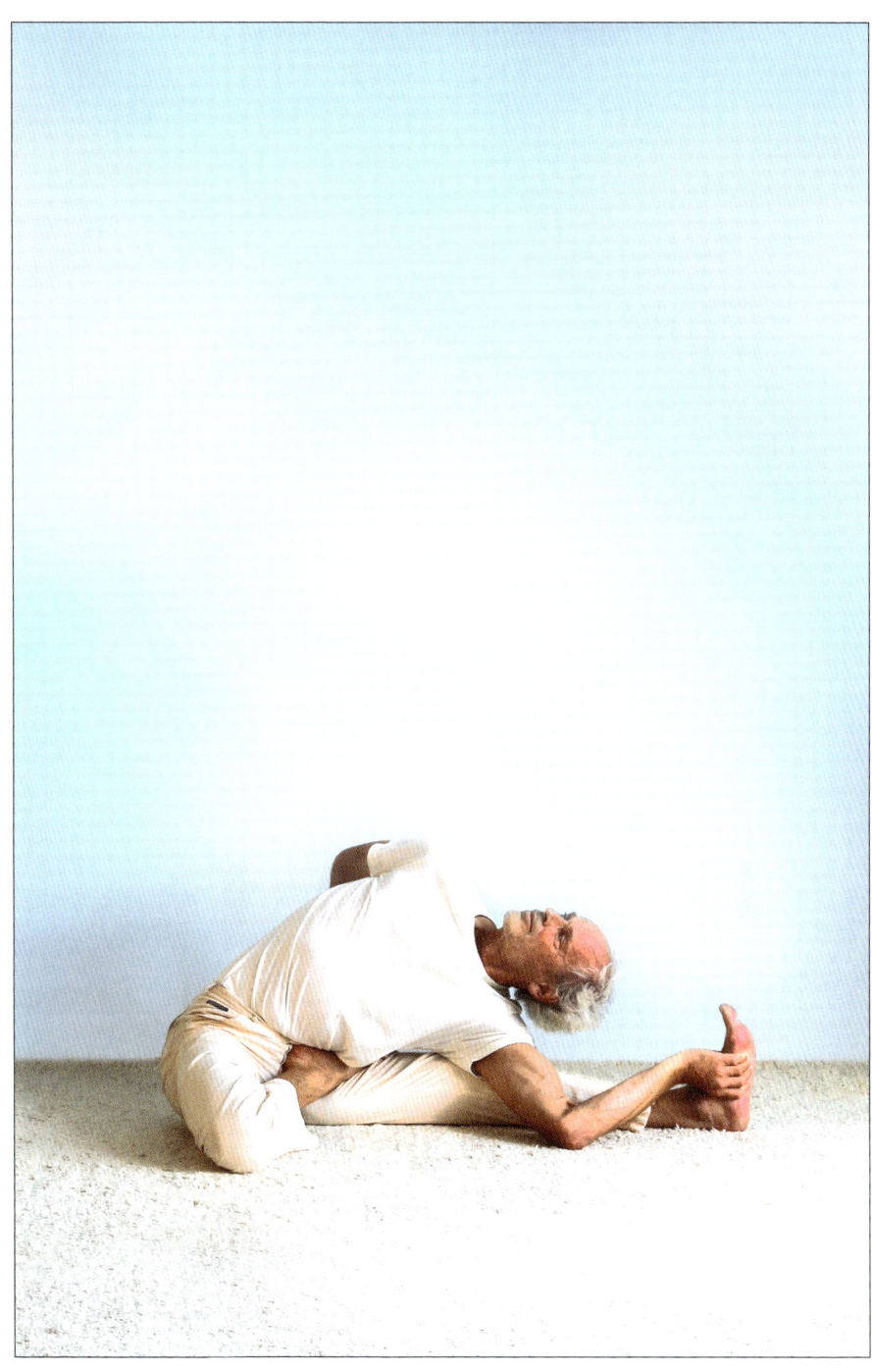

unconscious will-activity. This independently elected and activated will to mentally picture, in watchful presence, purifies all of the body's dull or dampened feelings and precisely because it remains peripheral and alert, it represents an effect of the fifth centre.

To practise

Bend the right foot into your groin and take hold of it with your right hand from behind your back. Raise your left arm and consciously observe the distance between your head and your hand. Then relax the whole body again before the movement lengthens along the ground into the maximum possible stretch. The movement has a conscious, subtly chosen pulling-force in the uppermost spine. Allow at least two minutes to do this and then change to the other side.

This subtly chosen pulling-force in the uppermost part of the thoracic spine, coordinated with clear mental pictures and careful movements, leads to a radiance of great light, shining like a star, which seems noticeable in the area below the neck.

Another worthwhile variation of this pose can be done from the end position by twisting the spine. In this *āsana* the third centre is implicated through the twist and at the same time a sensitive experience emerges because the body is opened outwards. The experience of periphery can be clearly developed into a subtle-feeling, for when this is experienced it instantly protects against sinking too deeply into the physicality. Quite particularly people suffering from depression should get to know this peripheral experiencing and further encourage it through forming suitable mental pictures. (picture p. 213).

Another variation, in which the connection to the second centre can be experienced, is the stretch directly between the legs onto the ground, *supta padma paścimottānāsana* (picture p. 215). Here practitioners experience themselves as unified but they do not experience this unification as sinking down into the body. The unification appears in a form that is more differentiated, highly sensitive, coordinated and open for the consciousness.

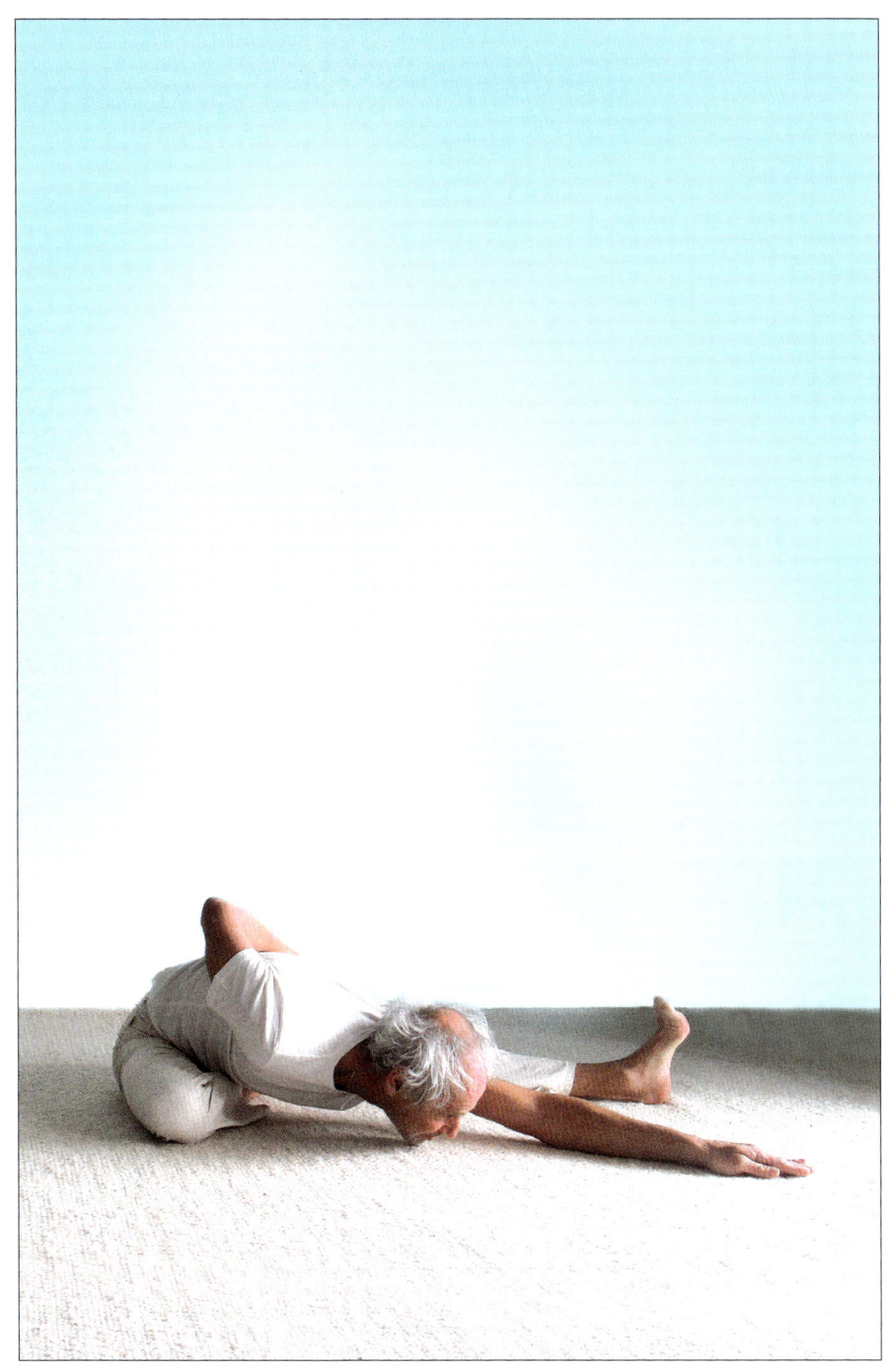

Water and the movement of gathering – *svādhiṣṭhāna-cakra*

Water gathers from drops to form a body of water or lake, from which it eventually rises up towards the air element, atomises into the finest of particles, and then, forming drops and rain in a coalescing movement, returns back again to its earthly starting point. For the external world this water element possesses the multi-layered tasks of irrigation, humidification and maintaining fruitfulness, as well as conserving the elasticity of living forms. Water constitutes the central life-element.

Seen from a deeper viewpoint, however, water possesses a quite specific movement, which it carries out not only in its gathering and atomising tendency, but which it accomplishes so-to-say in an inward direction. Water, or its more subtle element the ether, flows, from a gathering that is constantly renewed, farther inwards. Spacially this idea can hardly be conceived. The ether, however, which has already arrived at a centre, flows not only outwards, as one might usually think, but it begins to continue its direction of movement beyond the spacial boundaries farther inwards. This potential is characteristic of the ether and this is its particular, strengthening effect, which is ultimately reflected in a health-promoting, gentle, regenerative capacity in the body. The connecting, coordinating and mediating effects are rooted in that movement, which is able to detach from the external and lead into the internal.

The *svādhiṣṭhāna*-centre, which is located beneath the navel, is closely connected with the ether-force of the body and the strength of the immune system. The element of water, which is active in this centre, encourages flowing movements, which by mediating and coordinating, connect one's subtle-feeling both with the earth element as well as with the next element of air. The immune processes likewise take place in the watery element, and so the entire activity of this element is to coordinate, adapt and integrate.

The learning steps which students develop with the exercises here on this plane, demand a basic quality of natural trust in a matter or a thought. A thought or an idea are already at work before they have reached the stage of execution of an exercise. Practitioners now dedicate themselves to various forms of movement, try out the possibilities of thoughts in an interplay with the body and learn, through repeated practice of the exercises, to perfect and coordinate themselves better in the movements through clear, inner mental pictures. On the one hand they develop a very free feeling towards their own limbs, quite particularly towards the legs, which they release with a conscious reversal, to become a flowing instrument in the movements, and yet at the same time practitioners contract in the middle of the abdomen, or even in the sacral region, in a growing and fluid way. They can further this feeling of contraction through picturing the water element and its task of centring inwards.

The movements which are carried out in the individual yoga exercises acquire, with these mental pictures, a very natural and free aliveness, and this reduces the habitual forcing of muscles and generates instead a new coordinated flowing. The centre of the movement exists in the region of the sacrum and from there its path even continues farther inwards. A fine, centred and natural contraction flows inwards, while in the limbs, particularly the legs, a subtly felt, light and released flowing is experienced.

For advanced spiritual students, who want to develop the *svādhiṣṭhāna-cakra*, the challenge is to transform the so-called etheric body – because the *svādhiṣṭhāna-cakra* forms the energy-pole for the etheric body – and to keep this etheric body agile for the future, independent from the physical body. This is a very big challenge; it constitutes a comprehensive discipline of concentration-work and requires an enduring control of all thoughts and feelings. Alongside a trust in moral ideals and a dedication to these, students must generate these ideals themselves, represent them, realise them and turn them into the substance of their lives. This mastery, however, requires many years of practice.

A soul exercise

The picture and the meaning of the exercise

When the senses move outwards and touch their way along a form, consciously combining it in a rhythmic sequence, then as a result the human etheric body too will follow this movement inwardly. All outer sensing movements, followed by mental pictures of them, draw an inner image, which the etheric body actually takes up. If the eyes trace along a mountain ridge and perceive this ridge peak by peak, slope by slope, clefts and heights, an arousing is created inside because the etheric body begins to reproduce this movement.

Now, practitioners can devote themselves to different harmonious forms or objects and trace these in a clear, rhythmic sequence. Examples can be mathematical and regular curves, or also regular physical forms like for example a tetrahedron or an octagon, or they can dedicate themselves to forms in nature and trace the contours or lines with their senses. It is always beneficial when the sensory process moves along harmonious forms with conscious, perceiving involvement. On the one hand practitioners feel a newly strengthened order for the body-soul equilibrium resulting from the consciously guided sensory process; they feel how the outer movement, in its harmonious elegance and fluid dynamic, has a calming effect inwardly on the nervous system. On the other hand, they notice, when they remain in alert self-observation, how the sensitive effect directed to their inner, living, metabolically active will-life, and with this also to their regenerative etheric body, ignites pleasant, equilibrating processes.

This simple exercise, which can be practised at any time of day without effort or preparation, serves one's personal development quite particularly by supporting and encouraging an animated thought process. The etheric body addressed in this way increases its dynamic and lively flowing, it becomes stronger and, through its own fluidity, works back in a beneficial way on the thinking.

To practise

The drawing illustrated here, which shows a typical dynamic movement-process, can serve as an example. The drawing represents a kind of leaf-like form, which is actually very typical for the dynamic and connecting sphere of activity of the second centre. Picture this movement from the lower and central axis, moving up and out, but once it has reached its highest, most advanced point, moving sideways in a kind of rounding, and flowing back into the lower central axis. The farther the movement glides out, however, the bigger are the roundings of the returning, dynamic continuation. Follow the movement, as it is drawn, sequentially with your eyes. You will notice that this movement also works back on your inner, hidden feeling-life. In fact, the movements work on the so-called etheric body.

This movement, as it is sketched in the picture, can also be reproduced in the exercises, like for example in the one-legged head to knee pose.

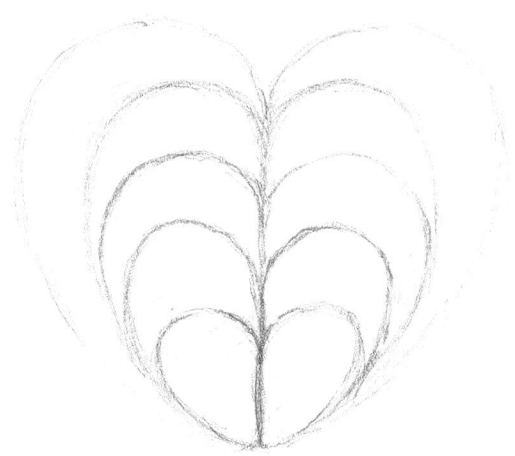

The standing head to knee pose
uttānāsana

The picture and the meaning of the exercise

Whereas in the classical head to knee pose practitioners work their way with an intensive movement closer and closer to a closed form, and discover an experience of "going-into-matter", the standing head to knee pose now describes an experience of "going-out-of-oneself". In particular, it is an elastic build up of tension based on polarity that is experienced in this pose.

The centre of this pose in energetic terms is deeper than the *maṇipūra-cakra*, it is in *svādhiṣṭhāna-cakra*, in the lower abdomen. Through the specific contraction in this centre, practitioners experience a duality with the gliding outwards of the arms. They experience this as liberating and like a step out of themselves, as if through the movement that glides outwards and flows forwards, a threshold of subtle-feeling could be stepped through and a new depth of experience could be grasped.

But after practitioners have grown far out beyond themselves, they nevertheless return entirely to themselves, into their own centre, and raise up one leg behind them to develop a new outward-gliding tension, *pratigamana eka pādāsana*. This end position, which is formed from the initial standing head to knee pose, *uttānāsana*, describes a polarity of centring and gliding outwards. This activity is quite strong, concentrated, unified and gathers itself at the centre of the metabolism, right where the second energy-centre is located. At the same time the legs glide far apart as a symbol that the personal life is not closed off, but remains stretched out between the monads of the worlds, between above and below. Nevertheless, practitioners go deeply into the contraction in the region of the sacrum and imagine that they are continuing beyond the boundary of the sacral centre to a flowing movement inwards. They experience duality in the rhythmic sequence, in the nature of "going out of themselves", both with the arms and with the legs. Gathering and centring lead to the experience of tension. During the practice, nevertheless, they always remain observers of these experiences.

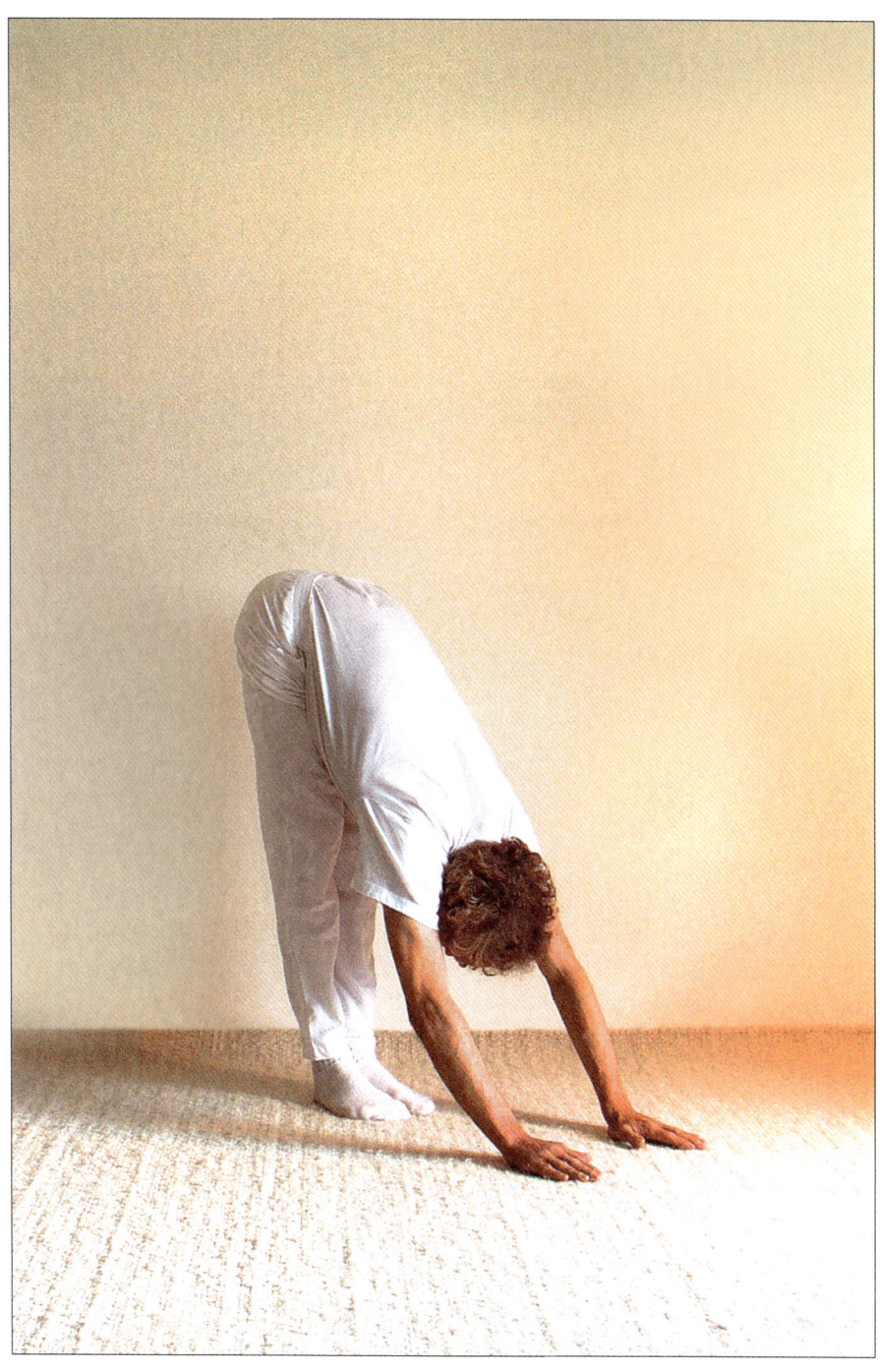

To practise

First begin with a simple movement, which can easily be experienced in the free breath, and which leads to an initial centring in the upwardly-rising leg region. This exercise is the standing half moon, *candrāsana*, and it conveys a light and centred bodily feeling by moving fluidly upwards, dynamic and narrow, starting from the legs with the ankles close together.

Then stretch far forwards and press your abdomen towards your thighs. The spine should glide forwards dynamically and at the same time should contract in the lower section. Relax the neck and let the movement happen with lightness and also intensity in the dynamic. Breathe freely for this. This is the movement-element in which the limbs glide out with soul sensitivity and the feeling of a free "going-out-of-oneself", while the contracting support and a drawing-together is retained in the lowermost spine. It is a very intensive experience of tension through the polarity of centring and gliding-out.

Then in the second part of the exercise, in *pratigamana eka pādāsana*, bring the hands next to the feet, take hold of your left ankle with your left hand and raise your right leg far up behind you. This leg glides upwards all the more dynamically the more you can find the centre in the middle of the abdomen and actively contract the muscles there, combining this with the mental picture of the inwardly moving ether. Hold this movement for up to about twenty seconds and then change to the other leg.

With the forms of experience of "going-out-of-oneself" and at the same time "concentrating-into-oneself", it is a case of pure subtle-feelings of the soul, in which the body only forms the aid to an experience. In this cyclical form of experience, rich with tension, it becomes clear that the movement can take place more naturally and beautifully when it is accompanied by a subtle-feeling of the soul, and practised methodically. The movement demonstrates a will-gesture, it is a direct expression of the will, but through imagining the potential flowing of ether, this will can now unfold into a more beautiful and noble aesthetic. The movement ultimately develops a growing freedom and no longer appears to be subject to the strains of usual muscular work. The body is like an instrument on which the music of the flowing etheric forces is played. Lead the movement rhythmically back again to the first position.

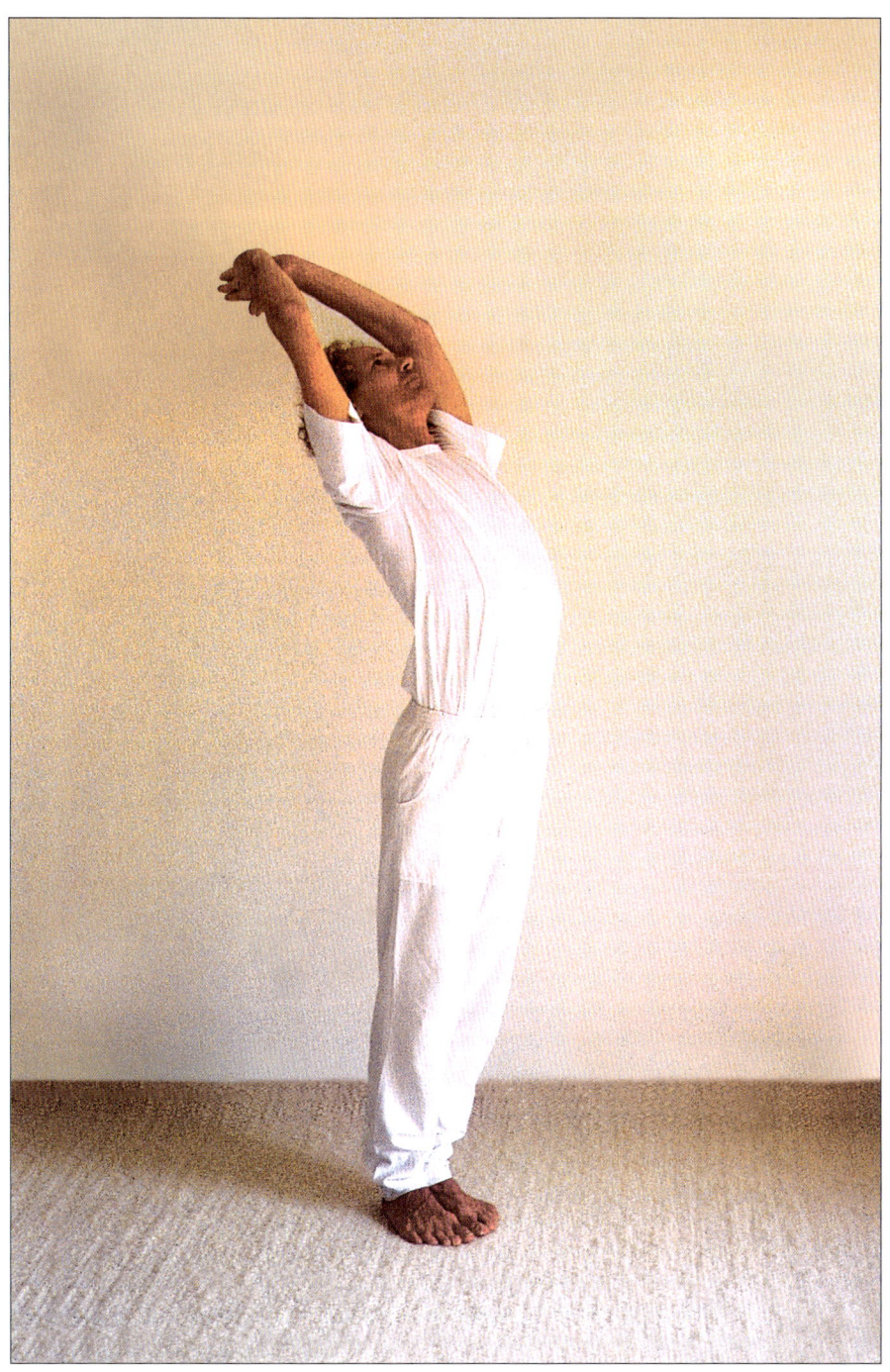

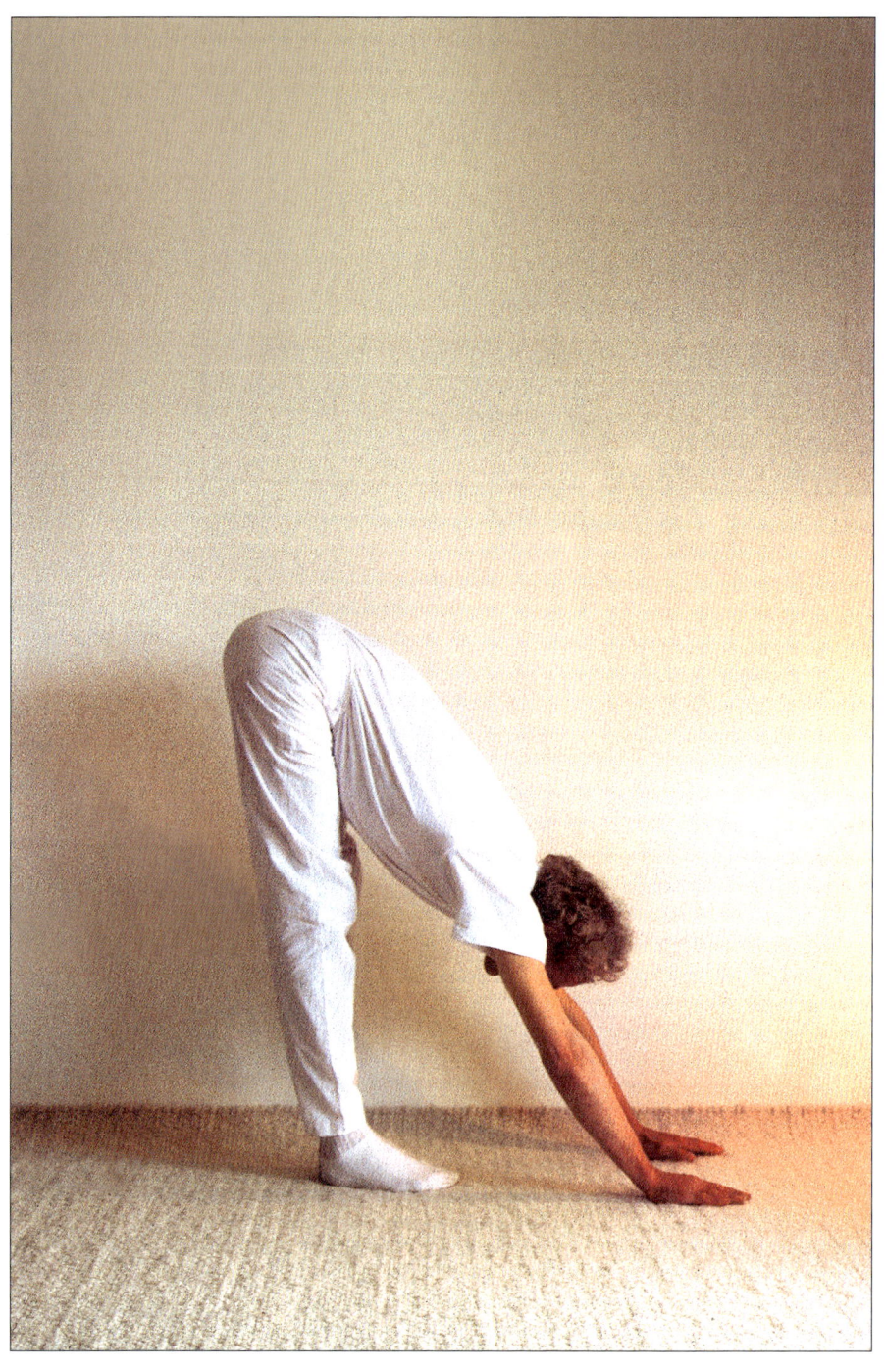

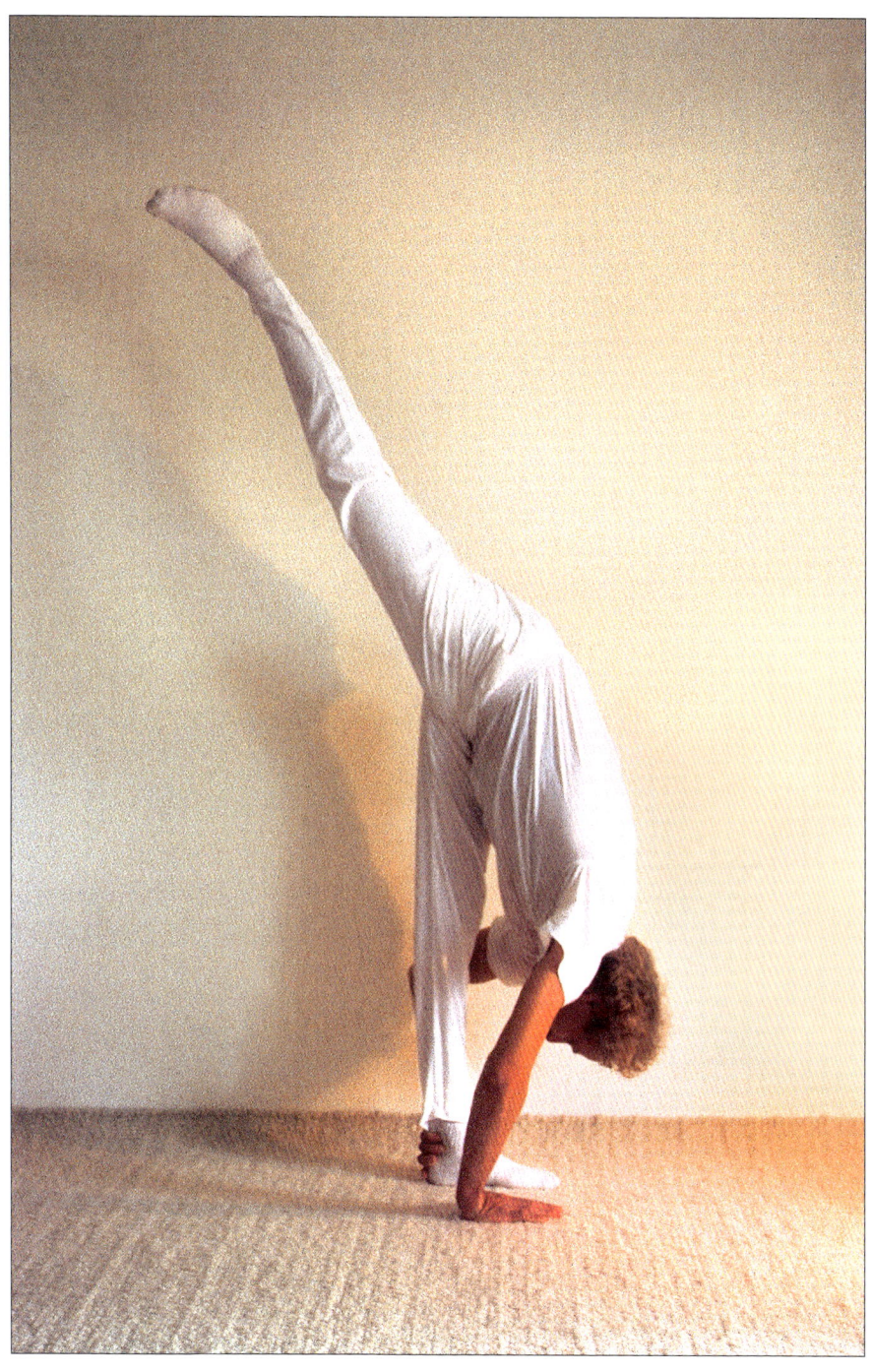

The locust
śalabhāsana

The picture and the meaning of the exercise

The locust is characterised by the sixth energy centre, but the start of the movement, where the strength is formed, is in the second energy centre. That is why the pose is described here in this section. In this second energy centre lies the seat of the life-body, or etheric body. Here is the energetic centre of all the effects that have accumulated from the forces of an earlier life and the past formed until now. In raising one leg, or even both legs together, with a vigorous action, which demands an extraordinary exertion, practitioners must move, to a certain extent, in a kind of independence in relation to their own physicality. This extraordinarily dynamic and vigorous action, which involves a collaboration between the arms, shoulders and back (see picture), naturally strengthens the will-life but at the same time it leads to a subtle-feeling of independence. Practitioners do not yet want to know the events of a past life, as that would require much more differentiated work of consciousness. They only want to feel this past life in all its heaviness through the bodily form and carry out a vigorous action to lift the body out, against this heaviness. The meaning of this pose lies in developing this initial, elementary independence. Independence is a sign of the locust.

Independence, therefore, means being free in respect of the impressions which come from previous life. Life that is past should not overload the consciousness with its heaviness, but rather the consciousness, out of the sixth centre, should oversee previous life, at least in a general overview. But to achieve this, practitioners lift themselves right out of their embeddedness by bringing the legs and hips up against gravity. This is an initial meaning of developing independence. But the development of a greater, really true and comprehensive independence can only take place when spiritual knowledge and experiences are further shaped. The exercise itself, however, opens up an initial sense for the nature of independence.

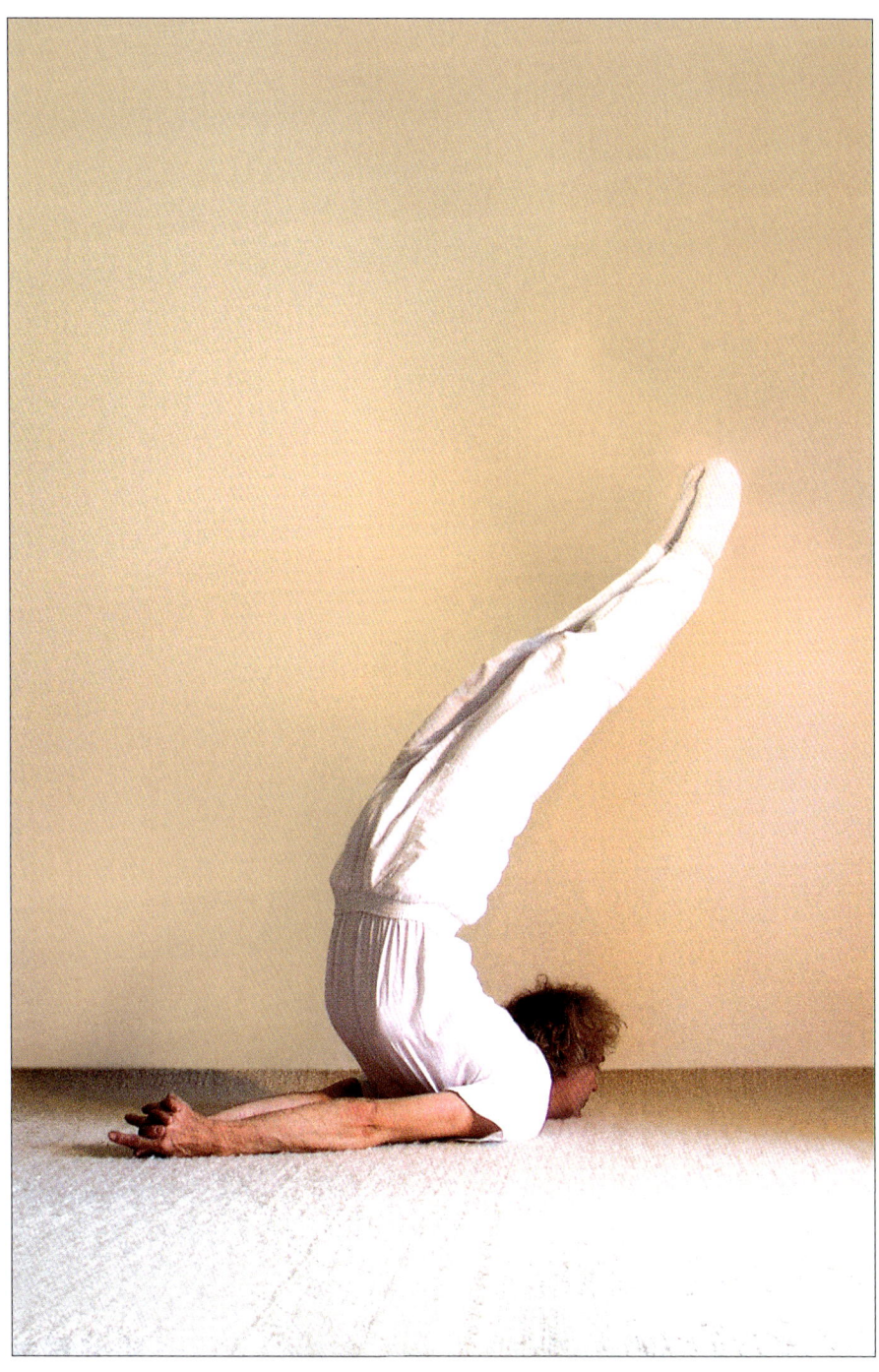

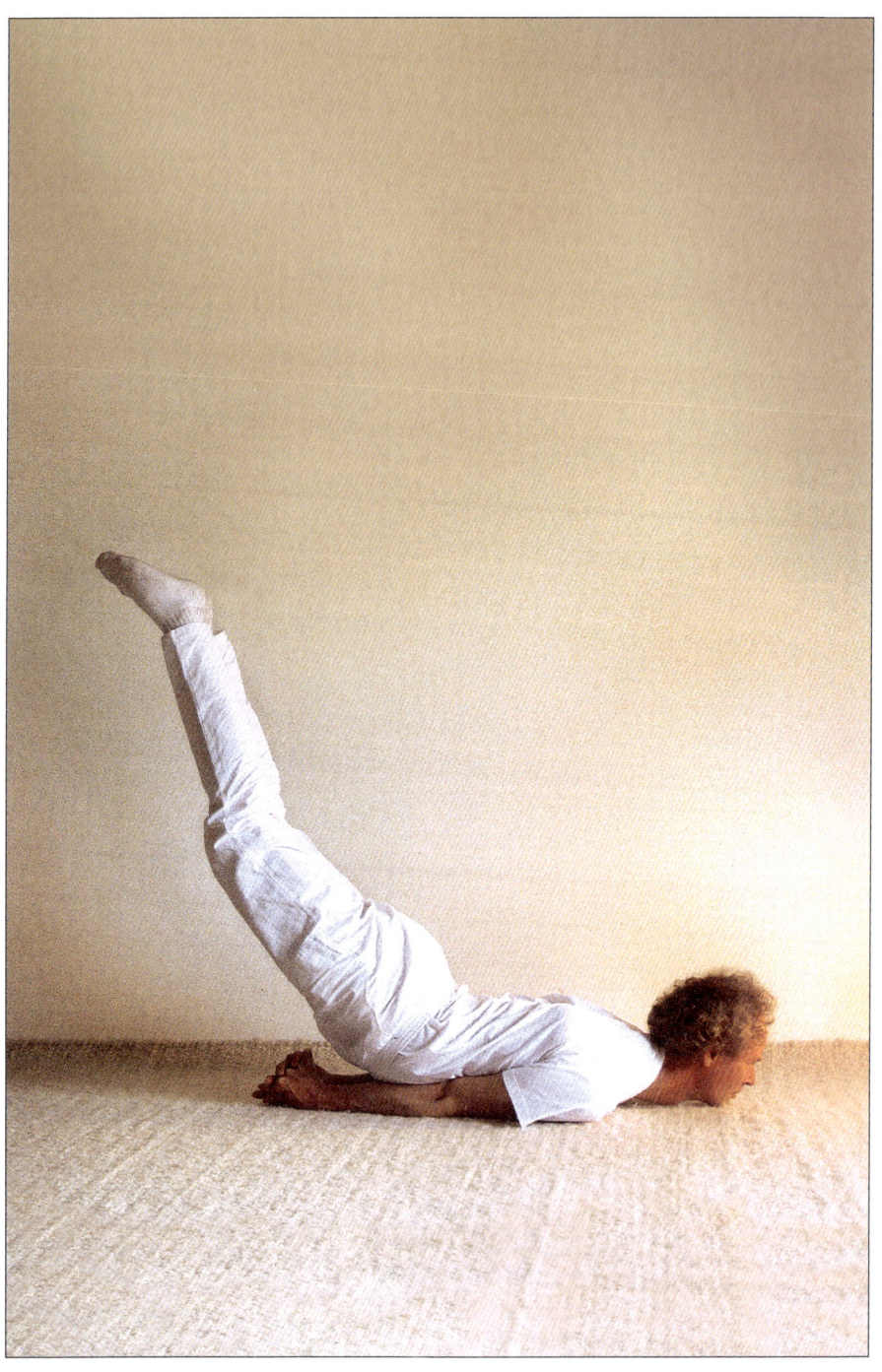

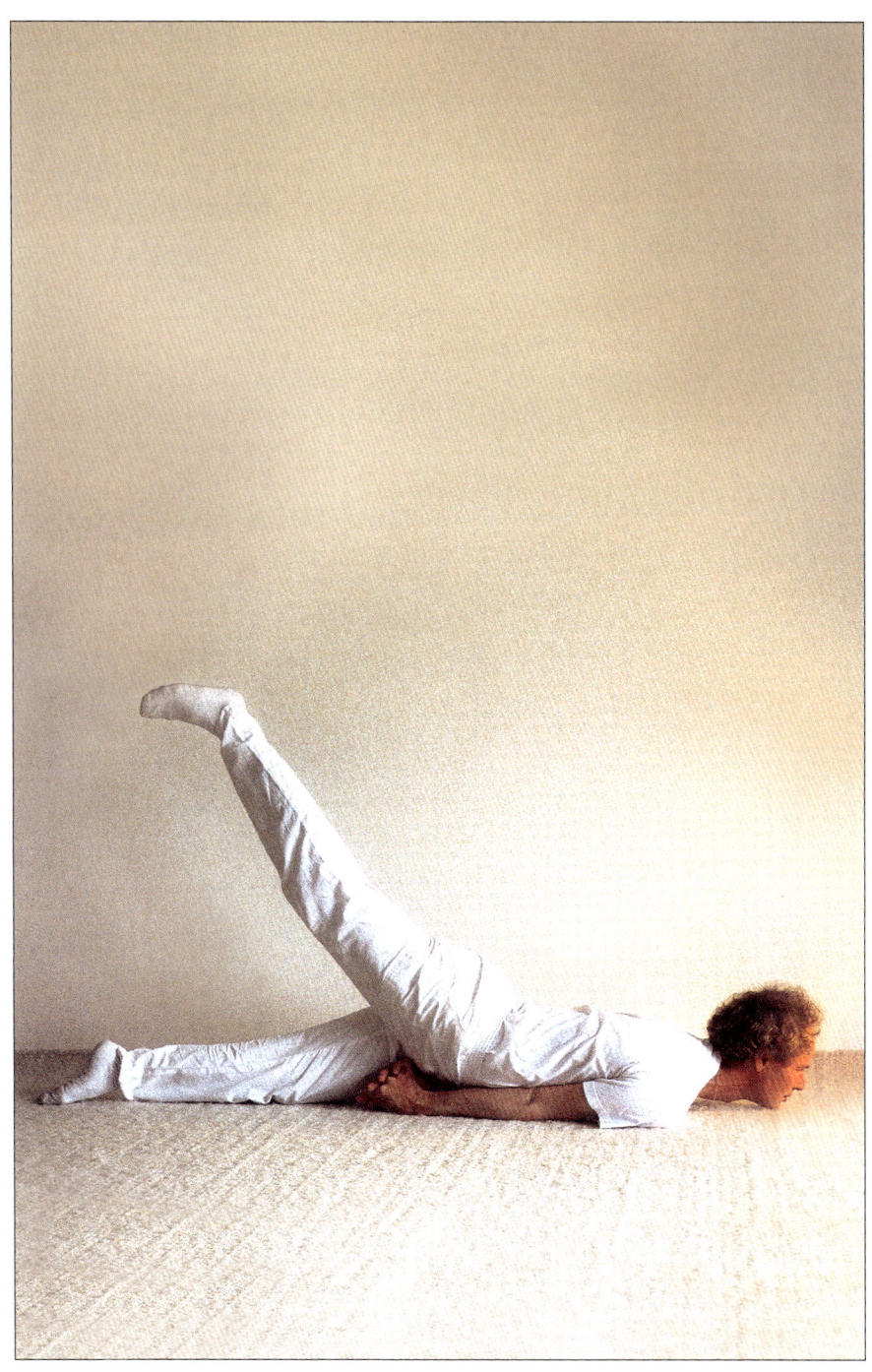

To practise

Lie on your front, interlock your fingers and straighten your arms under your body. For the half-locust, *ardha śalabhāsana*, bring your right leg upwards keeping it straight and consciously remain in this movement for about fifteen seconds. The hips should not tilt. Consciously keep the legs straight and then change to the other side.

In this movement a flowing feeling can also be created, which corresponds specifically to the second centre, if the leg, after it has been raised, is drawn towards the sacrum again. The whole body then glides into a pleasant closeness to the ground and into a lengthening, while with the pulling in of the legs the head lifts up pleasantly.

When it comes to the practice of the locust with both legs together, there are several variations regarding the height of the legs, from a lower level to the complete pose, *pūrṇa śalabhāsana*.

For this movement the spine must be flexible in all sections. If this is the case, then you can make a first attempt and bring your legs right up high. The breath remains free. Never use the breath by holding it in order to come up; it is even good if you pull the legs up strongly on the exhalation. By not using the breath to increase the power, the experience of the body also remains freer. Hold the position in the end stage for ten to twenty seconds, and then return to the relaxation position.

This gesture expresses a picture of the great, sublime strength of independence. The entire lower region of the body, together with the abdomen, rests lightly suspended above the upper body.

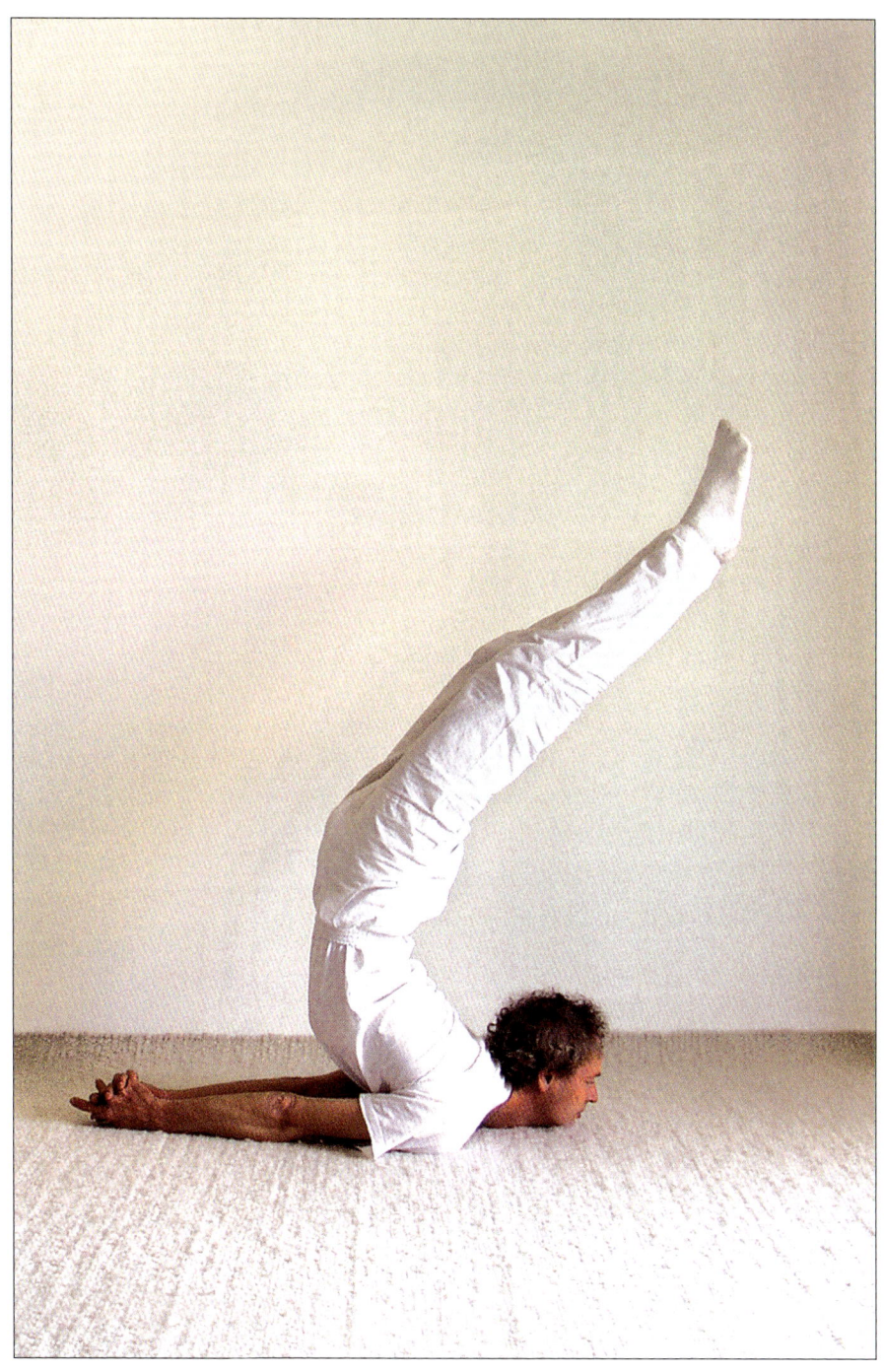

The wide stretch and forward-bending variations
koṇāsana, eka pāda paścimottānāsana

The picture and the meaning of the exercise

In this exercise the legs are highly engaged, while the upper body is carried by lightness and relaxation. The body stretches out widely and gracefully, not through powerful exertion from the back, but from a fluid collaboration between the limbs and the lowermost sections of the back. The meaning lies in developing a particular inwardness, which stands, as it were, in polarity to the wide openness in the limbs. Practitioners coordinate themselves from the back, which they lift, very carefully and cautiously towards the legs, release themselves from the periphery to some degree with their attention and seek a centre with a movement that runs backwards. Just as all circulating water-movements return again and again to one centre, so too practitioners turn in to the centre in the lower back. They experience themselves as unified and as one whole, by on the one hand entrusting the peripheral limbs to the free movement, and on the other hand centring themselves increasingly towards a bodily centre. The expansiveness of the limbs streams back into the centre in the lower back and becomes internalised in this centre. This course of movement is coordinated like a meditation, because it shows how the will takes itself back out of the limbs and how as a result that noticeable gathering is certain to develop in the bodily centre.

The exercise happens more easily as soon as it is combined with the imaginative-spiritual mental picture of the water element. This water element, with its tendency to internalise, gather and go beyond the boundaries of space, can open up a practical and concrete picture of meditation. The body is one whole and the ether streams through the body in all its limbs. If the ether does not dissipate through the outwardness of willed actions, but gathers inwards, a consciousness of calm and inwardness develops, and at the same time, through the thought, the capacity to observe becomes more alert and dynamic. So practitioners experience the conditions of their will in a concrete relationship, and they get a first, natural impression of the practical nature of meditation.

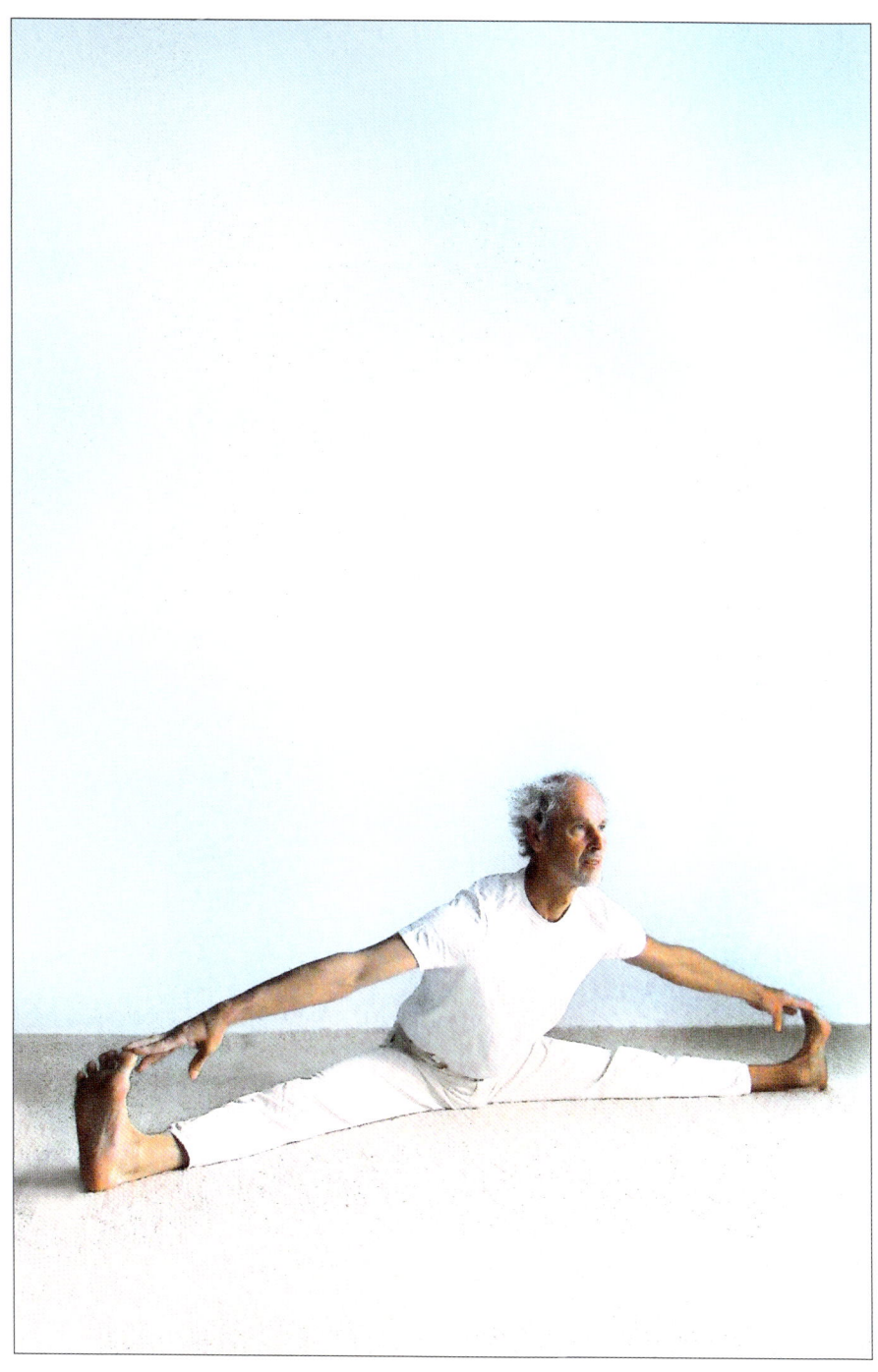

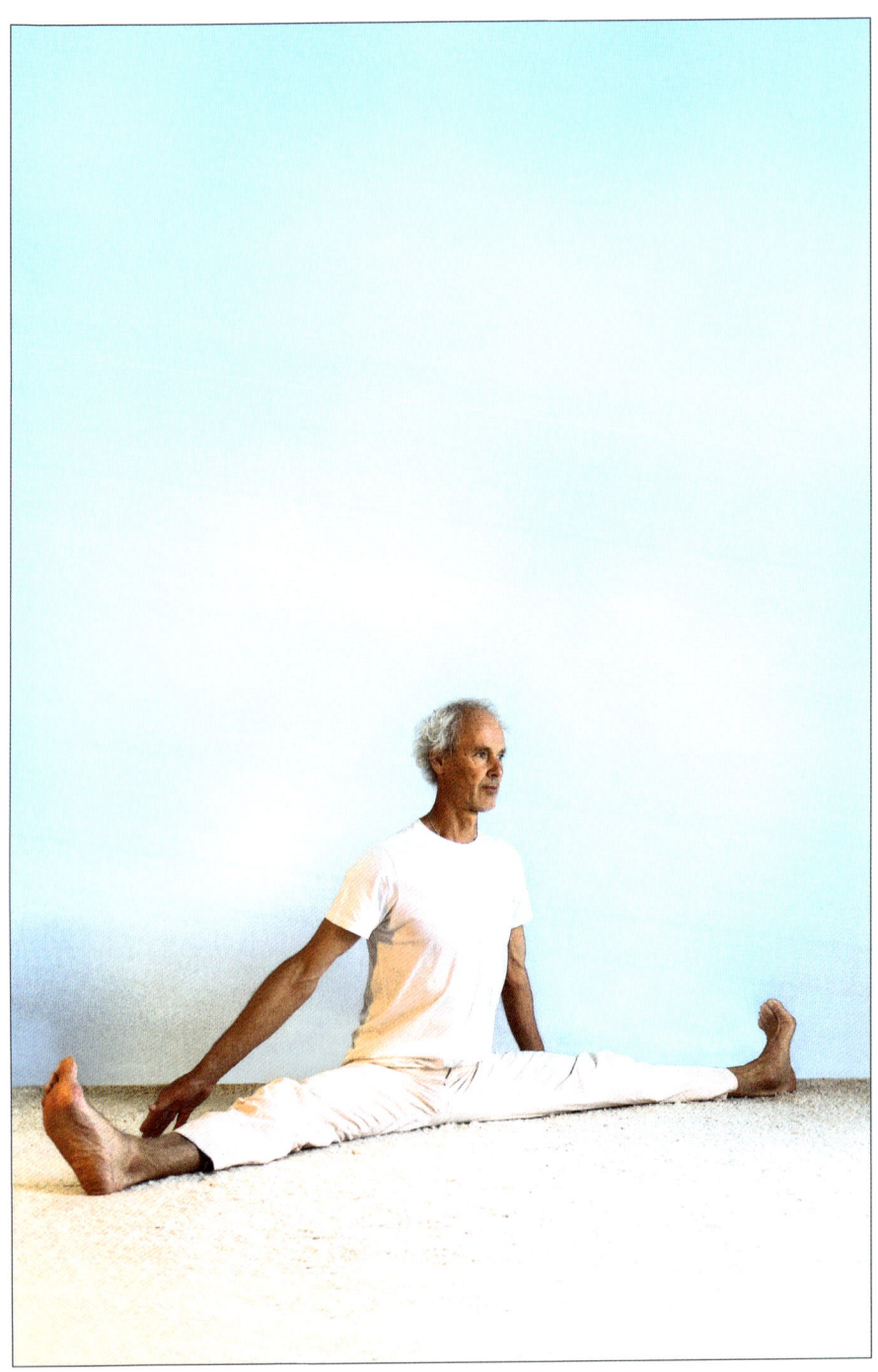

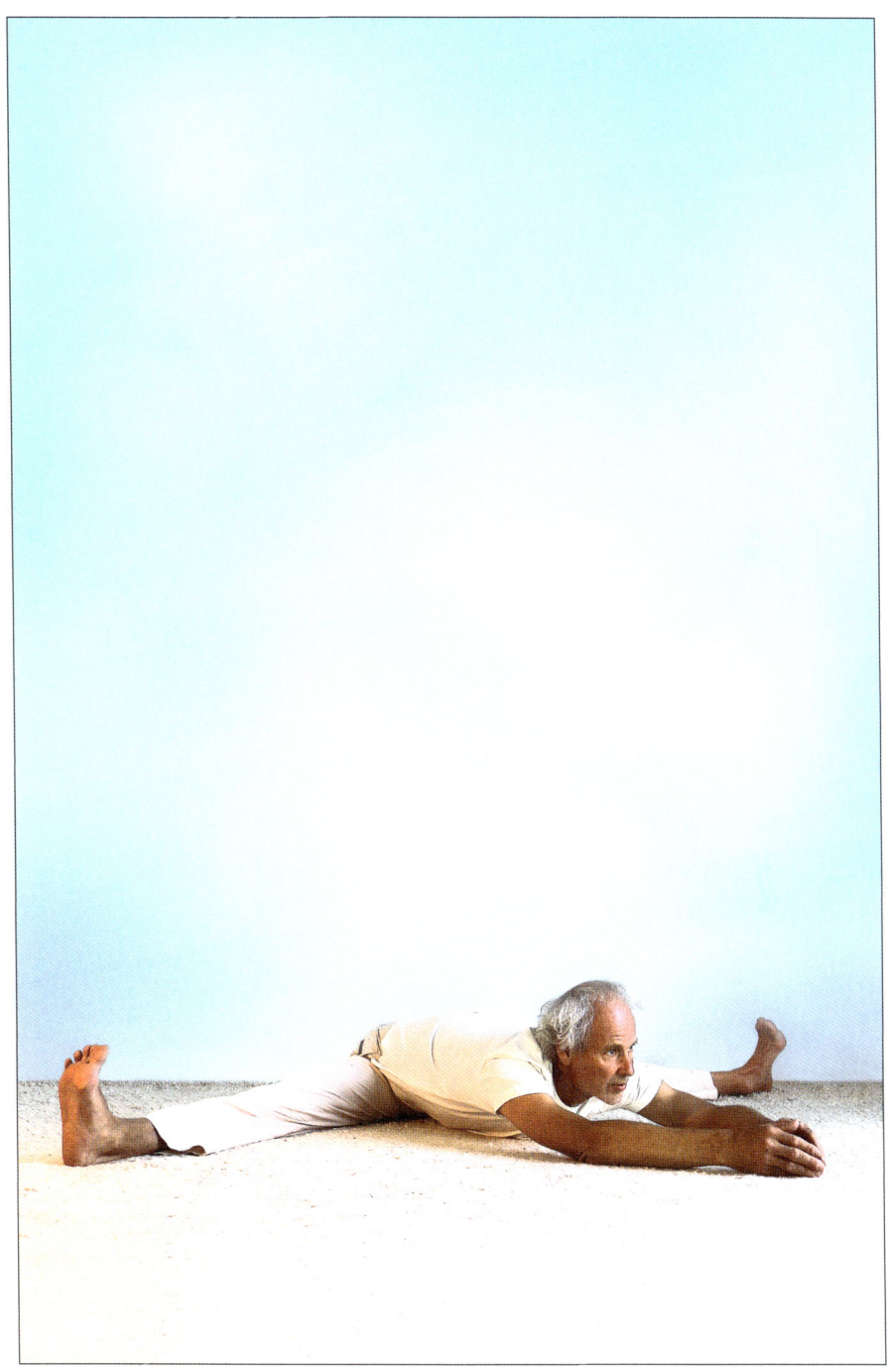

To practise

In the sitting position, bring your legs as far as possible into the spread form. Raise your upper body upwards. The arms are above the head. First coordinate the body. The upper body remains relaxed, the legs dynamically stretching, and the lower back should contract in the lumbar region. During the practice that follows, keep the feeling that the legs determine the form of the dynamic and of the movement out of themselves. The upper body glides slowly downwards in accordance with this leg-dynamic. The arms can move from above, down towards the toes like spreading wings (picture p. 233), indicating how the movement contracts towards the base of the spine, and so encouraging the converging and contracting force in the whole body.

Proceed consciously and slowly in the exercise, and avoid wilfully forcing. The upper body remains relaxed during the whole practice. You feel a contracting dynamic in the lower back and abdomen, which if it occurs properly in the interaction of the legs, assures a pleasant release of the upper body. Imagine that the contracting movement glides beyond the centre, further into the inner depths. Be patient while practising the exercise, so that you find the right coordination and from this build up the clear feeling of trust in this inwardly directed movement. The movement itself actually demonstrates a concrete inner depth.

The practice develops into a very dynamic and advanced form when you direct your arms forwards and, with a considerable force of contraction in the leg and pelvic area, move the body forwards. Gradually the whole upper body begins to align itself completely to the floor.

A few simpler, worthwhile exercises, in which the interaction between legs and back is equally noticeable, can be practised by taking the starting position for the one-legged head to knee pose, *eka pāda paścimottānāsana*. This position, in contrast to the classical head to knee pose, is motivated more out of the second centre.

Sit in the starting position and bend one leg inwards. The floor is now felt with the backs of the legs like a surface, and during this act of feeling, the legs glide a bit farther apart into the planar form along the floor. At the same time, however, a stream of subtle contraction happens from the

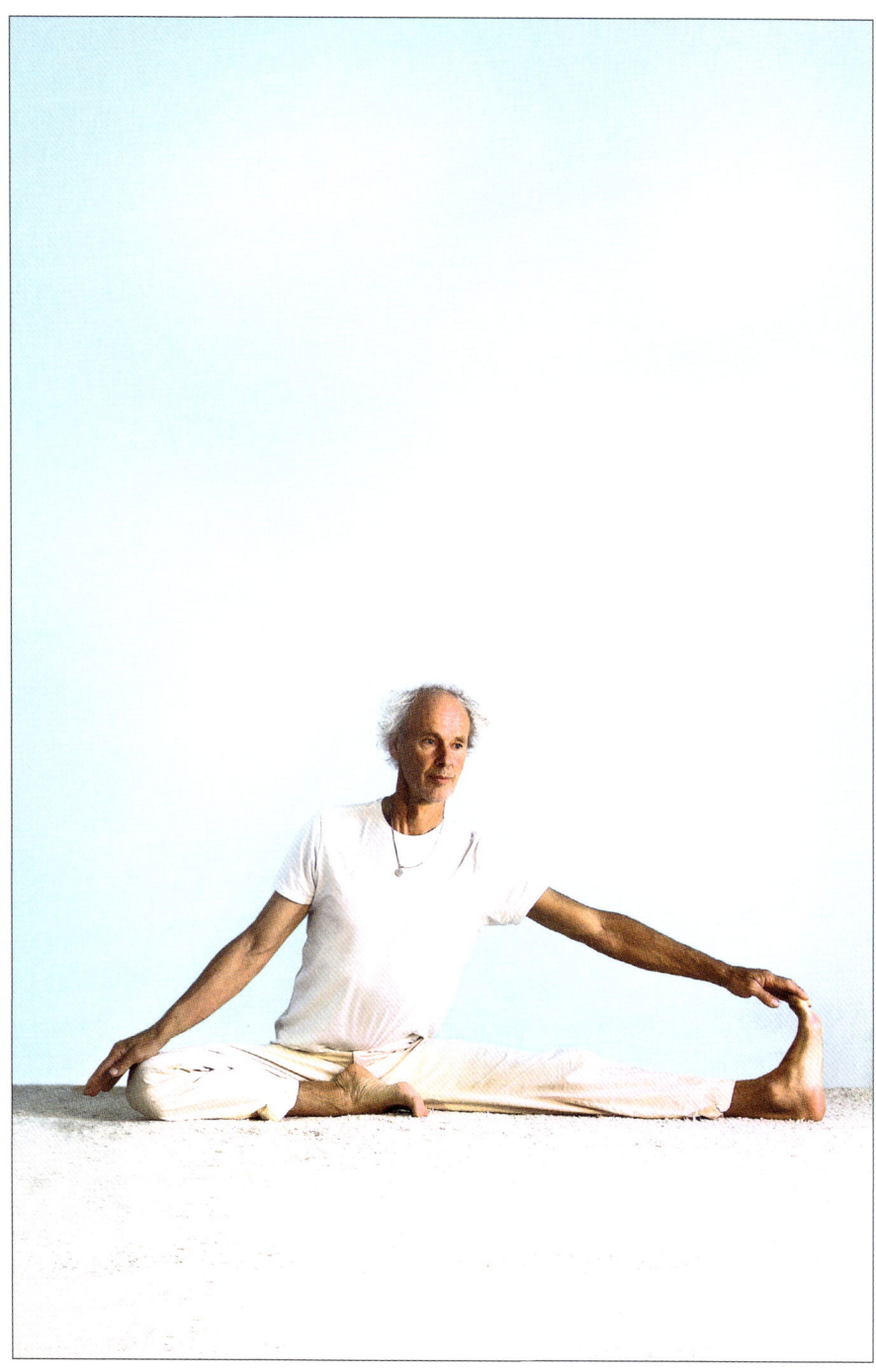

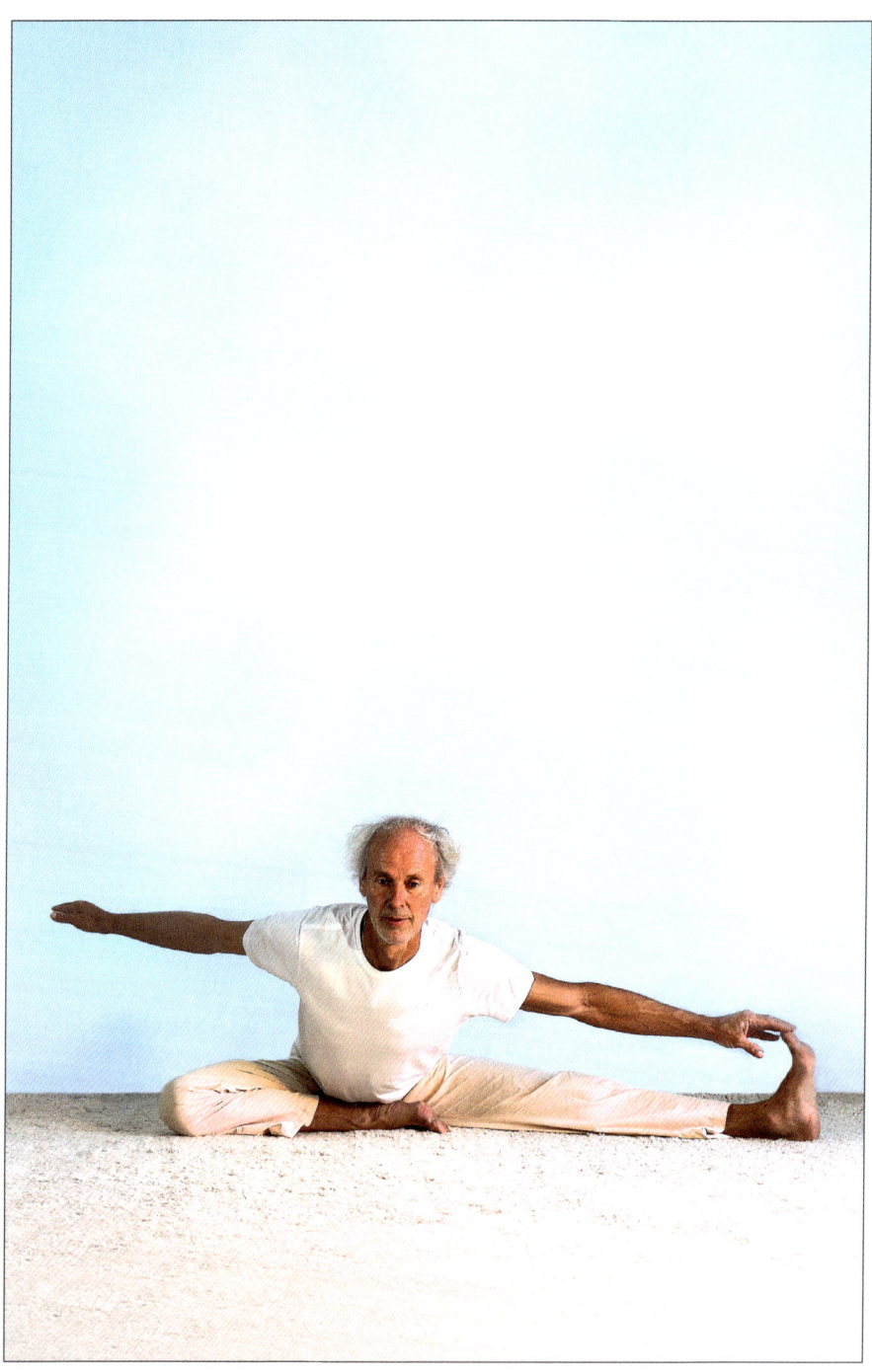

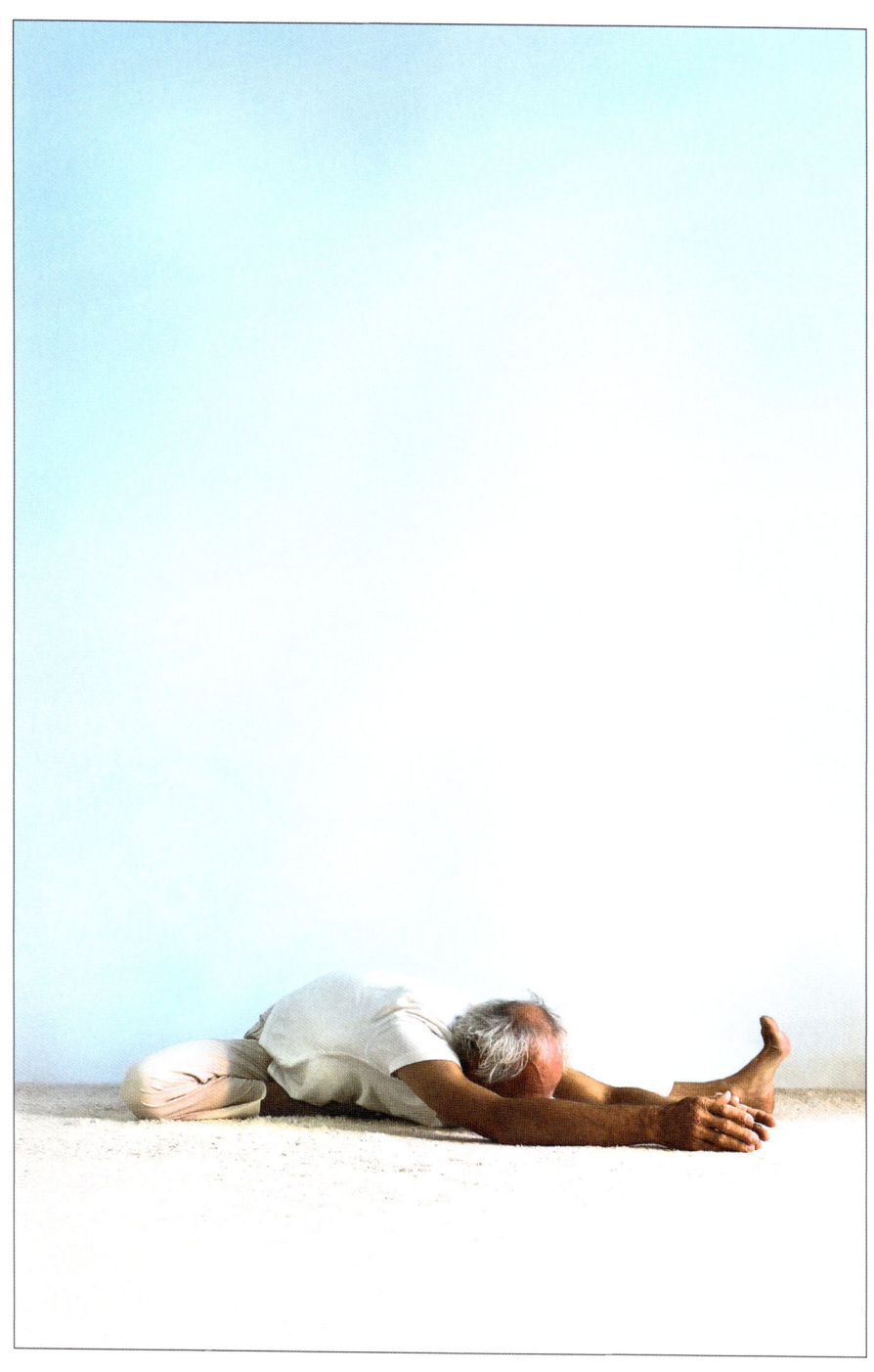

periphery back to the centre at the sacrum. This starting position allows a vivid feeling to penetrate into the consciousness, of how the leg-dynamic is connected with the upwardly erect and increasingly free spine.

Then glide far out forwards with the movement, while also contracting in the second centre. Deepen the movement by turning the dynamic back inwards, as if into an infinite centre. The body remains as if in a unified and inwardly centred dynamic. When the movement becomes centred inwards, it nevertheless becomes physically freer, as the consciousness perceives these forms of coordination in a concrete way, and does not sink into the bodily feelings.

Go as far forwards as is possible for you, and draw yourself into an increasing contraction. In this way the body becomes close to the ground and also feels as if related to the surface of the ground.

Once you have returned, after about another minute of remaining in the end position, you can once again try out some lively play with your legs, and then glide out into the movement between the bent and stretched leg. Again it is the experience of entering into a gliding-out movement in a sweeping dynamic, and of a gathered centring in the middle of the sacrum. The body approaches the planar form and experiences its contact with the ground.

Both sides are always practised alternately and perhaps up to three times. Gliding out, connecting back, depth in the sense of centring, and the experience of unity and of increasingly forming a plane, give the experience a very smooth and connecting character.

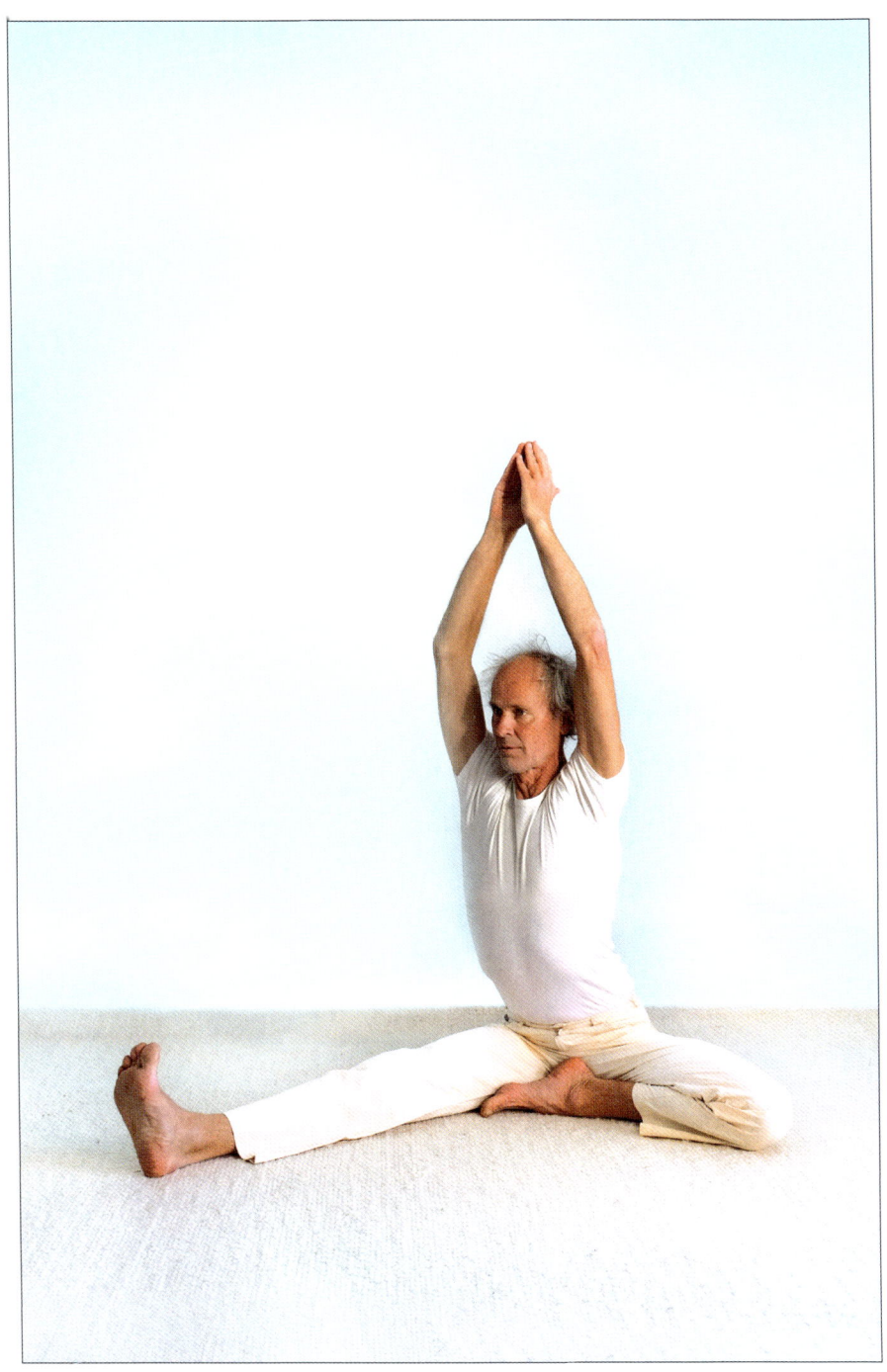

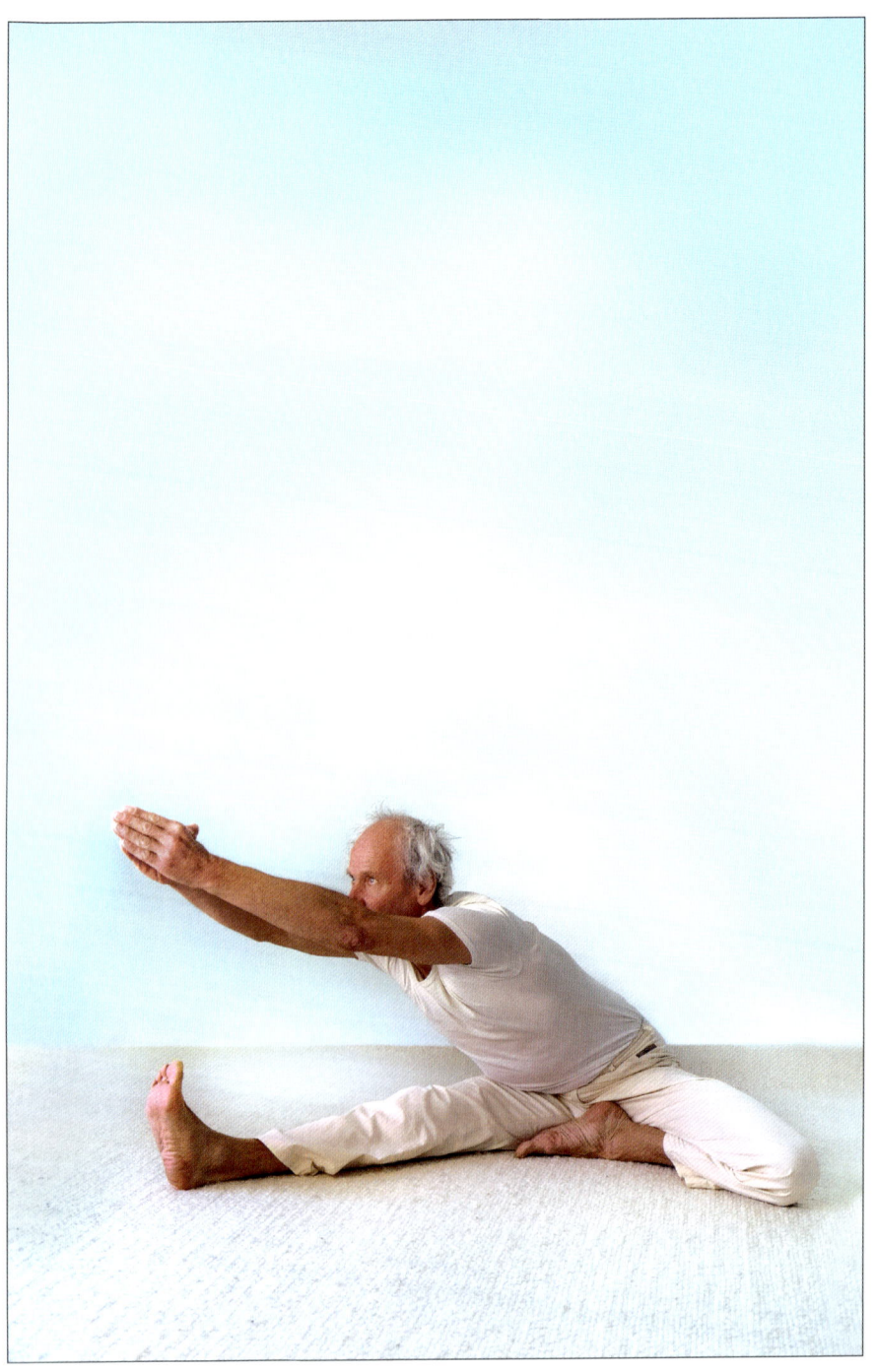

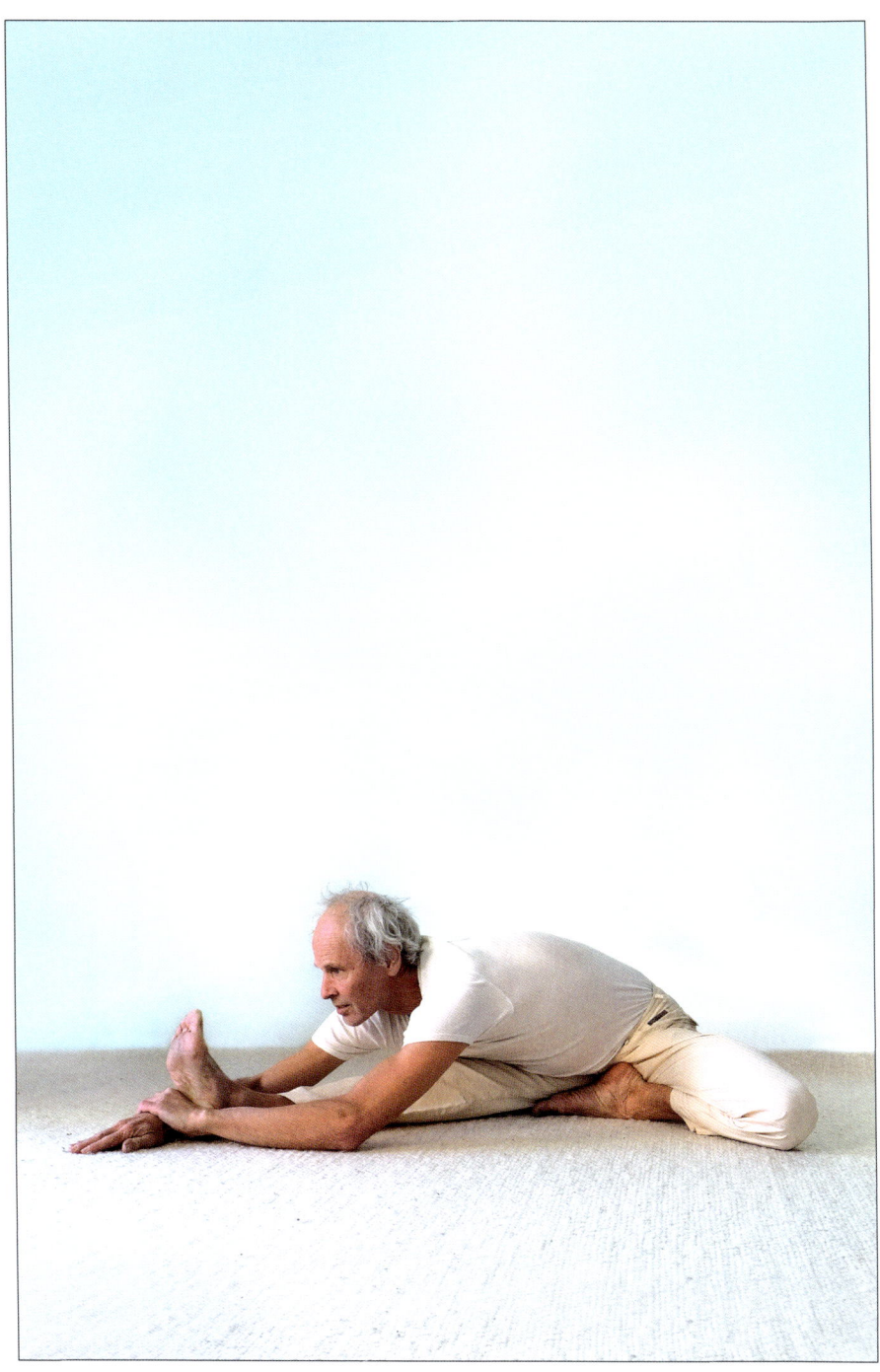

Developing a force of consciousness free from projection
ājñā-cakra

The *ājñā-cakra* in the middle of the forehead is represented by the important hormonal gland, the pituitary gland. The pituitary gland governs most of the hormonal processes via an encompassing circuit that regulates the other endocrine glands in the body. The forces that the hormonal glands receive are managed by the subtlest etheric thought beings, by actual, independently existing entities. The etheric body has here in this mid-point of the forehead its fire element, out of which the most subtle, shaping and organising creative forces of thought are set free.

During the exercises, students now get to know the etheric nature of the thoughts in a direct and absolutely real way. In perceptibly feeling, they no longer perceive the thought to be a mere abstraction or something supposedly cerebral, rather they feel with the thought a so-called living entity, an independent etheric existence. When they sense this entity as such, this gives them an initial feeling for a spiritual reality and also for the reality not only of thought beings, but also of their own consciousness, which connects them with these thought beings. The human being is the creator of the different thought beings, and so brings into being their wished for existence.

After this process of differentiation, consciousness and recognition of the reality of the thought has been carried out to some degree, and students no longer see mere abstractions in the thoughts, and in the emotions no longer mere temperamental surges, but behold all stirrings of the thought- and feeling-life within these free and existing modes of existence of their own human nature, practitioners can now become conscious of their own I, their possibility for I-activity. For now they can form these modes of existence into mental pictures and work to form and organise shapes out of the free fabric. They get to know the mid-point of the head as the central place for the activity of consciousness, the actual place of work for the various creative beings. The consciousness becomes active in the thought substance, shaping, perceiving and executing. It is not a thinking in the sense of materialism, in the sense of a mere mechanical involvement that from now on forms the benchmark for the practice, but rather a perfectly free, detached contemplation and productive thinking, which is understood approximately like a kind of creative capacity that is accomplished through the consciousness. With this thinking activity, however, the error should not ensue that aspirants on the path think they must now bring into being purely thoughts that no-one has thought or used before. They are far more like people who take a work material from the surroundings and learn to reproduce, process and shape this material in free availability. This free and shaping activity, which is free from projection and exhibits a direct, creative activity out of one's own thinking and thus out of one's own I-activity, is the learning aim that accompanies the development of the fiery mid-point in the head.

The development of a force of consciousness free from projection, with a free perception of the thoughts as existences, is rather difficult for beginners, for it requires a first "stepping out", or what could be expressed as a certain form of asceticism from the natural and automated chain of thought processes. In the ideal sense, the thinking must become simpler and clearer, instead of wilfully more embroiled and complicated. The path to the simple, however, may sometimes be considered as the more difficult one, as it takes place against the usual processes.

For those who have progressed, this centre proves to be the fiery, radiating mid-point of the consciousness, out of which pure concentration proceeds, detached from the body, and via the freely available thought can pervade the space with warmth, shape and light. A true action of love and a creative force of love shine out of the centre of the head.

A basic exercise for developing the mid-point in the head

As already indicated in the introductory chapters on the sixth centre, aspirants can carry out a simple soul exercise, which they only perform mentally. For this they imagine an equilateral triangle; then they move on and imagine, of around the same size, a square, and then finally a circle. This picturing activity should take in all about a minute.

In a second step, aspirants now move on to formulate a question, which is of specific interest solely as a question. One could also say that the aim of this second stage of the exercise is not to find an answer but only that the question as such finds the way to its manifestation and also that the consciousness becomes conscious itself of question as a creative process.

What differences exist between triangle, square and circle?

As a rule, habitual readers will tend to transition immediately from the question to an answer and will add a range of thoughts that enable them to support this answer. For example, they will say that the triangle has different angles from the square, and the circle has no angles and that is what makes it different in every way from the first two figures. However, the task was not set to give an answer to this central question at all, rather the basis of the task was to create the question as such and to manifest it sufficiently in the sense of forming a thought.

On this basis it now becomes clear how easily and automatically the will runs away with the thinking, so to speak, and how with this the initial primary thoughts of working to picture the geometric figures, and formulating the question about the differences between the figures, receive far too little creative and concentrated attention, owing to the urge always to find immediate answers and ultimately also evaluations.

Now if observers remain in the mental picturing of the figures, and if they just create the question with some calm persistence for two or three more minutes as the exercise proceeds, and if they then dwell in these thoughts that they have established, then they will notice that with their sense of thought they have now started to actively create. The triangle, the square and also the circle now appear as if pictorially before their inner sense, and the question too, if it has actually been formulated adequately, seems like a specific, creative form itself. Practitioners experience these processes like first quiet revelations of the spiritual world, and they sense how these individual figures, and also their question, open up to them a spiritual reality. The geometric figures actually reveal themselves in the quietest intimations as realities, which in the spiritual world demonstrate an existing order.

The exercise can now be practised with many further and different objects. The essential thing for the process is that aspirants do not gravitate into an intellectualism or into a premature, disconnected evaluation, but rather that with the creative formation of a real, mental picture of the objects, perhaps paired with an analogously formulated question, they gain an elevated consciousness. They keep wilful and emotional grabbing far removed from the exercise.

With this kind of exercise, practitioners learn to perceive and develop the mid-point in their head.

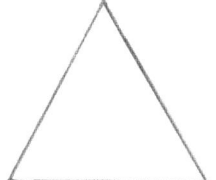  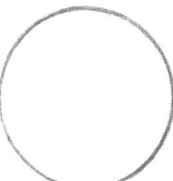

The sitting twist
ardha matsyendrāsana

The picture and the meaning of the exercise

The head, in the light of the thoughts and radiating sense organs, watches, in wise overseeing, over the remaining physicality. The thought steers the sensory processes. Just as the head dwells perfectly freely above the tensions of the physicality and the specific form adopted by the limbs, and yet directs with the senses the dynamic to be performed, so equally should the thinking be involved in wise, clear observation and direction, and yet not be entangled in the action. The thinking should remain free from emotions and free from the clutches of the willed gestures of the body. This freedom of the thinking, with simultaneous activity of the will and subtle-feeling, symbolises the high and sublime mystery of the sixth energy centre. A purity of the soul is expressed in the wise and free overseeing of the light around the head, particularly when the consciousness is alert and creatively active, and at the same time also leading the intended movement-dynamic, through the limbs, into a forming. The sitting twist depicts this free and yet creating activity of thinking, which oversees and regulates the perception processes of the sensory stream, and therefore the sitting twist denotes the high significance of purity in the thinking. This steered thinking activity bestows a purity for the sensory life. Purity and expansiveness in the head are expressed in the image of the sitting twist.

To practise

The simplest way of leading the body into an upright twist happens in the sitting position with out-stretched legs, *vitata matsyendrāsana*. Sitting with your legs straightened out, lead your arms up and starting from the sacrum stretch the spine actively upwards. Pay attention to the clarity and consciousness in the head. Then lead your arms down to the floor to your left and at the same time also twist the spine in all its sections to the left. The head is also included in the twist. Remain in this twist for about a minute with alert overseeing of the head. Then change to the other side by taking your arms up again and carrying out the movement in the same way to the right.

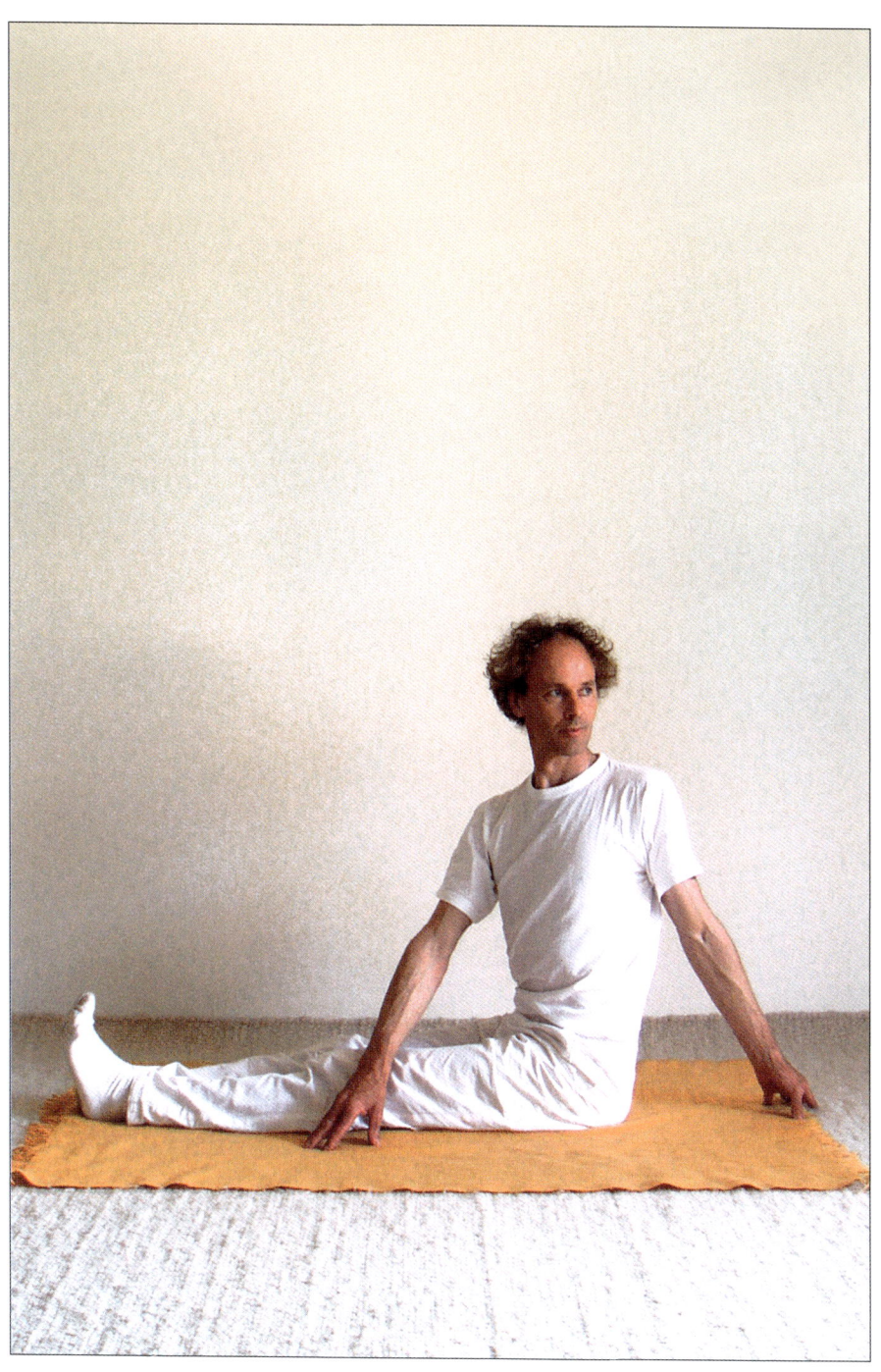

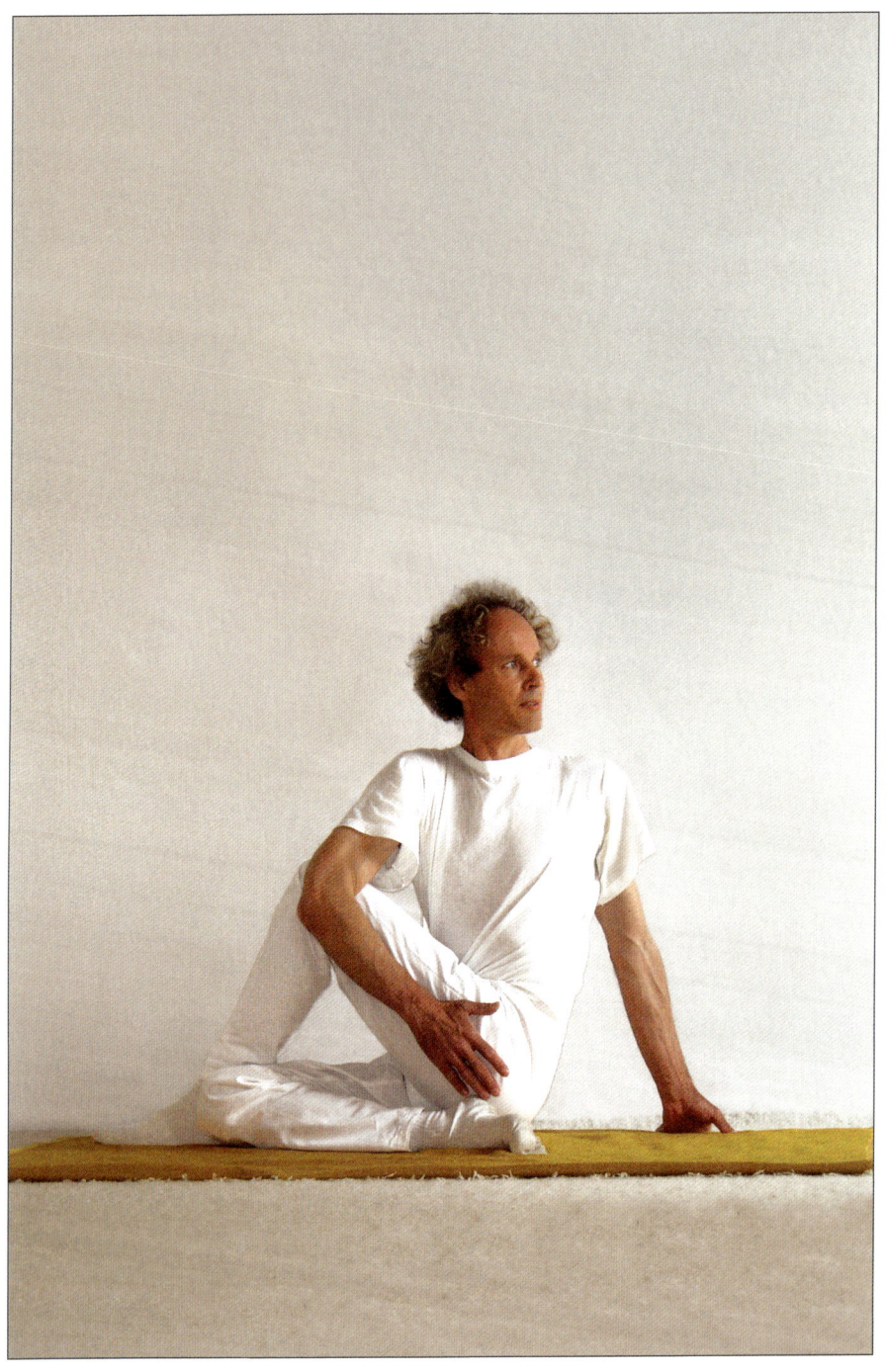

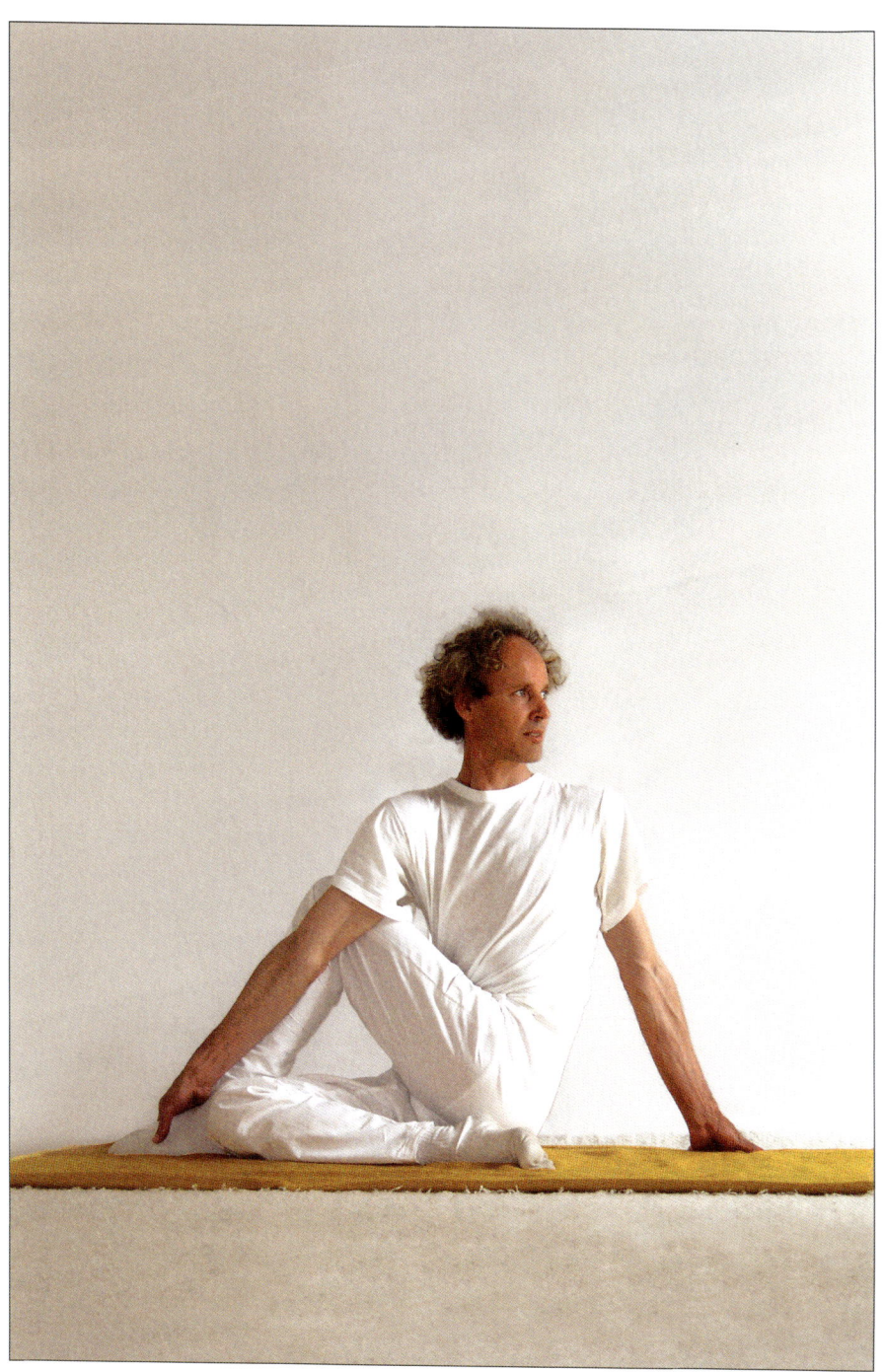

A form of practice closer to the actual sitting twist is to place one leg, bent up, over the other, actively straighten up the spine again out of the lower regions, and out of the overseeing of the head initiate the twist. Here you press the left elbow, together with the forearm, against the right knee in order to shape the movement into the twist. The body is gradually led into the desired form of the ideal. During this preparatory exercise, which can take up to a few minutes, the head should remain clear and the thoughts expansive. Pay attention during all the sitting twist positions to the clearly formed and already pre-existing mental pictures so that with unerring thoughts you can enter into the subsequent stage of shaping the exercise.

For the ultimate stage of forming the half sitting twist, *ardha matsyendrāsana*, you can bring your left arm beyond your right knee to reach for your foot and hold it firmly. The spine straightens up out of the sacrum and twists in all its sections, up to and including the head. The shoulders remain as relaxed as possible, and to retain the balance the right arm can provide a gentle support on the ground. Out of the thought, a concrete form develops.

Afterwards you can change sides and practise on the other side for the same amount of time. Give yourself time in all the sitting twist exercises and avoid forming the movements in too forceful or fixed a way as this would give rise to the danger of damaging the vertebrae or over-stretching the ligaments. The sitting twist demonstrates the harmonious way of proceeding in which out of a conscious thought, precise work comes about, and this is reflected in the form, that means in a specific bodily gesture. The thought itself, which lies at the beginning, motivates the movement, but itself remains free from the movement. Through this the image emerges of expansiveness and purity in the thought.

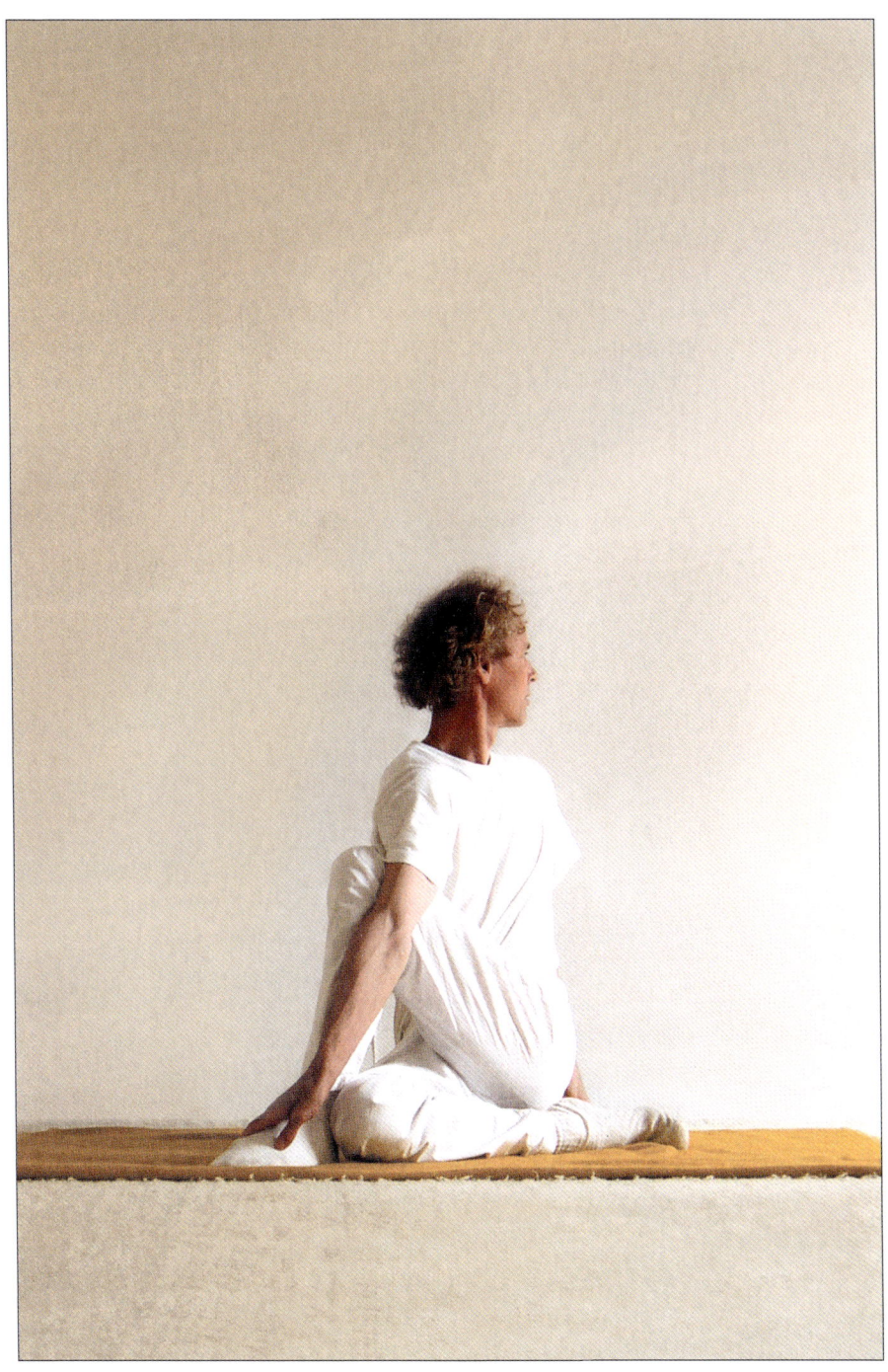

The headstand
śīrṣāsana

The picture and meaning of the exercise

In this *āsana* the body rests upside down and in a graceful, vertical form, on the head. Already from the picture, as well as from the practice of the dynamic phase, in this pose all energies are centred onto the region of the forehead. Dynamic, concentration, uprightness, shaping-force, firmness of purpose, and clarity are expressed in this *āsana*. The headstand can therefore be designated as a typical exercise which emphasises more the masculine qualities of life. Just as the shoulderstand emphasises more the etheric nature of dynamic uprightness, so in contrast to this the headstand expresses more the stringent, assiduous *āsana*, shaped more out of the form of the thought. Practitioners experience the vertical line particularly intensively in the inverted form, as this form is inescapable in the headstand and also moves into consciousness through the inversion. The vertical line reveals the nature of the thought, which in itself is concrete and clear and represents a celestial power, a spiritual substance itself. In this symbol, which can be vividly experienced, lies the meaning of this graceful *āsana*.

To practise

For the practice, preparatory steps can support the development of a feeling of form out of the thought, and an order that is experienced in the form. One of the most pleasant preparatory exercises for the headstand, which creates a centring in the solar plexus and gives an idea of the vertical extension, is the lying triangle on the ground, *supta trikoṇāsana*. Although this pose appears completely different from the headstand in the character of its expression, there is nonetheless a certain similarity in the character of its subtle-feeling. A clear form with ordered centring characterises both poses. To practise, lie on your back and leave your shoulders relaxed. Raise one leg while the leg on the ground remains stretched and dynamic. Pay attention to the centre in the upper abdomen, out of which the active extension flows into both legs. This centring gives a first feeling for a healthy distribution of tension and a centring order through the developed form.

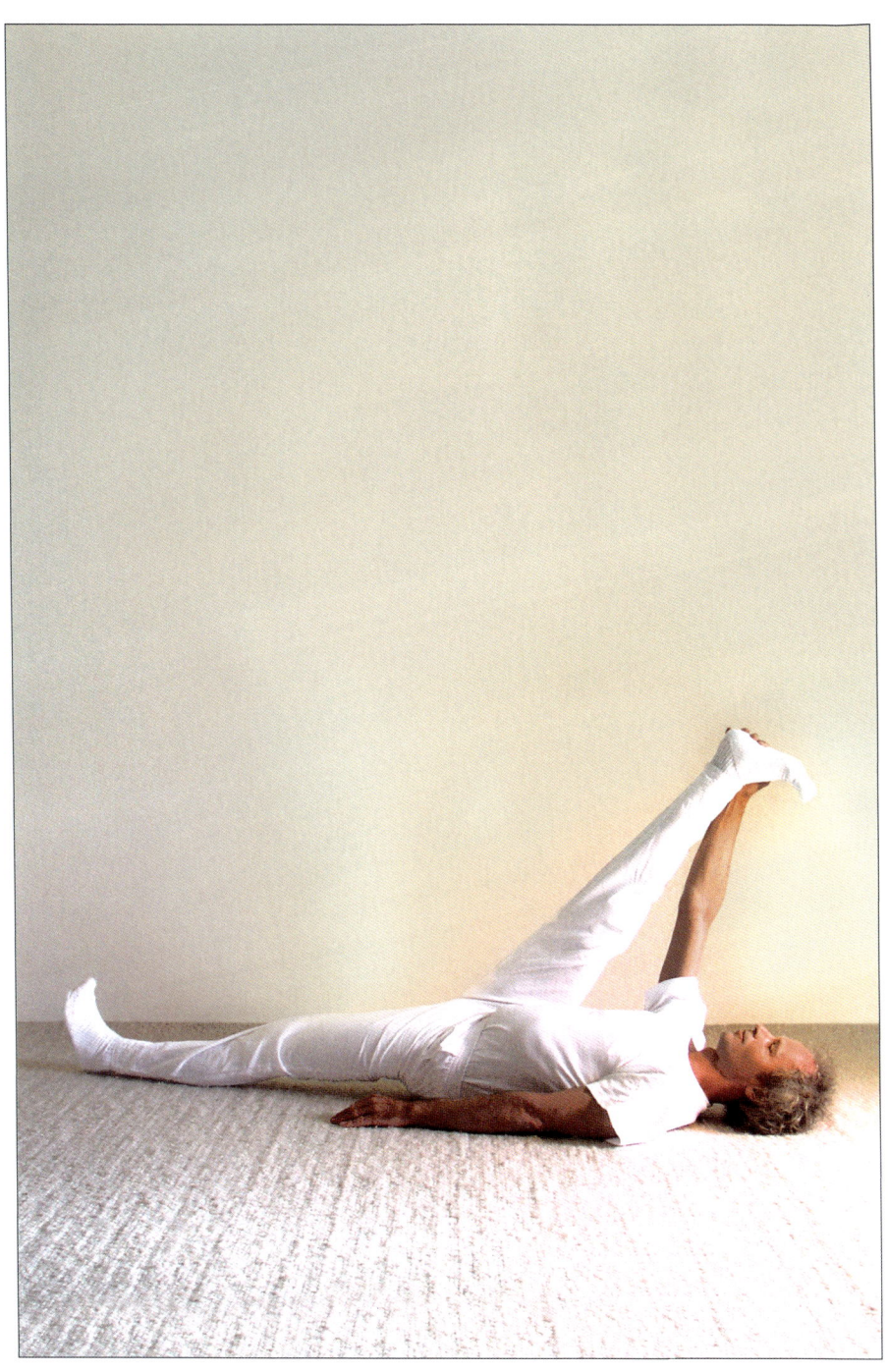

255

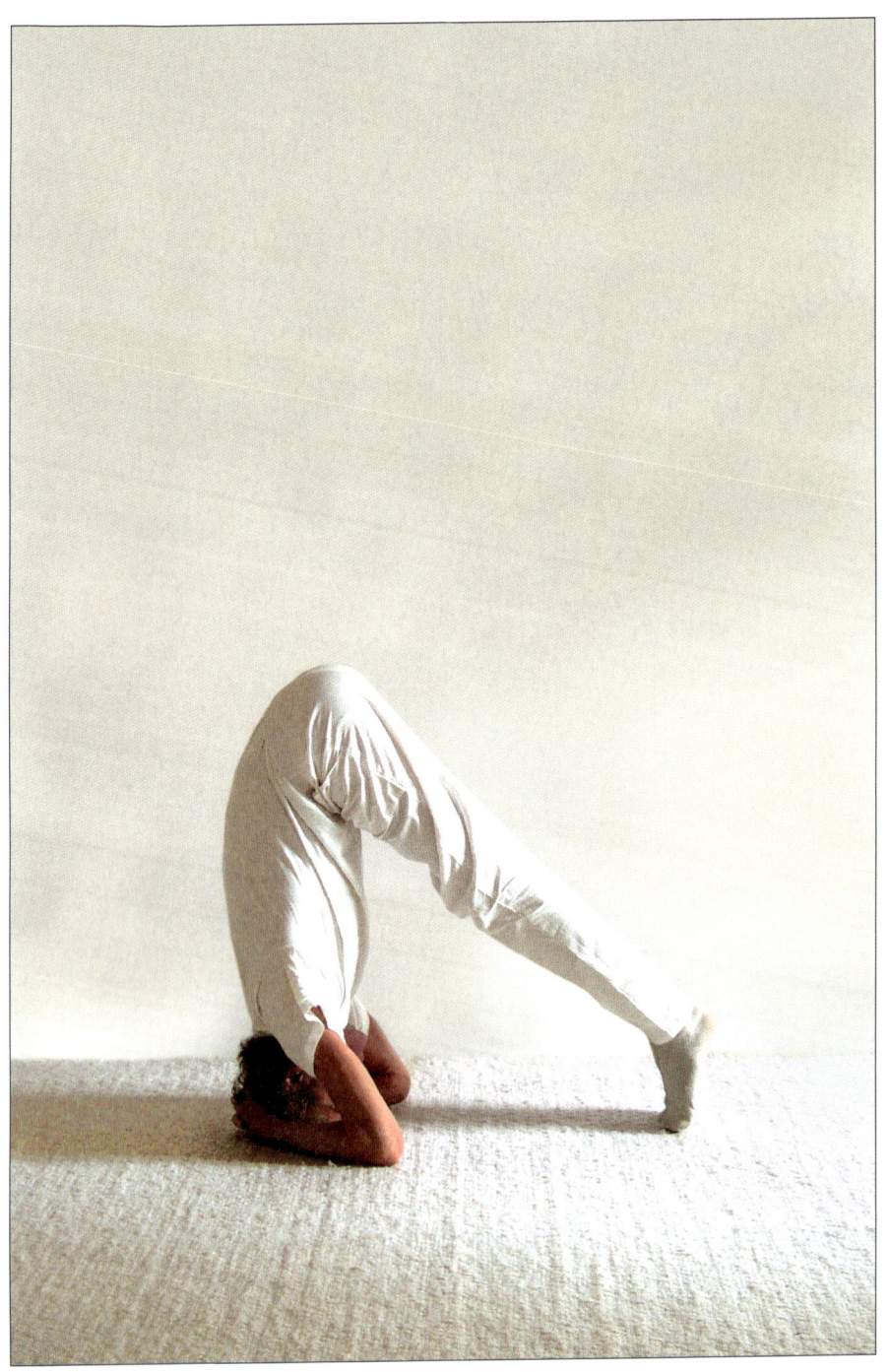

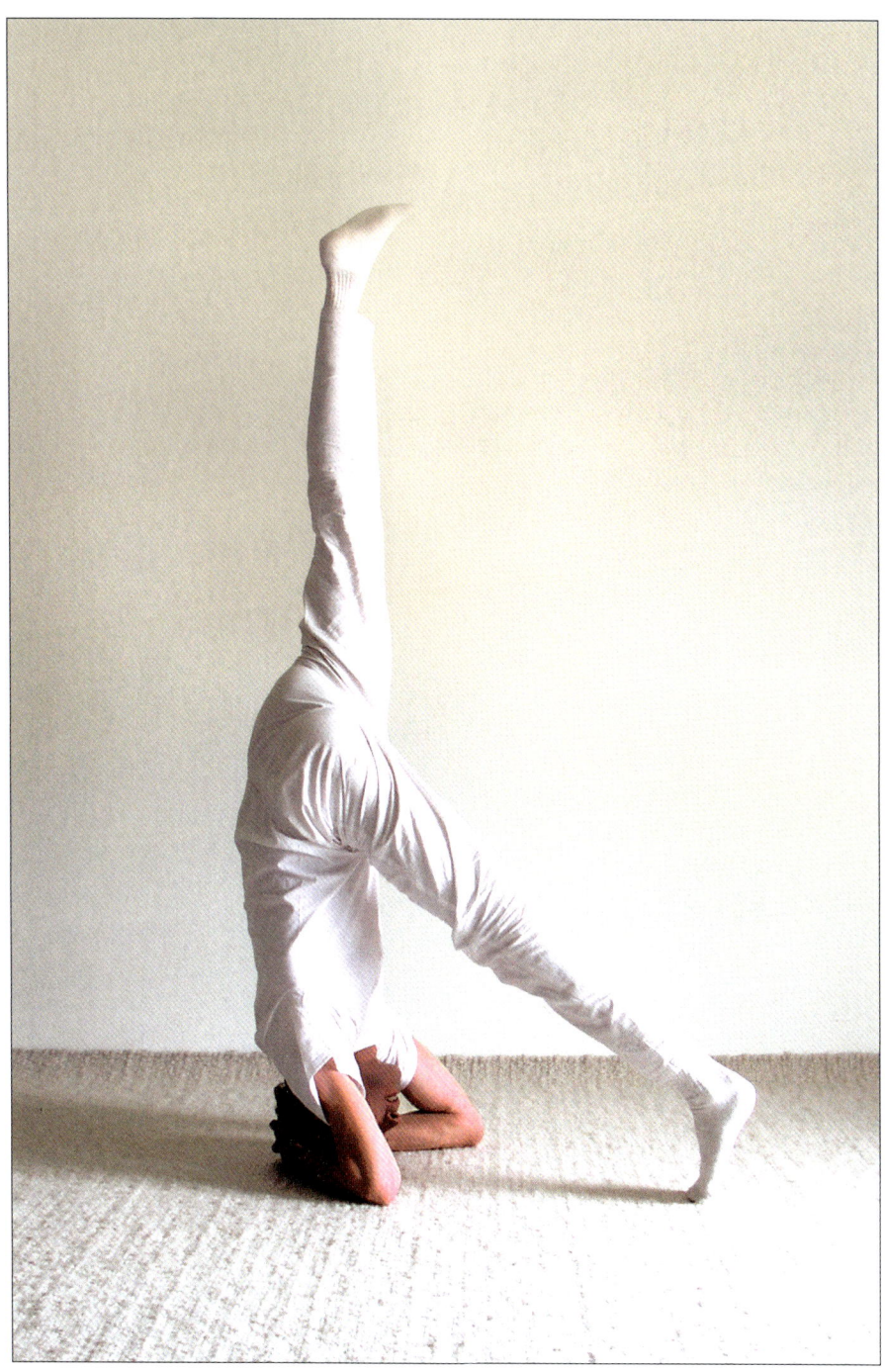

Then kneel on the ground and mentally prepare yourself for the inverted posture which seeks its end position in a vertical line. Place your elbows shoulder width apart on the ground and firmly interlace your fingers. Then very consciously place your head with the crown on the ground, so consciously that you perceive the closeness of your head to the ground, and stably clasp the back of your head with your interlaced fingers. Now straighten up your hips directly over your head. This is the first preparatory position, which paves the way for straightening up into the vertical inversion.

A next step is to raise one leg up vertically. The other leg still remains outstretched on the ground. The pose is called *eka pāda śīrṣāsana*. It is a graceful gesture which allows the uprightness to come into closer experience. The experience is always of the form developing out of a clear and concrete consciousness.

To take the headstand into its end position you can either raise the second leg or come back again and go into the vertical with both legs together. An initial tentativeness in straightening up can be overcome with time and with some practice the headstand acquires a stable assurance.

Avoid kicking up. If you fall, draw your head in and roll down on your back. With high blood pressure, illnesses affecting the head, or spinal problems in the neck you should practise the exercise very cautiously or if necessary omit it. In the initial stages the headstand can usually only be practised for a few seconds. With some practice and experience, however, the exercise can be held for up to several minutes in the static phase. A useful variation arises from the headstand through lowering alternate legs (picture p. 257). Finally come back rhythmically out of the position.

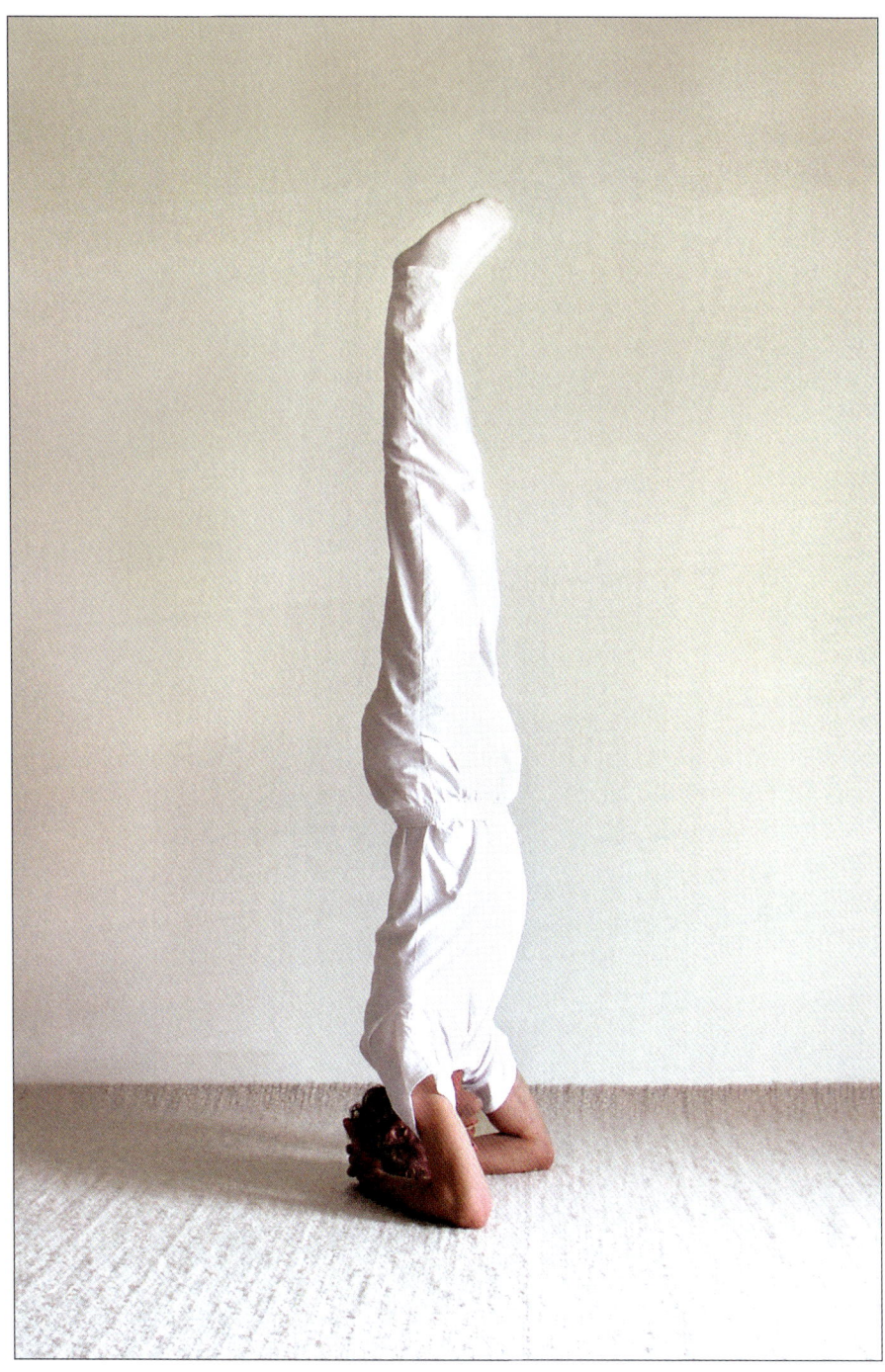

The cobra
bhujaṅgāsana

The picture and the meaning of the exercise

The cobra can be compared with a blossom of self-forgetting, which seems unobtrusive, as it builds itself out of the creative forces of free thoughts. The body actually does not raise itself to a mighty gesture of uprightness out of mere will-power, it rounds itself, curves and builds itself in a graceful backward bend, and finally rests in still, overseen openness in the sensitive space. Devotion and self-forgetting, which arises through a conscious, overseen and created thought-life, are signified by the exercise. It is self-forgetting in a well-considered self of thought.

To practise

The body lies on its front, the feet are closed. The hands lie under the shoulders directly by the collarbones. The movement now begins from the neck and grows along the back down into the region of the sacrum. First lift your head, form the upper thoracic spine and then the middle part of the thoracic spine into the stretch, and with gentle support of the arms raise the body further and further up into the stretch throughout the spine. The strength should be actively applied, chiefly from the spine. The arms themselves only give the body some accompanying guidance, so that it does not tilt forwards and the individual movements can more easily be coordinated.

During the exercise remain conscious of yourself in the forehead region. The sensitive consciousness of alertness and overseeing can be felt quite particularly when the static phase, that means the highest movement in the cobra with the farthest stretch throughout the thoracic spine, is reached. This position is accompanied by intense calm.

The cobra itself describes a graceful image. The body is not broad, the legs remain narrow, the shoulders are also slanted slightly backwards. Not straightening up high but stretching through is of most significance, for the body is not only lifted up into a greater plane; far more it is shaped through its entire length in the movement and becomes smaller again, for

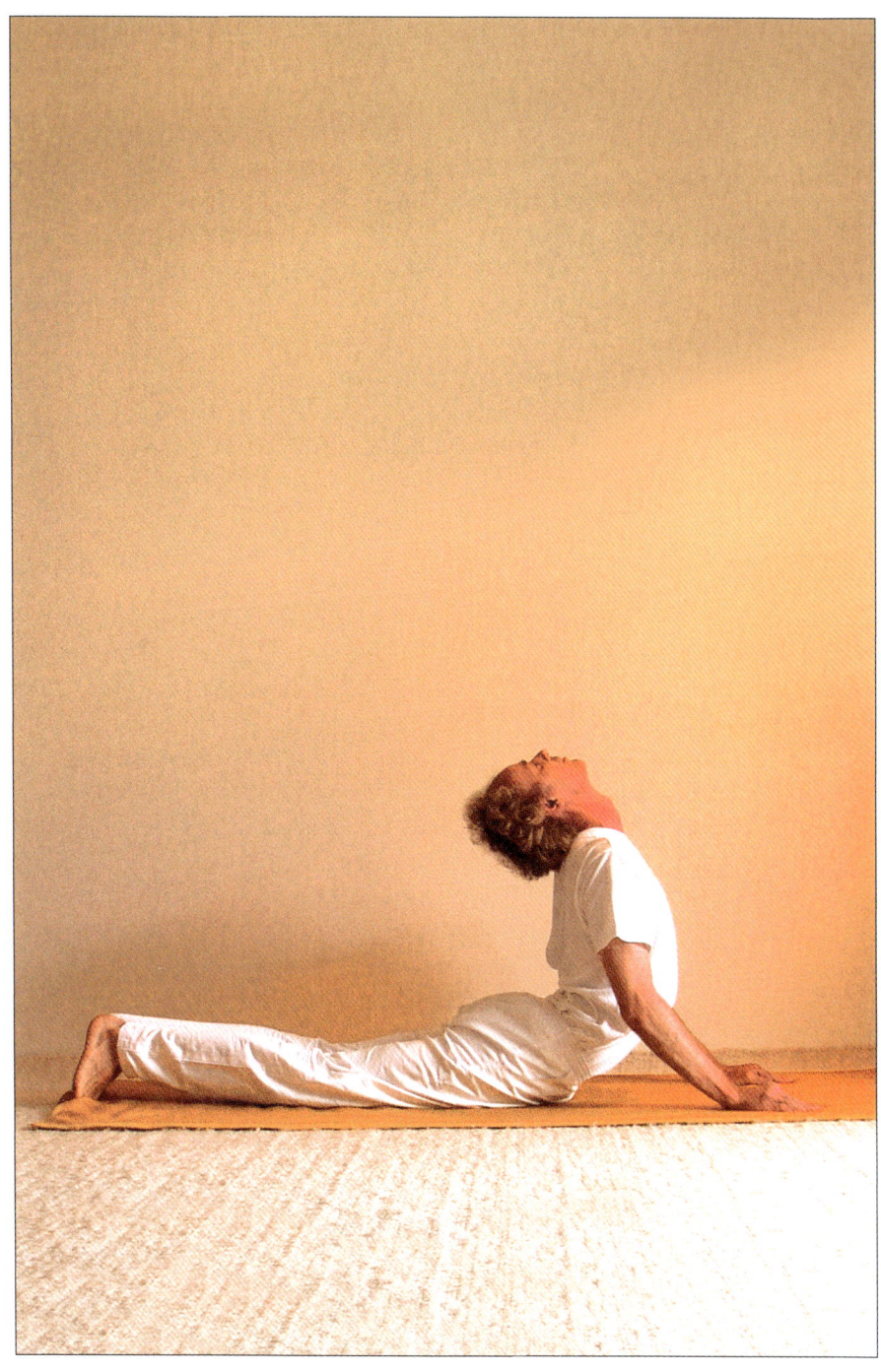

backward bending reveals a consciousness of meditative devotion, and a contemplative, pleasant humility is expressed in the pose.

For very practised and advanced students the basic pose can be developed further, to the king cobra. In the king cobra a sublime devotion and self-forgetting is revealed. As a rule it can only be achieved after many years of practice. Young people who have not yet awakened to a mature "I" can sometimes do the king cobra in a playful and more childlike way. The aim, however, is to experience the movement in an expression of maturity and consciousness. Therefore, the work with this exercise is connected with an encompassing, lengthy and multi-faceted discipline, coupled with a path of study for spiritual development.

Backward bending is easy to master in youth, as the spine is still very supple and the metabolic forces flow in a very unhindered and regenerative way.

All movements in which the spine bends backwards happen not primarily with strong use of force, but with calm relaxation of the mind, which forms the basis for the relaxation of the body.

Noble devotion and meditative openness are expressed in the forms of movement. The body recedes in its vital dominance, it becomes less obtrusive and affords a great space for edifying, new possibilities.

This releasing of material or vital dominance is what backward bending symbolises. In order to learn the noble art of backward bending in its stylish expression and in unobtrusive perfection, the novice must first of all learn to release themselves from the materialistic forms of thinking and learn an edifying thinking. Then even in more advanced years the supple, devotional backward flexion becomes possible again.

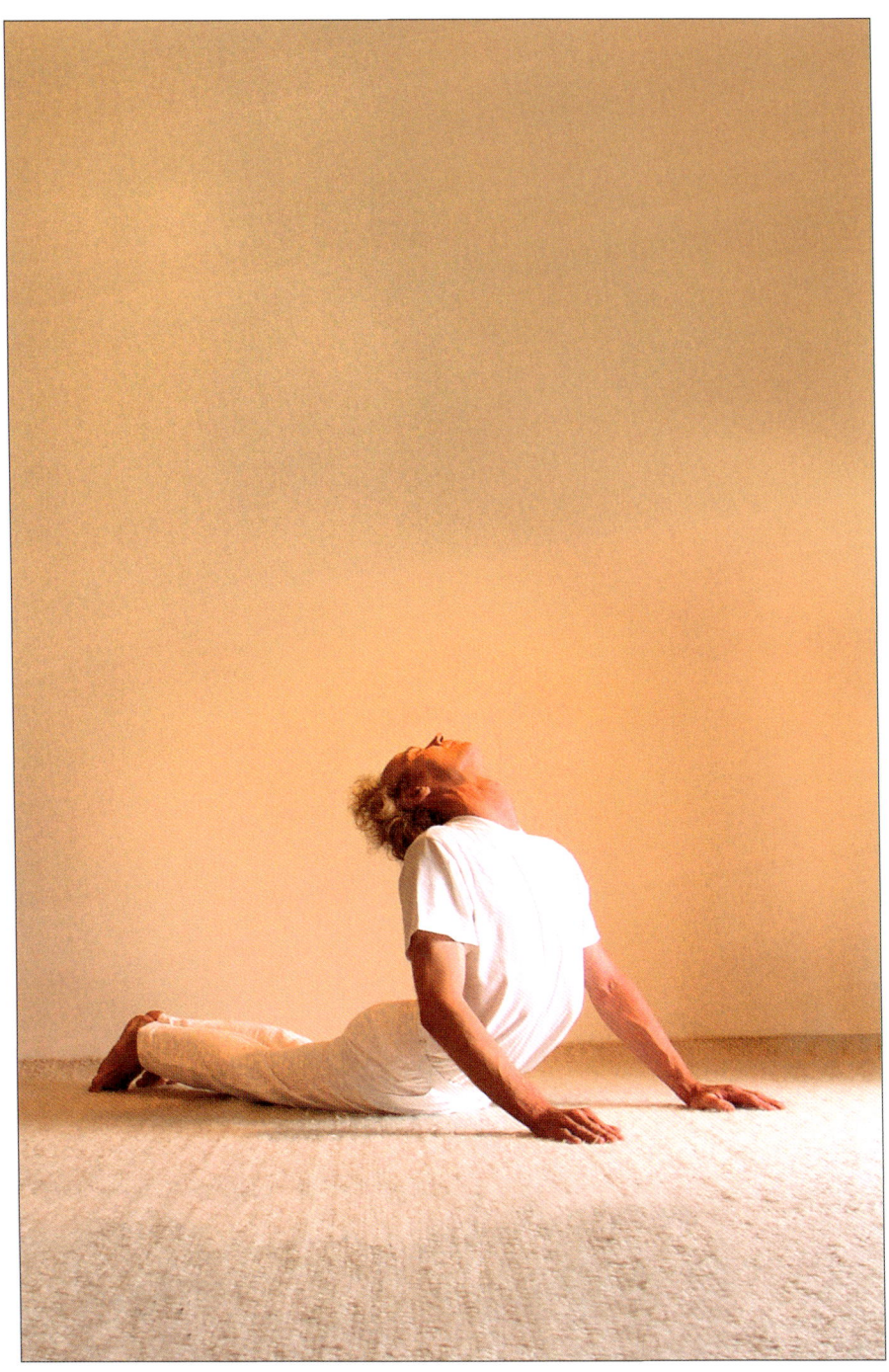

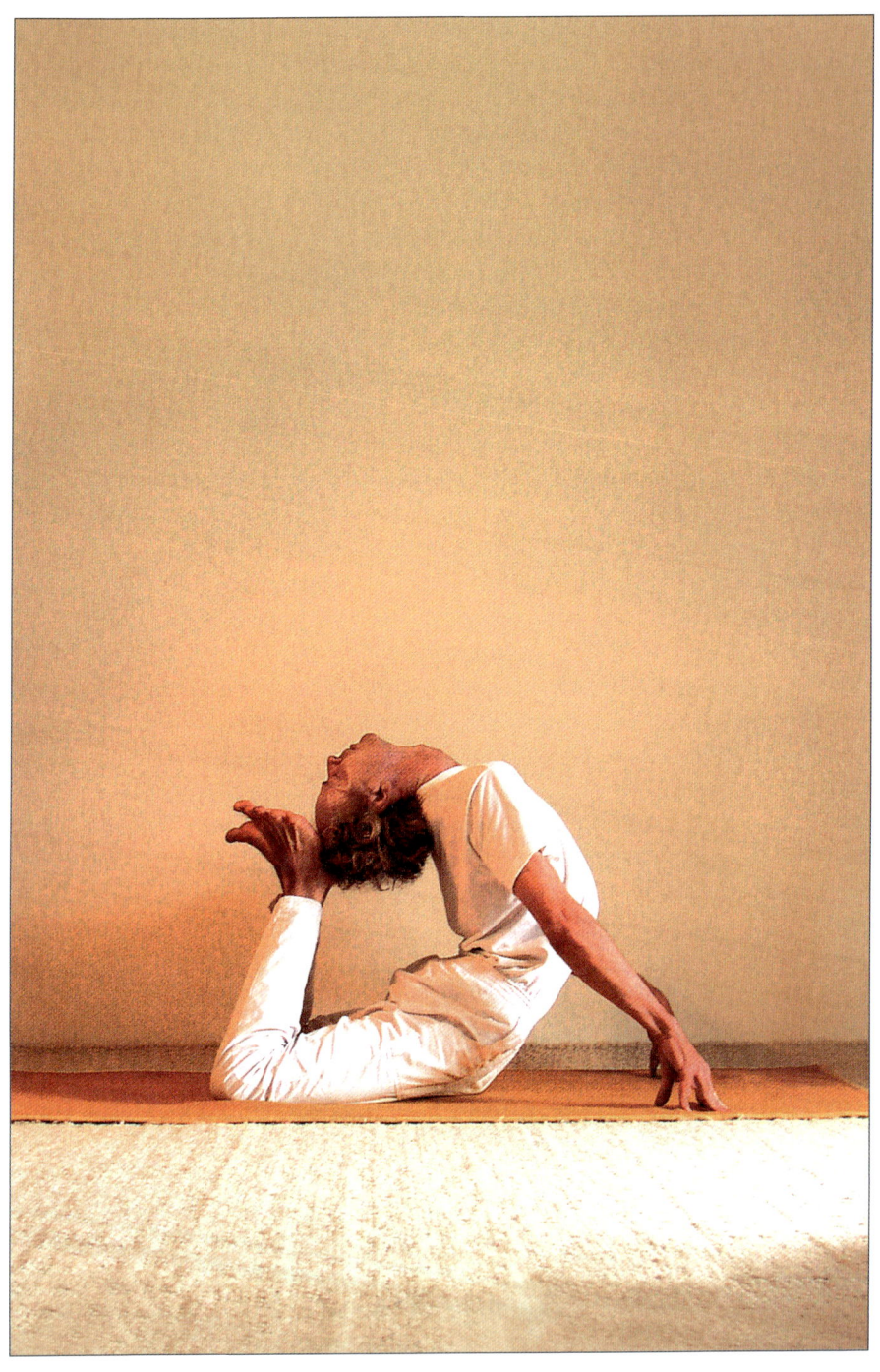

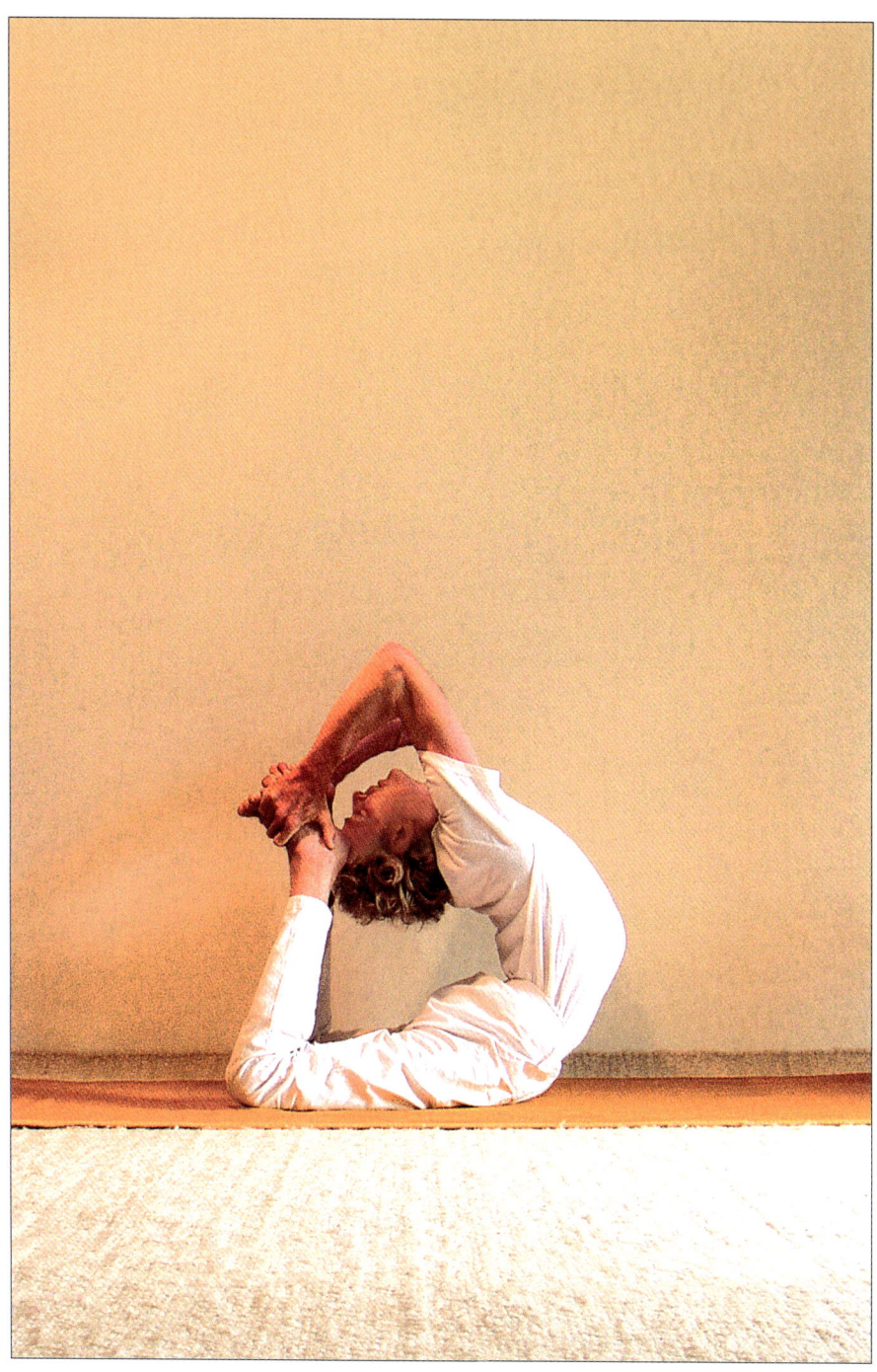

Encouraging primordial strength and developing a freely available decisiveness – *mūlādhāra-cakra*

Primordial strength, which usually develops in the first seven years of life, from a physical perspective is connected with the healthy morphology of the organs and their harmonious metabolism. The organs form the kind of protein specific to the human being, and they must display the necessary firmness, structure and form for this activity.

Decisiveness is a particular, intensive force in the soul, which is conditional upon the primordial strength in the organs, and in turn is more easily ensured when a productive, free way of dealing with wishes and needs in respect of the world of the body, and also in respect of the earthly world in general, is developed. Wishes are will-impulses, feelings too are often motivated through the will from the unconscious realm of the body. Now, however, these unconsidered will-impulses, still unclear in their direction, should become led into the purest and clearest direction possible through a very careful and exact differentiation.

An alive and dynamic expression of lightness and of bodily independence awakens in the practice with yoga exercises when, through our own independent decision, the strength of the will is directed towards the body and towards matter, and at the same time holds back the subtle emotions of a habitual feeling of expectation, of sentimentality or of clinging desire. The breath becomes purer and lighter, freer from the desiring powers of physical or emotional dependency. A purity develops in the breath in the form of integrity and independence. With a soul-attitude where the body is managed with a free will, in fact with free emotions, the quality of the breath expresses itself with a sensitive gentleness, which gestures a new and open space in which ultimately the feelings also express themselves creatively as they take form.

One might assume that the earth element, which has its home in *mūlādhāra-cakra*, would be weighed down with a certain heaviness. The earth element, however, is light and pure, clear in its contour and orderly in its form. It gradually recedes in itself and in its form, and gives itself to the current of the times. Only that takes itself to be important which inflates itself in its desire for the world and seemingly declares this matter to be the most important scenery. So it is the irrational importance given to the material world that allows this world to appear so very oversized in its forms and phenomena. In reality the earth element is like calm silence, as it has already left itself to its own form, and that is death.

The primordial forces of the body and the organs are, however, particularly strengthened when progressing students dedicate themselves with full consciousness to the content of the spiritual school, and actually study the *kāma*, the clinging desire that has settled in the emotions or even in the energies of the body, and ultimately learn to order it through a greater, more concrete discipline, directed from pictorial thinking to creative feeling and to clear, sequential and unemotional action. Practice remains concrete and guards against emotional influences. Through dedication to content, thoughts and also to exercises, which up until now have not been rooted in one's own experience, and which describe a higher dimension of existence, a challenge is simultaneously presented to the will, with which indirectly, and that is the notable thing, not directly but so to speak through an alternative spiritual route, an inner force is fired up in the metabolism, which ultimately adds to the firmness of the whole bodily interior and of the personality structures.

In relation to the physical exercises, practitioners learn to dedicate themselves to their own bodies in a way that is now free from emotion, by learning to free themselves from the habitual, desirous urges of their own nature and from the usual feelings of sympathy and antipathy, and with clear, dynamic intentions, entering into the exercises giving them form and shape. On the one hand they listen to the body, to its signals, to pain, resistance, stiffness, weakness, or particular feelings of inclination, enthusiasm which are generally taken to be positive, but also to the feelings of reluctance, despondency, depression, which are usually judged negatively, and yet they remain in an attitude of decisive determination to form the result that they ultimately want to create with the *āsana*. For example, they hold the exercise for a time period they have set themselves at the outset, as long as health or a major impediment does not really prevent them. The intent to purposefully carry out an exercise without accoutrements, according to a clearly formed idea and a newly developing feeling, is another aid in strengthening the inner metabolic forces.

Mūlādhāra-cakra is the mid-point of the physical body and it can be equated with the deepest will, and this in turn can be equated with the innermost nature of desire itself. It is the centre of the physical body. As spiritual training advances, its perfected development requires a very strict discipline geared towards self-control and self-mastery. An immaculate purity in acting and an implacable aim directing the thoughts, as well as a truly body-free, creative force in the feelings, which requires exemplary control of the emotions, are in the long term necessary, so that this centre can translate its innermost strength and will into action. This perfect mastery, however, is hardly achievable for students, and therefore the introductory thoughts about learning to differentiate the substance of desire and recognise the element of earth, which by its very nature wants to find the repose of its earthly being, suffice as an initial and also good working basis.

The earth
bhūmi

The picture and the meaning of the exercise

This simple exercise, which is not typical for classical yoga, gives a basic idea and subtle-feeling for developing the will with a consciousness free from the body. The earth element, which is subject to gravity and transience, is perhaps best experienced when a complete freedom and relaxation is developed in the entire middle and upper body. The upper body is given to the earth, or in other words the upper body is released in the most intensive way from all tensions and left to hang, so that it seems to fall downwards as if it were dying. For this reason the exercise can be assigned to the essence of the earth.

The gravitational force, that can be measured in the earth's atmosphere, is arguably a very hard, almost violent force, for when we observe falling bodies we notice how through this mighty movement towards the centre of the earth, matter can be smashed into pieces. Gravity is the visible movement of all physical bodies in the earth's atmosphere towards its centre. On the other hand, however, the phenomenon of gravity is an exceptional, glorious and beneficent movement, as it does not concern the human soul, but only physical matter. Both the physical body as well as all physical objects can fall down, but the soul, in a kind of counter-movement, extends into ever expanding and greater spaces. One cannot therefore speak of a fall of the soul; at the most one could say that the soul reaches into wrong and disharmonious connections and as a result the whole person ends up in too strong an attachment to physical circumstances.

From a complete letting go, new ether forces develop, or from a real process of release, or death, new steps of will result. The soul meaning lies in this subtle-feeling, which is consciously created with the exercise, and in consciously experiencing the body pictorially.

To practise

Practitioners start in a natural standing position. Beginners can bend their knees a little, while for the more advanced it seems advisable to keep the knees almost completely straightened. The upper body is brought down and forwards into a hanging position. Gradually the head, the neck, the shoulders, the arms and finally the chest and thoracic spine become entirely given over to gravity. Within a holding time of about two to five minutes a feeling of complete letting go should be created; a feeling of almost indifferent relinquishing of any fixedness or tension in the upper body. The idea that everything in life is over and with this the will can now be conclusively relinquished, determines the feeling in the hanging upper body.

While the breath remains completely free, and through the conscious idea that the tensions in the upper body subside, a feeling actually comes about of perfect hanging in will-less self-surrender. The consciousness, however, remains alert and even creates this feeling of letting oneself hang. In the complete calmness the body is experienced pictorially.

After the exercise has been done for some time and the feeling of being detached has come into effect, the will can now be seized anew and with this the hands are gradually taken up over the head and the spine builds itself up into a thorough stretch, particularly in the middle region (as in exercise on p. 223). This straightening up concludes the exercise for now.

This basic exercise is particularly suited before the leg pose, *utthita eka pāda hastāsana*, or also before the horse, *vātāyanāsana*. A feeling of applying one's forces, out of the unbound and body-free regions of the will, which comes about when a good picturing activity motivates the exercise in new and unbound ways, is produced through this preparatory *āsana*.

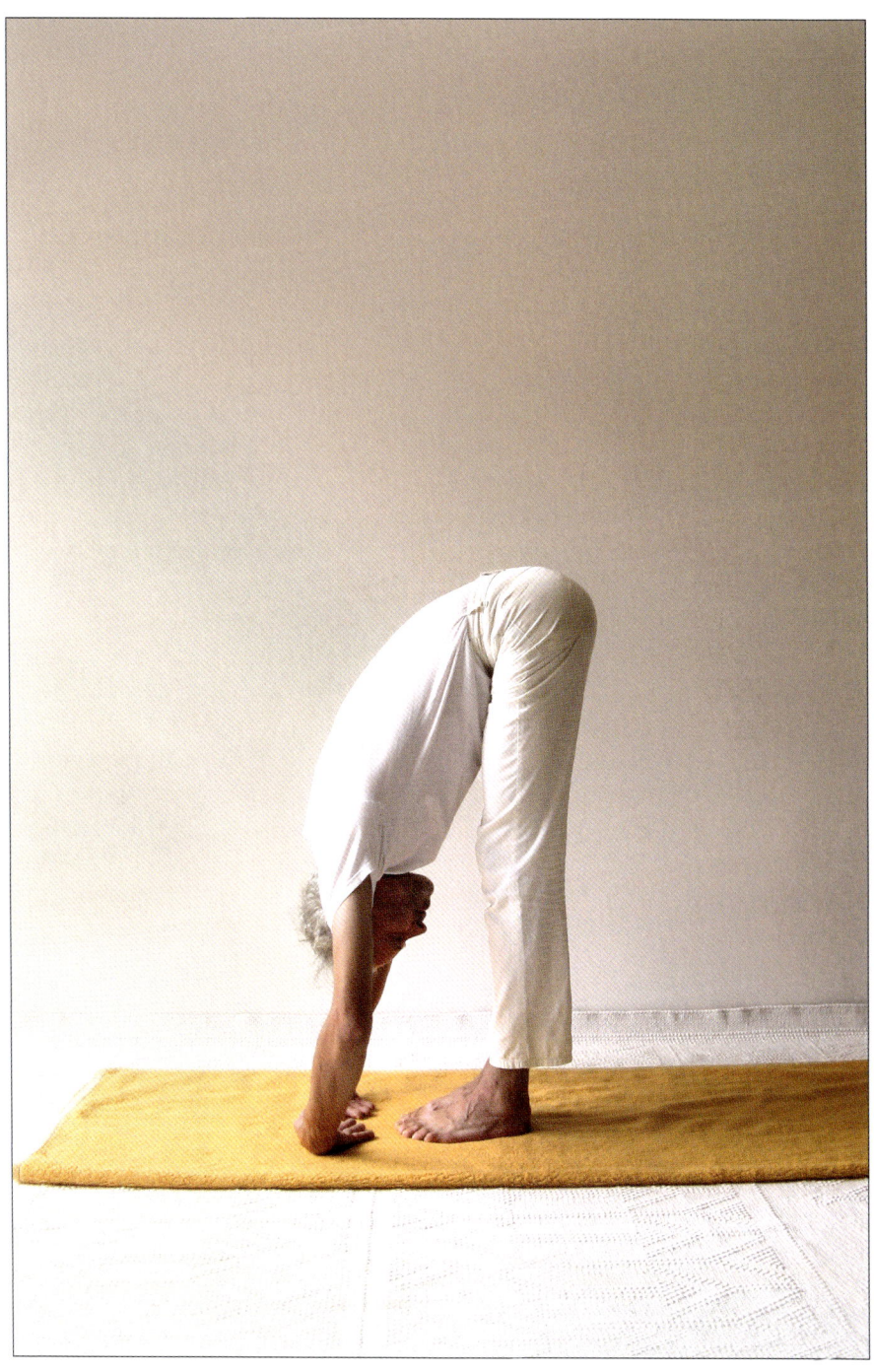

The leg pose
utthita eka pāda hastāsana

The picture and the meaning of the exercise

The graceful and challenging upright leg pose stimulates the whole body's capacity for uprightness. The centre for uprightness lies, in the first instance, at the lowest end of the spine. Practitioners seem to straighten up both with the legs and also with the back against the pull, heaviness and resistance of gravity. However, on clearer and more precise inspection, this uprightness happens not only through an outer, wilful effort against gravity, but even with a decline of this wilful effort. Although the body itself straightens up gracefully with the legs, in its earthly being it contracts to a mid-point, so to speak, and the person becomes noticeably more unassuming. In this effort to straighten up, which occurs through a contraction in the mid-point of the body or in the lower two energy centres, lies the outstanding and instructive meaning of the *āsana*.

Furthermore, from a deeper esoteric perspective, an inner soul picture is marked out through this movement. The legs are usually the natural walking instruments with which earthly citizens stand and move around on the earth. From a cosmological perspective however, which is related to the inner picture of the human being, the legs are not just walking tools for earthly life, they are far more the direct organs of expression for the action and power of the heart. The heart itself is the centre of the personality and the legs are the organs of expression for the acting forces of the heart.

Now in performing *utthita eka pāda hastāsana*, practitioners enter into an increasing upward dynamic by practising this straightening up not solely on a level of training the body and will, but by learning to leave the body in peace and bringing themselves into a contracting dynamic in the lower centres. Instead of striving only upwards with the will, at the same time they enter into their own body, seek the mid-point in the lower centres, and become conscious that this mid-point of their body is also at the same time the mid-point of the earth itself. The will seems to draw back with all its forces into this mid-point. At the same time, a free sphere opens up with newly awakening ether forces, and practitioners learn to place the upwardly directed leg more and more into the vertical, until they can even take hold of it with their second arm above their head, forming a closed, unified circle. Thus practitioners span between earth and heaven, between something below and something above, and they firmly hold the raised leg with their arms to form a circle. One could say they become a universal heart and experience themselves in this form as if etherised, like an etherised world-axis or like a heart become vertical. The arms and the raised up leg, which together enclose the head, describe a so-called polygon, a kind of regular, many-sided form. This many-sided form also looks like the symbol of an etherised heart, which is elevated and lies closer to the free space of the cosmos. With one foot the body touches earthly ground and with the other foot it projects into the free space of the cosmos.

This pose leads to an experience that the first and seventh centres belong together. Both spheres, that of the earthly being with its transience and that of the whole cosmic circumsphere, become noticeable for practitioners as soon as they focus on the movement in the reverse direction described here. When in the movement they centre towards the mid-point of the earth, the movement attains an elegant freedom, and the legs, which are a metamorphosed expression for the heart, are freed from the influences of gravitational forces.

Straightening up one leg precisely in this way, with a mental picture with which one turns to the mid-point of the earth, particularly encourages the ability to take hold of one's own will in a new freedom, use it without claiming space, and apply it in the world without power. Thus the exercise itself leads to an extraordinary skill and elegance in the way the thinking is approached and opens an insightful view to the higher worlds. It shows how a far greater and more elegant action of forces can come about, an action which is truer and freer in world-creation. The leg glides upwards, almost as if in weightlessness, when the centring to the earth element in the body, and with this to the mid-point of the earth, is practised and mentally pictured.

The exercise itself, because of its character, can only be practised in a concrete way; it tolerates no emotion or sentimentality. This concrete way of forming and approaching the body is another characteristic of the earth element.

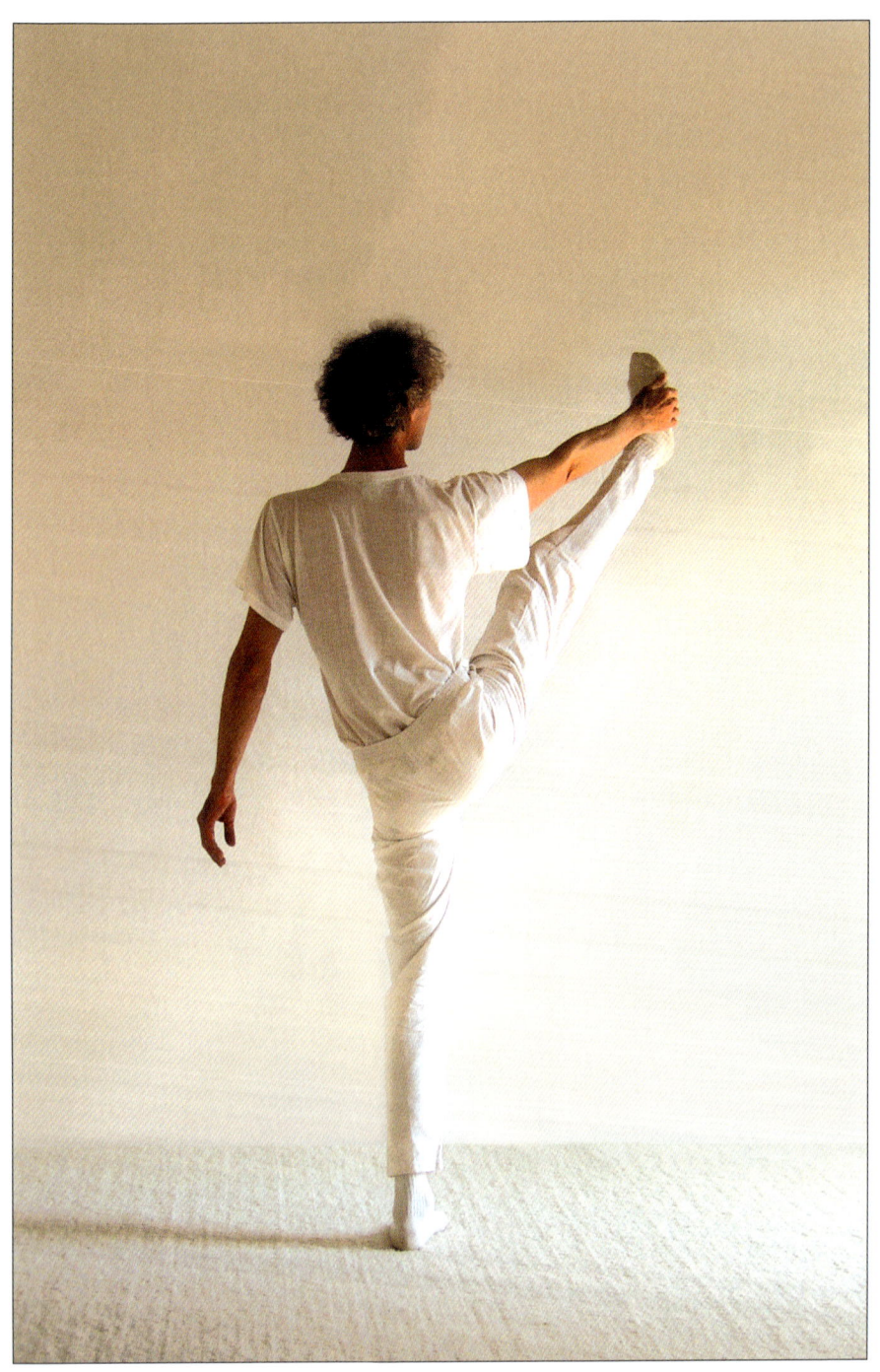

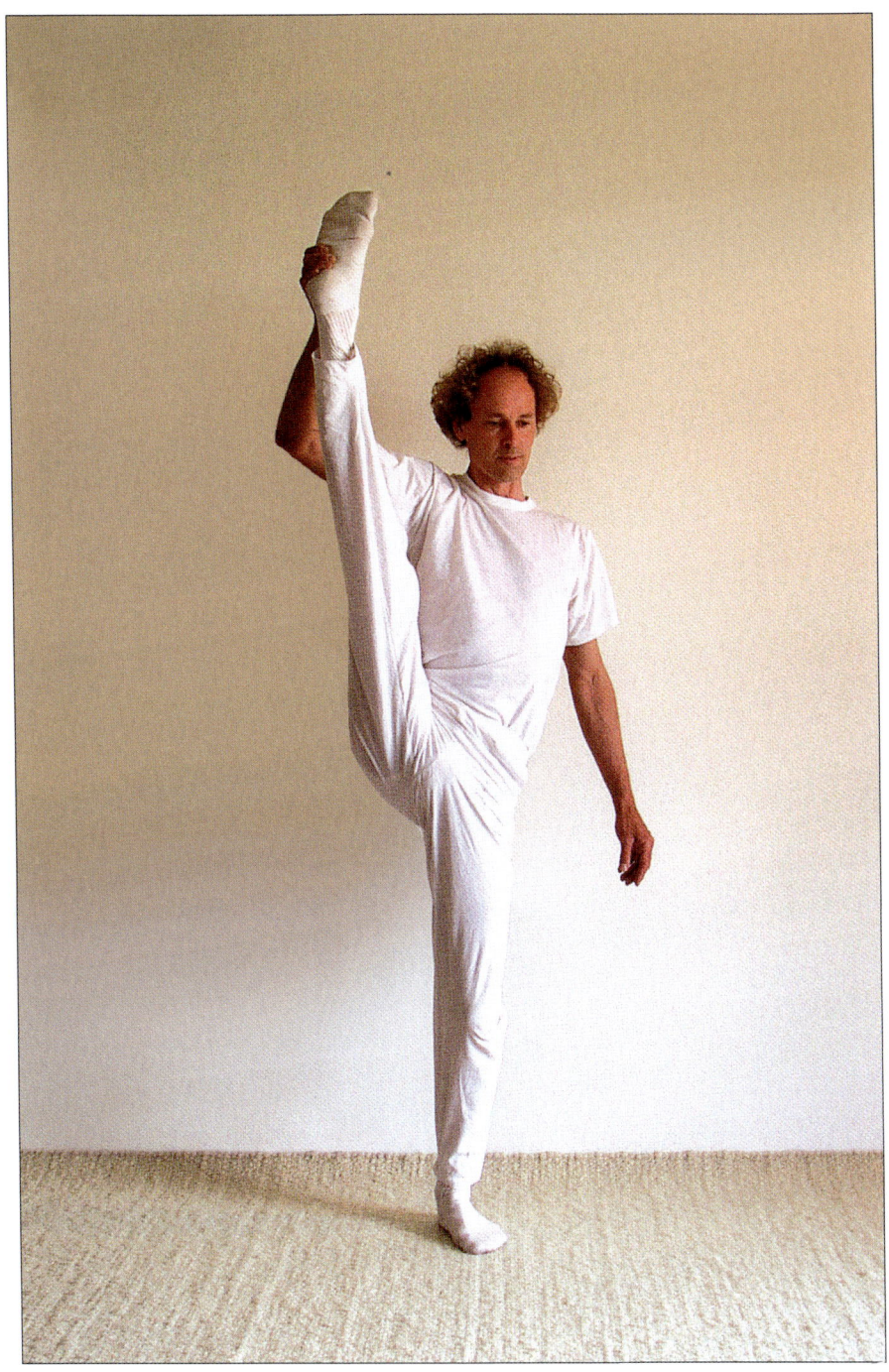

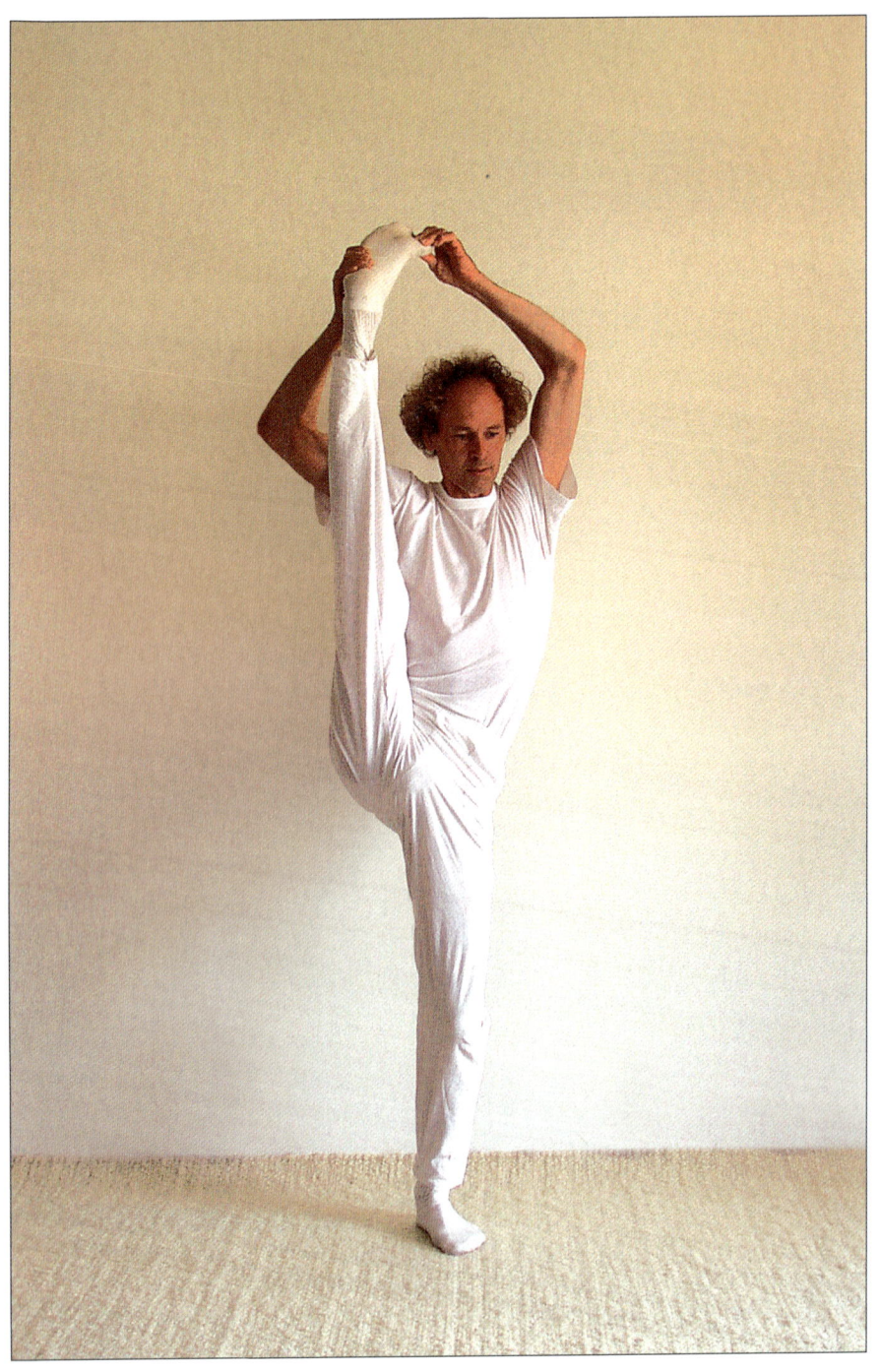

To practise

Let us remember that with every *āsana* not only is a physical position adopted, but the consciousness is immersed in a particular, specific subtle-feeling, gets to know this subtle-feeling, and realises it in an artistic picture expressed through the body. To practise it, therefore, the picture of the pose, its form and the dynamic of its movement must first be carefully studied.

Then stand firmly on your left leg and with your right hand take hold of the outside of your right foot and guide this foot up, letting it be carried as much as possible from the dynamic of the lowermost back. Leave your upper body, neck and shoulders as relaxed as possible.

In whatever position is possible for you, now keep your attention focused on the two lowermost centres, i.e. on the region of the hips and sacrum. In this region a muscular contraction should come about, however not just mechanically by applying force, but with the mental picture that the body draws back into this region, making itself more centred and smaller in this centre. The upper body bends as little as possible, for it is the legs themselves that aspire up into the vertical dynamic. The uprightness originates from the lowermost spine and from the dynamic being released, which flows into the legs. The breath constantly flows freely, the eyes are open in all stages.

With increasing practice of this in fact inverse centring, a centring to the mid-point of the earth, you can lead the leg further upwards into the vertical and you will notice how with this the upper body also aspires from the lowermost back into the vertical (picture p. 275).

Once the leg is vertical you can take hold of the toes and in a concentrated dynamic, directed towards the mid-point of the earth, you can hold the position for up to twenty seconds. The body is experienced like an elegant, upright and vessel-like Papyrus. It actually looks open like a vessel (picture p. 276).

You will very quickly notice a feeling that with increasing uprightness you do not really slip into ideas far removed from the earth but, quite to the contrary, you become more rooted in the ground and in the mid-point of the earth. This subtle-feeling is an effect that comes from the right mental picturing connected with practical realisation of the exercise. The first and seventh centres work together in the exercise.

Always practise on both sides three to five times. Short breaks in between to relax and concentrate are highly advisable as the exercises are very strenuous.

As this leg pose is relatively difficult to do, older people and those with less confidence can practise an easier variation, which comes close the basic feeling of the movement. Once again, stand in an upright position and lift your right leg up, bending it. Lift it up as far as possible, with your arms form an upwardly opened triangle and in doing this leave the whole shoulder and neck region relaxed. Hold the position for up to half a minute and then change to the other side. Always go into the position rhythmically, in an ordered and concentrated way and after holding it for half a minute also return again in a concentrated way.

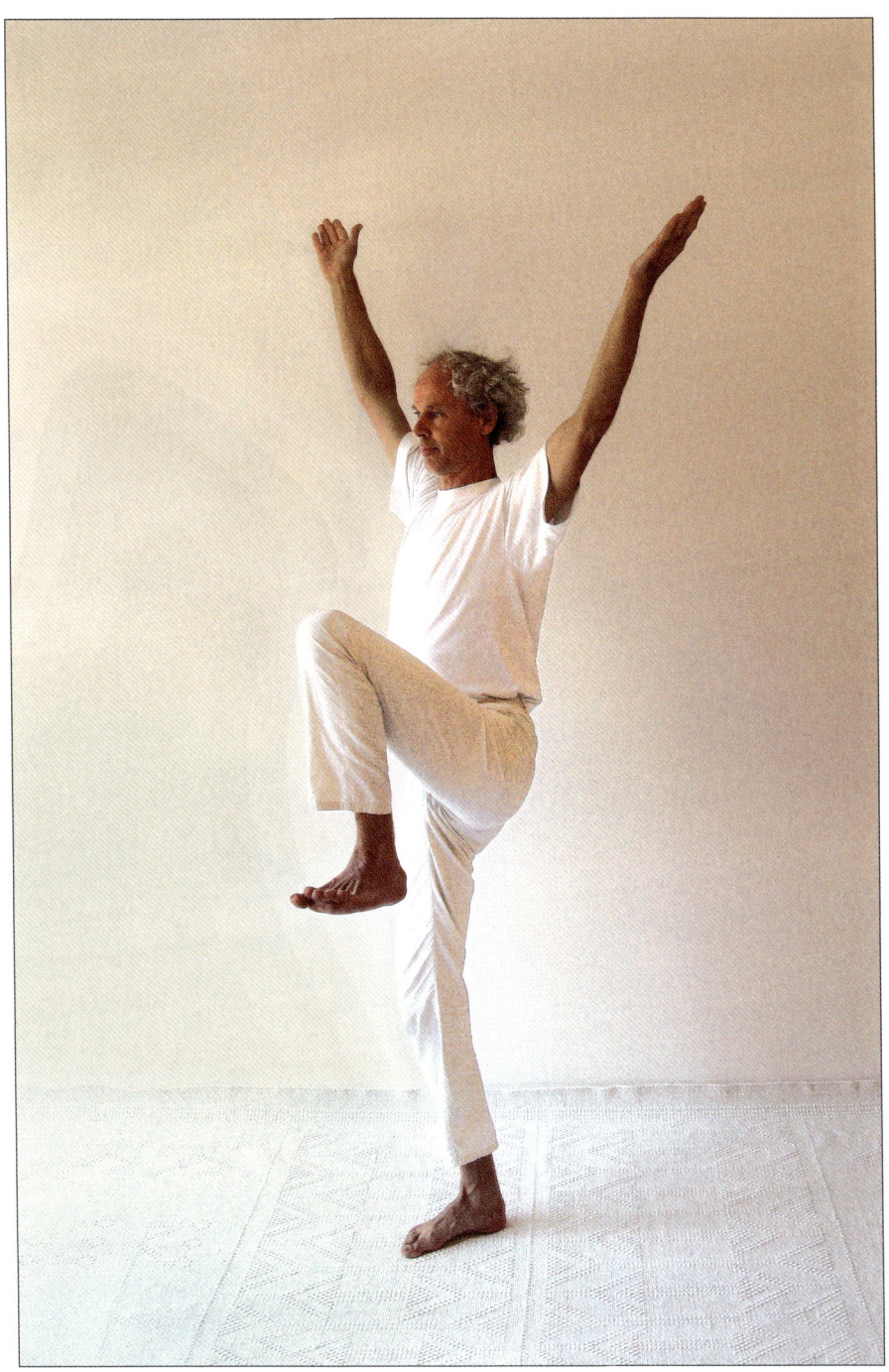

The inclined plane
pūrvottānāsana

The picture and the meaning of the exercise

From a relaxed, supported position with straightened legs, practitioners lift up the torso into the farthest stretch possible and in a big stretch through the legs they press the soles of the feet flat onto the floor. The body is extended into an almost horizontal plane. This horizontal plane is like a contrast to the vertical extension and therefore is of a fundamentally different nature. The horizontal plane is a symbol for the earthly world, while the vertical orientation reflects the celestial dimension of the human being. Here practitioners consciously enter into the tension throughout their body and hold themselves stable in the horizontal, exposed state for a predecided length of time.

The movement itself attains its lightness through the fact that practitioners become conscious of the body and experience it in a kind of "tension without being tense", or as the Bhagavad Gītā says, in an "action in inaction".[11] This perfectly free movement seems like a great contraction of the body to its own mid-point in *mūlādhāra-cakra*. It is in this aesthetic lightness expressed by the movement that the learning step and the meaning of the exercise lies.

To practise

Begin with a sitting position and with straightened legs on the floor. The hands support the body with the fingers pointing backwards. At first keep your head upright and mentally prepare yourself to tense the whole body, to stretch out your body into the horizontal plane. For the final stage of the pose, decide upon a duration of at least half a minute, or better still up to a minute. Breathe freely, without fixing the breath, and to begin with remain relaxed.

After a short period of composure in preparation, lift up your body in a big movement and then let your head fall back at the neck. Continue to breathe in a free flow and press the soles of your feet flat onto the floor. Maintain

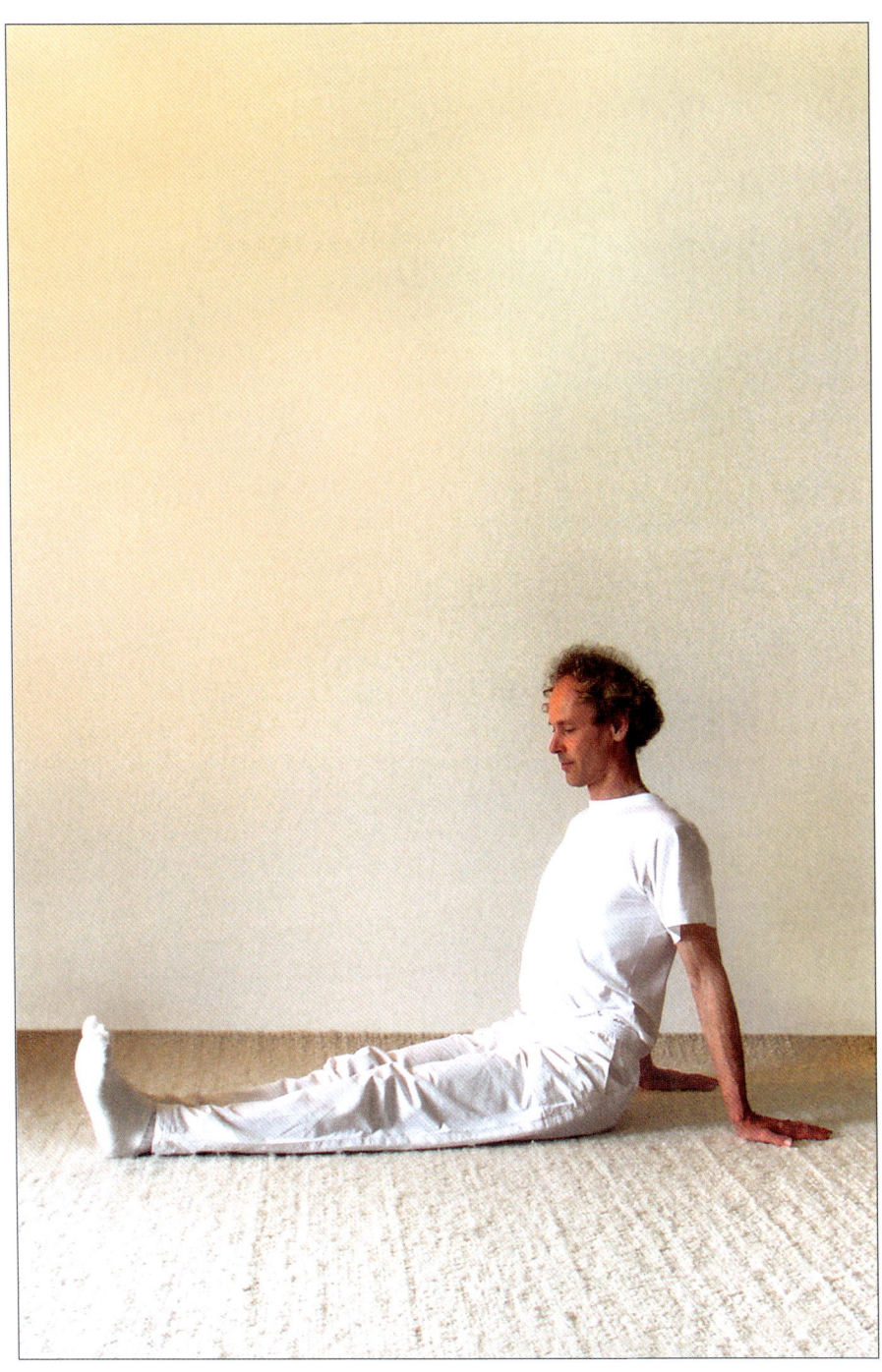

a calm clarity and serenity during the exercise. The body, in its extended state in the horizontal plane, can easily be considered as a transient stage of development.

After the exercise relax for one to two minutes lying on your back and let the picture of the pose work back on you.

With the practice of these particular, demanding poses, it soon becomes clear that with the *āsana* you use the body like a tool or instrument, and with the help of this body you penetrate, via the actively formed, subtle-feeling, into a specific state of soul. You do not enter into the fleshly-bodily interior, as is wrongly the case today in general yoga disciplines, but rather into the light, free soul experience independent from the body. The body itself actually takes on no more than a functional character. It reveals the actions of the soul, the thoughts that have been thought, the feelings that have been animated and realised, but it remains more the body, which on its plane is dependent on the higher carriers of the consciousness and spirit. This differentiation is exceedingly important: Practitioners do not gravitate towards a particularly stimulated bodily feeling, they do not sink into their interior world of flesh and organs; they use the body as an instrument. In the way that a musician uses a musical instrument and, with the help of the sound that the instrument produces, listens to the piece of music, so with conscious, subtle-feeling, via the wilful action with the body, practitioners enter into the perceiving and knowing of the soul and thus experience themselves freely beyond the body. They practise with the body but do not slip into this body with physical dependency or psychological ties. For they lead the movement to an experience that is more subtle, of a new kind, and free from any emotionality. If this understanding and discernment about the body and the quite differently oriented inner world of the soul is achieved, a great creativity with freedom and altruistic love for life can awaken.

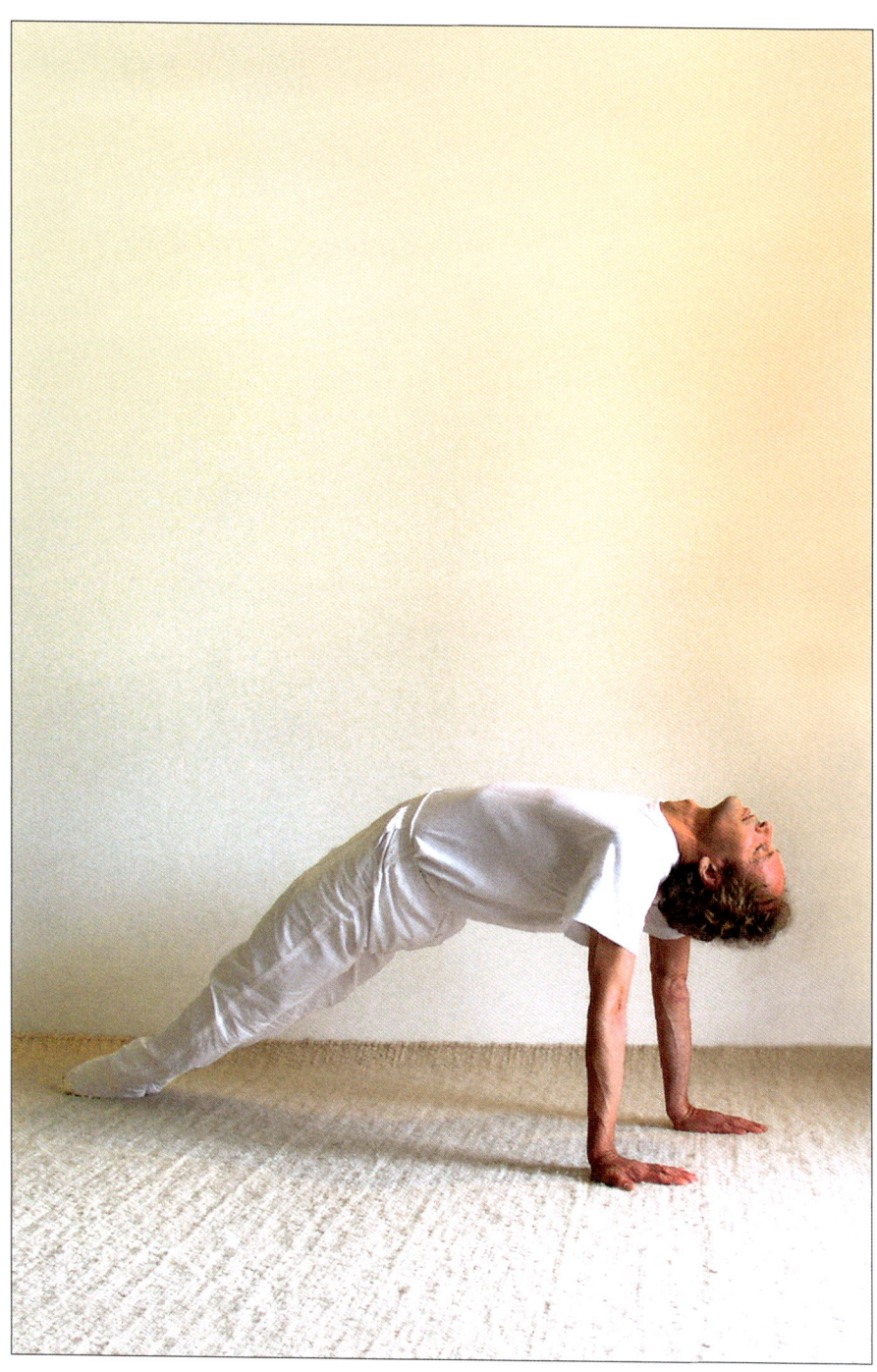

The peacock pose
māyūrāsana

The picture and the meaning of the exercise

The peacock, like the inclined plane, also depicts an extension into the horizontal plane, but now in a completely different way. Here the head is part of the horizontal line and the body seeks specifically its centre on the supporting hands. A specifically directed, deep entry into the inherent and yet consciously tangible dynamic of the will is expressed in this form of movement. In a precisely calculated distribution and transfer of tension, practitioners enter into the horizontal line. As expressed in the picture of the exercise, practitioners now feel more deeply into their own incarnation and into the sphere of earth. The peacock is an expression for a deeper entry into incarnation, an expression for the path of the soul which seeks the depth of earthly existence.

To practise

The first centre is characterised by the abundance of decisiveness. In this exercise, in a way almost similar to the inclined plane, this soul meaning is expressed through the fact that practitioners move from a state of calmness into the movement with its exact use of strength. From a clear overview, relaxation and preparation, the specific, finely-tuned movement-element follows, which through its targeted dynamic leads instantly to the static structure in the pose.

Start in the simple kneeling position. Mentally prepare yourself by picturing the exercise. Then place your hands on the ground a little in front of your knees with your fingers pointing backwards. Bring your elbows as close together as possible and then place them supportively in the pit of your stomach. Then immediately lift up your head and transfer your bodyweight as far forwards as possible. Once you have reached the farthest point of transfer forwards you can stretch through your legs and go into the horizontal plane.

Because of the exceptional difficulty of the exercise, an easier alternative is suggested, which emphasises less the centre of strength in the lower back,

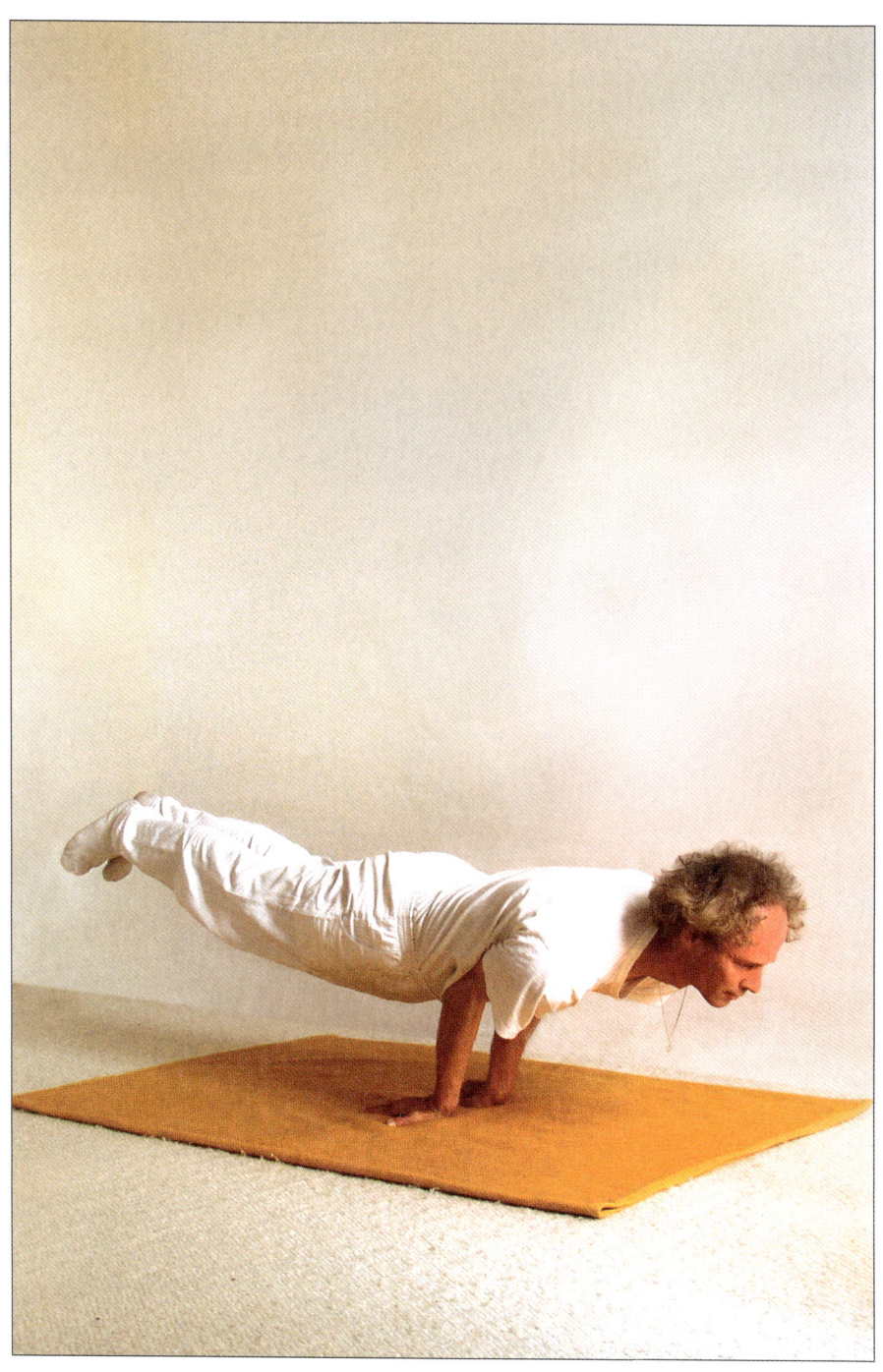

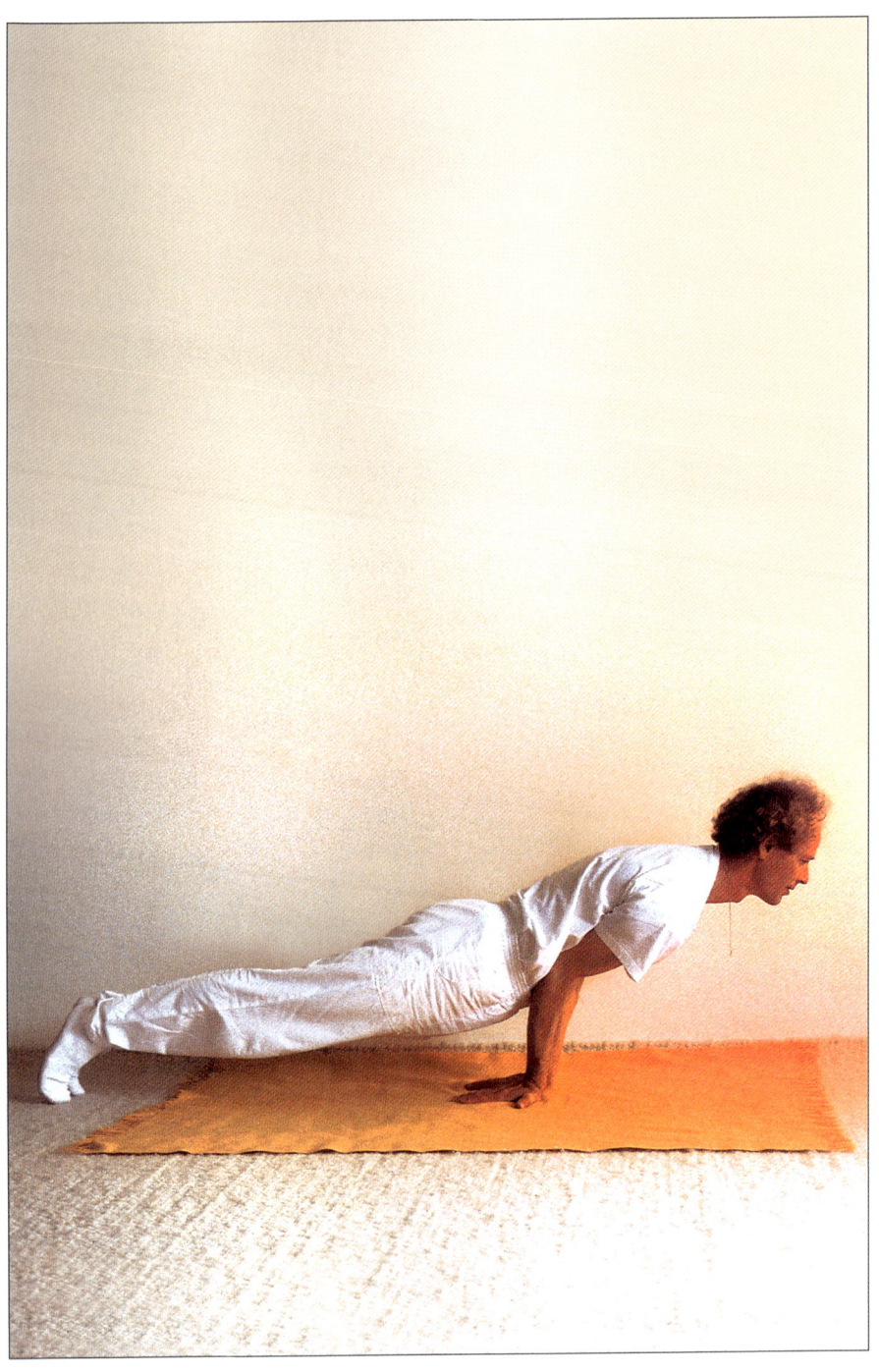

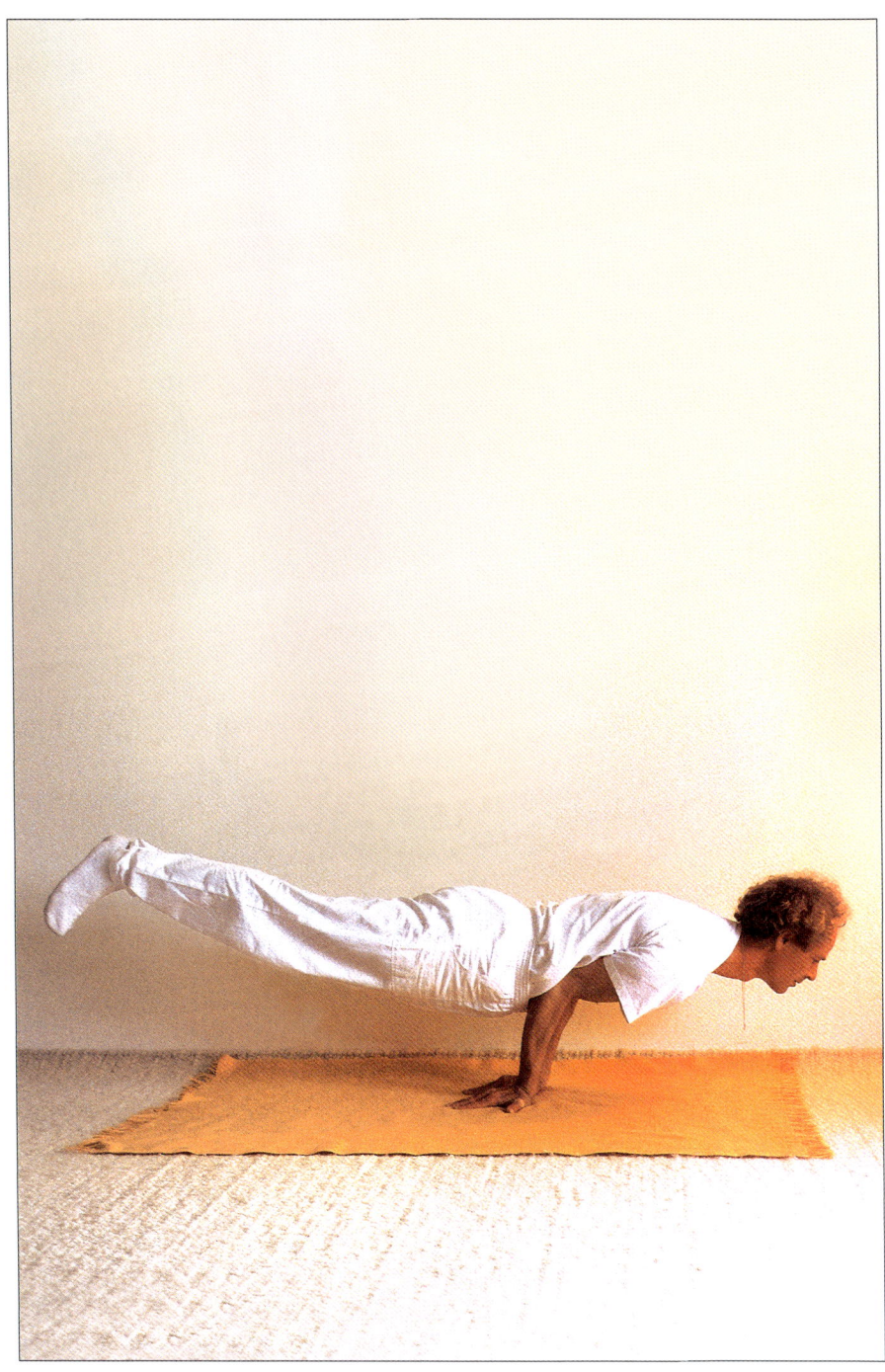

but rather shows how the exercise is lifted out of gravity and thus out of any forcefulness (picture p. 291). The centre of the force is the lowermost section of the back, where the spine is rooted in the pelvis. Starting from this section, the free, light, dynamic force of straightening up occurs, elevating the upper thoracic region, the neck and the head, and including them in the movement. From the lowermost centre, *mūlādhāra-cakra*, the exercise ascends to the uppermost centre, *sahasrāra-cakra*. The peacock begins to soar.

The point where the force is centred, resting in the lowest section of the spine, rises up and seems to dissolve as if into a free, airy, and also limitless spacial sphere. The following illustration can demonstrate this experience of a force that becomes free within the "etheric lightness".

To carry out the variation of the peacock, practitioners support themselves on their lower arms as before, transfer their weight forwards, place their chin on the ground and with a skilled movement, either first with one leg or else with both legs together, they swing up into the air. Paying careful attention to the balance, they lead the movement as far upwards as possible. Only when the legs are almost moving in a vertical direction does a feeling arise of soaring upwards.

Another variation, which is also somewhat easier than the main pose, is the peacock in lotus. It is necessary to master the lotus. However, because the centre of balance can more easily be brought forwards, this position is recommended for anyone who has less strength in the arms and shoulders.

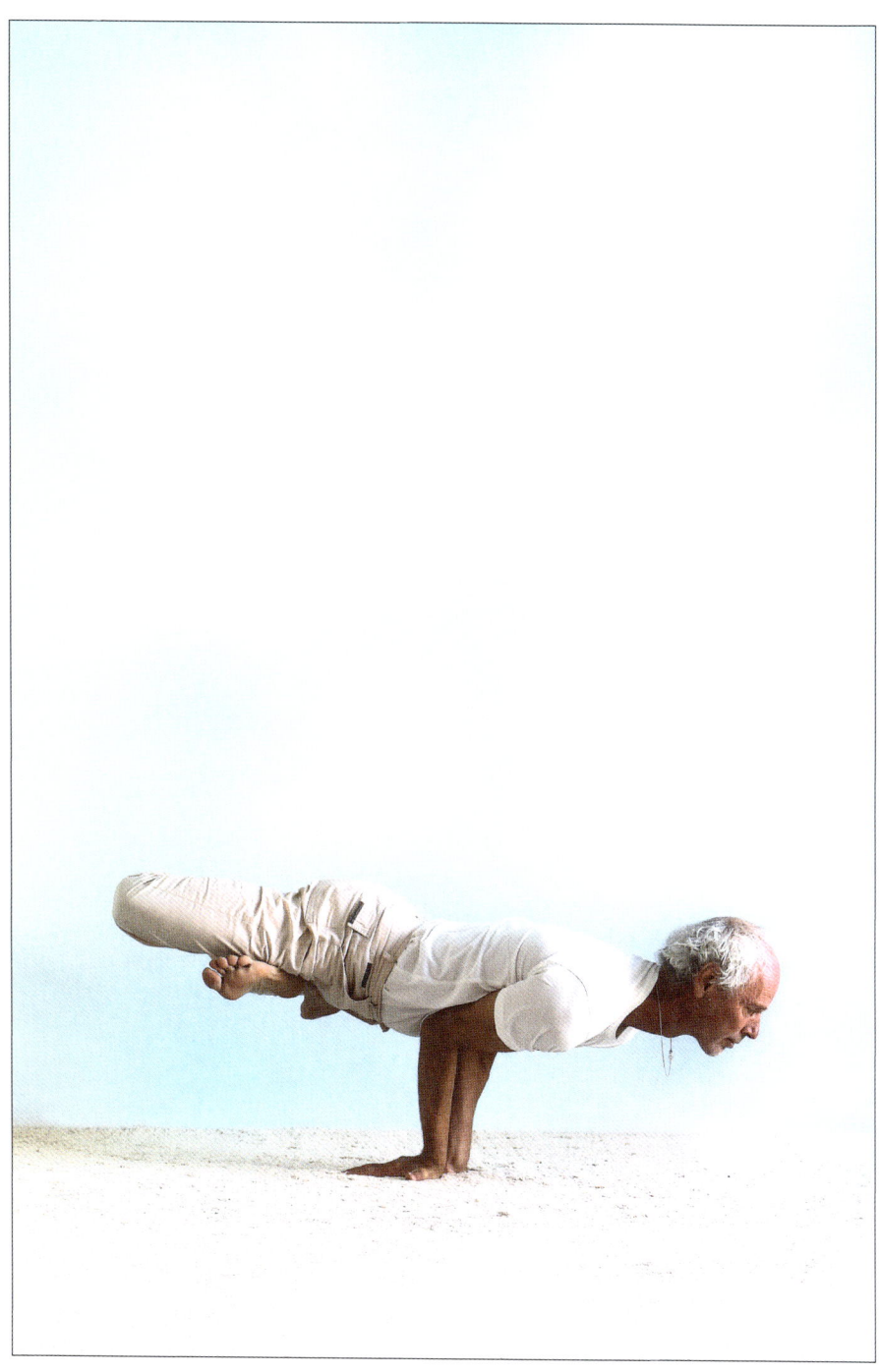

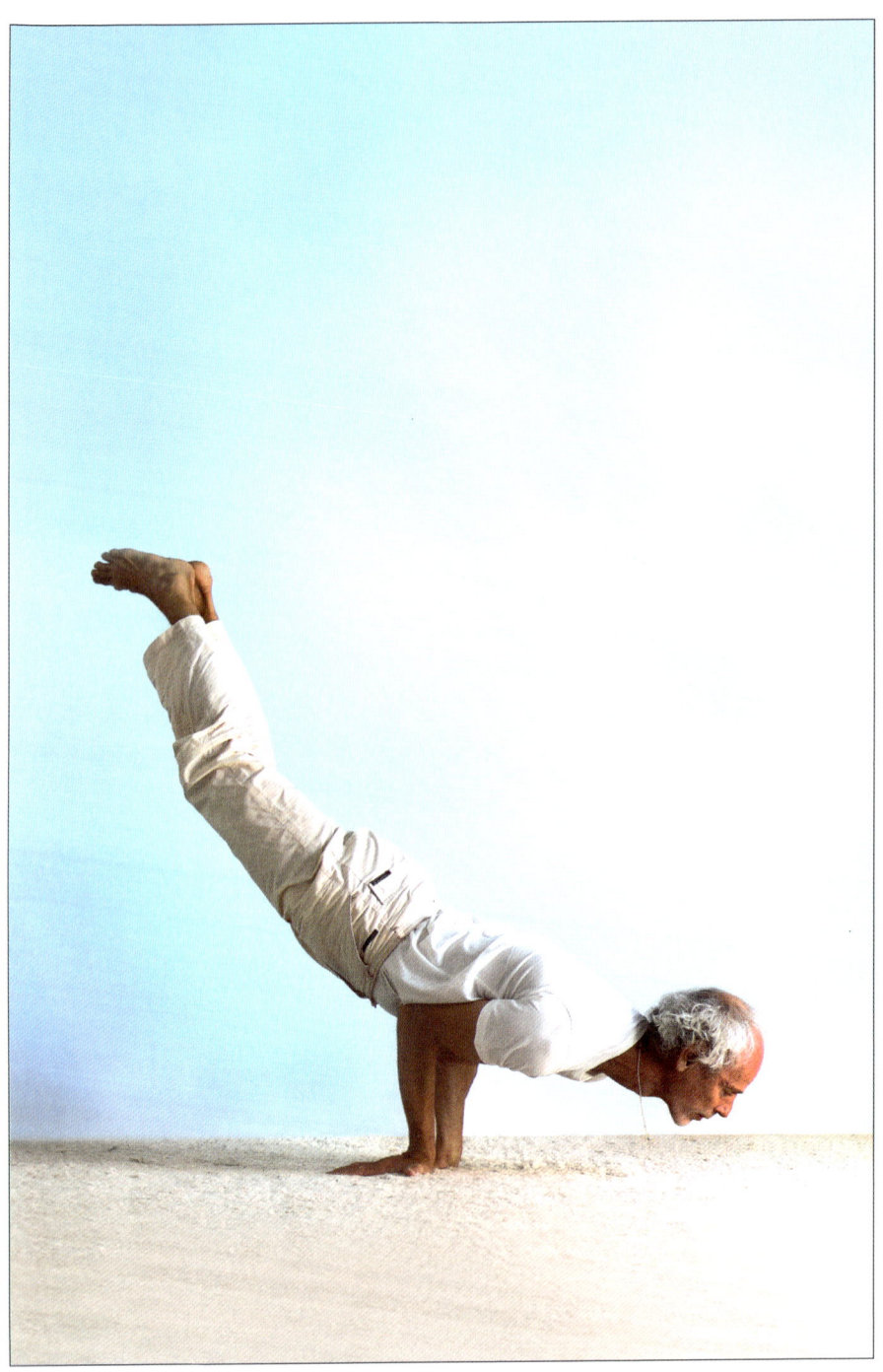

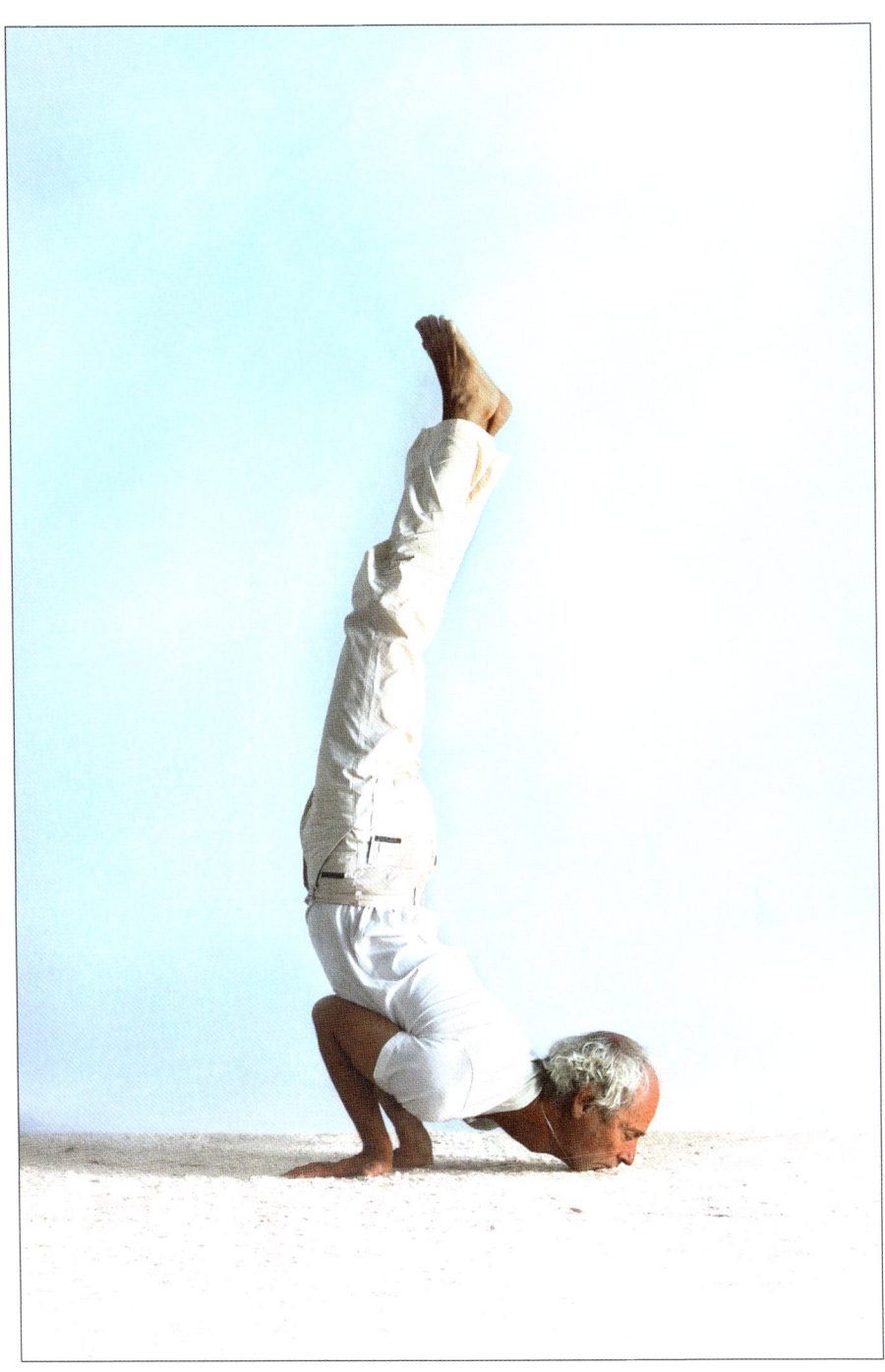

The development of complete freedom from the body – *sahasrāra-cakra*

In the seventh *cakra*, in *sahasrāra-cakra*, the region of the crown of the head, lies the hidden potential for complete freedom towards personal, bodily experience. Here at this stage a basic principle of the soul-life, which is characterised by a different kind of desire, can be recognised once again and in a kind of comprehensive form. In the soul, human beings are not what they have outwardly achieved by way of titles and results, but what they actually send out to the world through thoughts and feelings. A basic premise can also be the fact that the human soul is always at the place to which it has directed its true attention or defined its real objectives. When the personal being thinks of an object, then in reality it is also at the place of that object. But if the concerns are related to the personal ego, the attention lies in one's own narrow circle of personal I-feeling. A thought directed sincerely and comprehensively towards another person leads the soul over to that person. In the soul, therefore, human beings are actually that concrete content that they think, feel and resolutely want. The soul is not limited to the body, it travels in a constantly moving dynamic, and a fluctuating extension, to the most varied areas of interest.

This learning principle of developing a concrete soul content which is thinkable, true and imaginable, should now be verified once again in the practice. Aspirants study the most varied spiritual content, elicit concepts of spiritual life and then research these right into their profound meaning. Their mental-picturing skill develops a deep relationship to the individual symbols of an exercise or an expression, which is given through artistic revelation, and hence turns to the different objects. The consciousness will attain the possibilities which it itself inwardly accepts, strives for and ultimately develops, consciously or unconsciously. The soul will live in those feelings that are born through the work out of the inherent forces of the object. For example, the consciousness develops a sense for a true, ethical aim worth striving for, and with time, through this development which it strives for or, better said, even desires in vivid feelings, perceptions and insights, it can express this ethos in life and in the exercises. Desire is made concrete and filled with warming soul content. Through the practice, the consciousness becomes experienced, and with this also the desire, as a symbol towards the aspiring aim. Aspirants experience soul existence through the identity of consciousness, and through making concrete the essence itself that is in the process. In this way, through the meaningful soul content, they become able to lead life step by step out of passion into the glory of the conscious freedom of the soul. This is the spiritual meaning of *yad bhāvan tad bhavati*. Human beings, corresponding to their inner orientation, also outwardly become that same being.

The first energy centre, *mūlādhāra-cakra*, affords the gathering process, the anchoring of structures, of forces of form, and builds the primordial substance in the organs; the seventh centre, *sahasrāra-cakra*, now enables the direct, warming permeation with spirit, which can penetrate right into the physical body and with this into the primordial substance of the organs. Both centres work in mysterious and hidden ways together and form the deepest region of the astral body and with this that configuration described as "will". When aspirants learn to build up meaningful content according to a spiritual truth, and to apply this content to the exercise or also to life, they always work from above to below, penetrating their will with warmth, stabilising it and healing it.

The first centre gives structure, strength and stability in the thought, the seventh centre now enables the greatest freedom, *mokṣa*, and leads desire not away from the world but rather leads it towards a higher and clearer law. In the seventh centre the universal justice of eternal transcendence is accomplished.

The fire of lengthening
dīrghāsana

The picture and the meaning of the exercise

Action directed to the earth is expressed symbolically in a horizontal line, while action directed to the spirit depicts its image in a vertical line. A thought, understood in a very pure sense, rejoices in its own asceticism. The fire of asceticism always strives to extend lengthways as far as possible, while the addition of earthly interests also sets the thought into a horizontal line. Although a thought does not necessarily strive away from the earth, does not flee from the earth, it nevertheless causes an extremely vertical action, as the thought itself remains true to its spiritual realm. The thought itself is spirit. What lives in the thought, and ultimately creates its authentic expression in verticality, is the fire element [12].

The beings of Saturn on the one hand form mineralising processes which reach right into the bones, and on the other hand give human beings a structure, which tends into the vertical line and in this way represents the extraordinary and intensive inclination towards spiritual life. Long and thin, the body rises up as if it wants to fix a space right through the whole cosmos. The thought, one could say, is right up high and also puts its feet downwards, it is lifted out or even lifted up and at the same time in its movement it reaches right to an earthly footing.

To practise

Take the natural standing position with closed legs, raise your arms above your head, come up onto your toes and then with a good but not strenuous stretch move as far as possible into the vertical line. Grow in this position and remain there for up to a minute with calm, free observation and free breath. You experience yourself in the vertical form of being upright and of the greatest possible upward space. An inner, hidden fire should express itself in the movement.

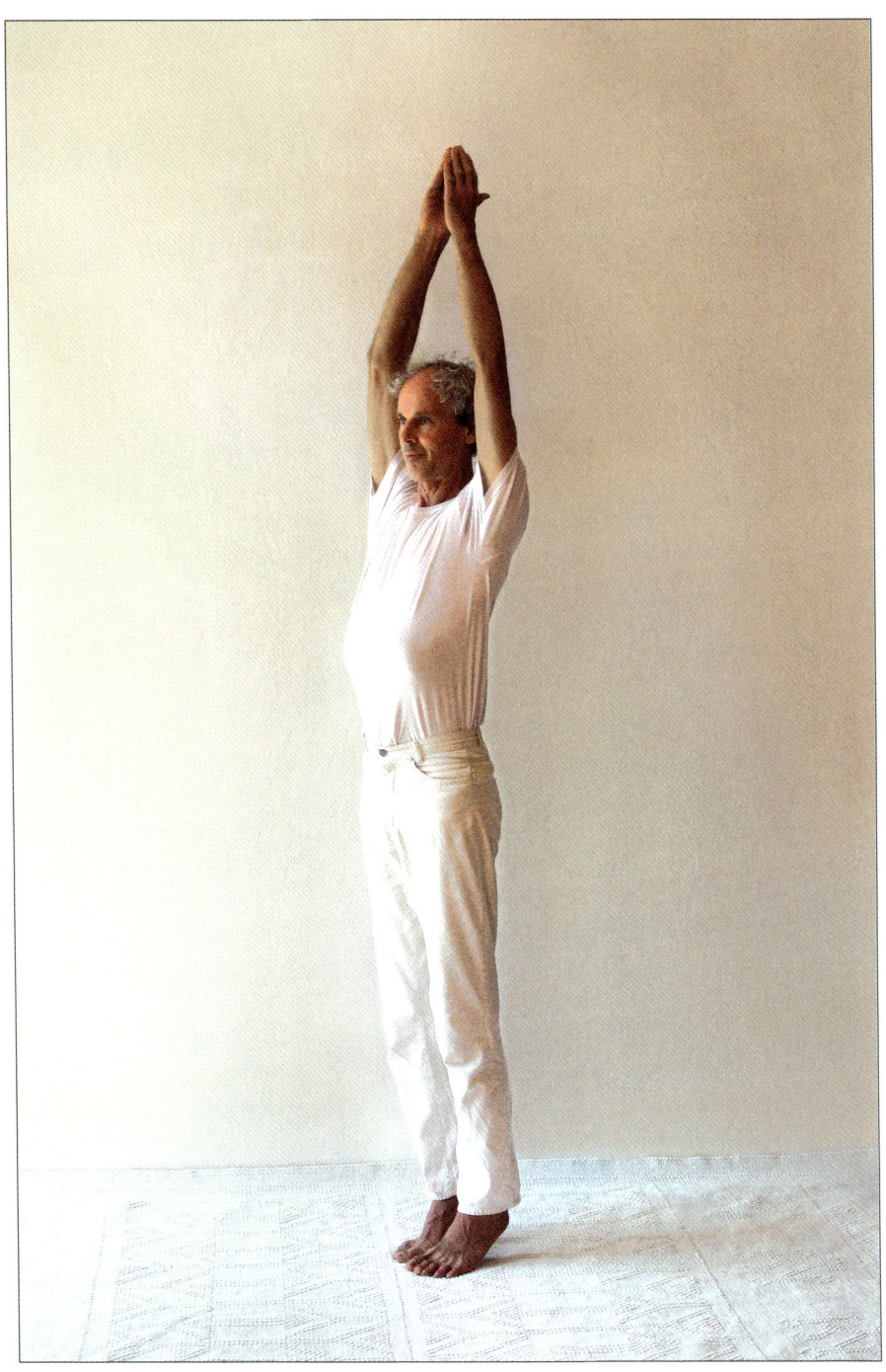

The lotus
padmāsana

The picture and the meaning of the exercise

In *padmāsana*, the classical lotus pose, practitioners express the direct, peaceful calmness of the body. The body itself draws back into a unified and in itself unobtrusive position. It is close to the ground, yet at the same time upright and the head can be raised effortlessly. The calmness and composure, which is particular to this pose, bestows a subtle-feeling of freedom from earthly conflicts, passions and turbulence. The thought processes, which take their first expression in the etheric sphere, as well as the subtle-feelings, which tend more into the astral sphere, can be perceived freer from the body in this position. It is in this calmness, alertness and uprightness, with concurrent release from the body, that the meaning of this exercise lies.

To practise

There are various sitting positions which are advantageous for meditation or for a concentration exercise. The half lotus, for example, is a preliminary stage towards the full lotus. Here one leg remains under the thigh while the other leg is bent into the groin. The knees are on the ground. If it is possible also to bring the second leg over the first then the full lotus can be practised.

Work at this exercise slowly, patiently, less through intensity but rather through repetition. For the West too, the lotus is a suitable pose that can be adopted for mental exercises, as it promotes a centring of ether forces towards the head. However, do not revel in this position, but include concrete thoughts for your practice. At the beginning it will only be possible to hold the lotus for a few seconds, but with time the joints can get used to the unusual form and the lotus can be held effortlessly.

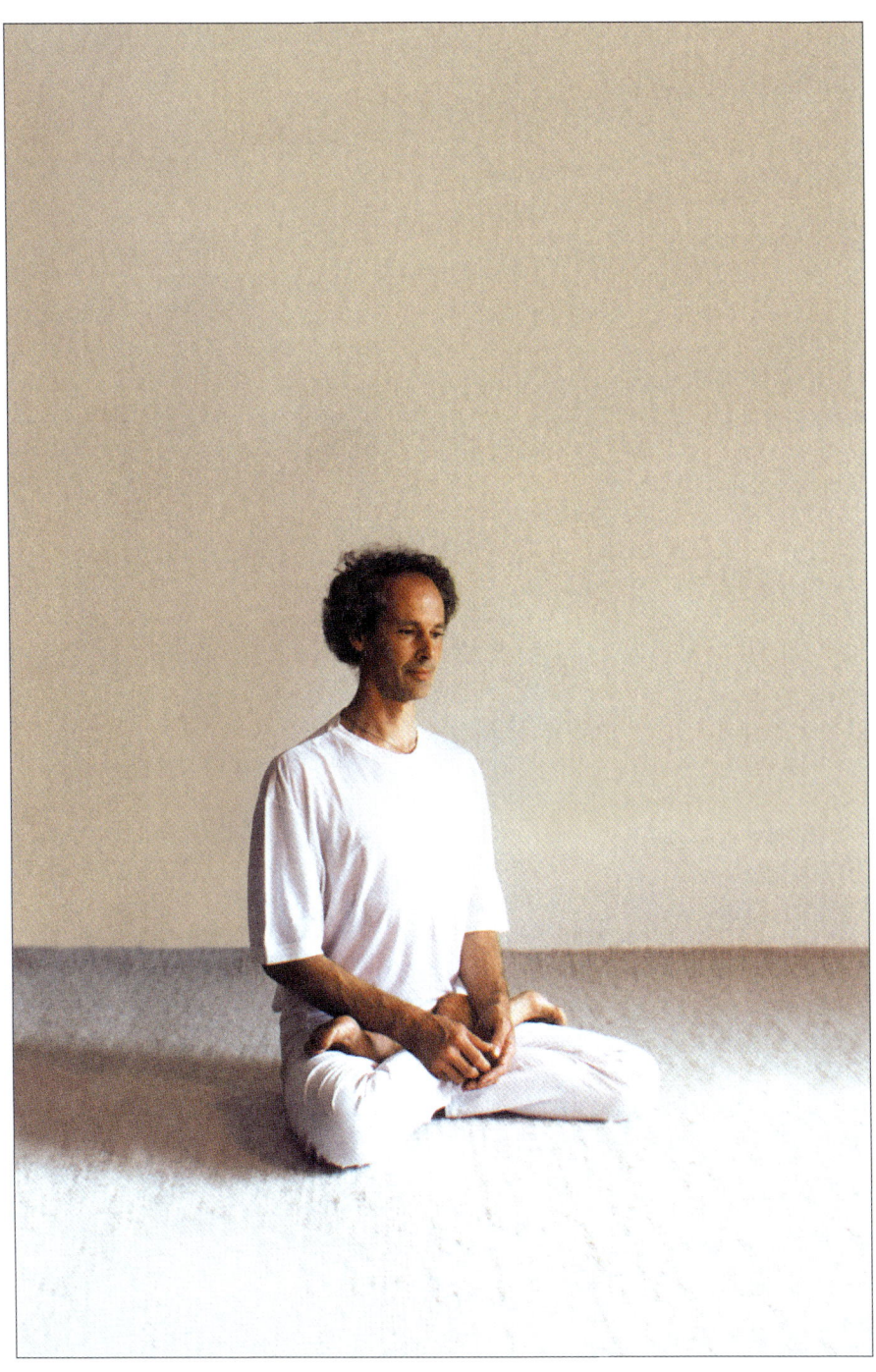

The half diamond
supta vajrāsana

The picture and the meaning of the exercise

From the normal kneeling position practitioners lean slowly backwards, support themselves with their arms, and gradually come closer to the ground. They experience a growing feeling of tension in the legs in this movement, which may well even become painful. With increasing proximity to the ground, however, they experience the pleasant, subtle-feeling that the body is connected to the horizontal streams of life, and they soon feel themselves to be part of an earthly surface. In this way, they leave the normal, three dimensional and upright sitting posture and in lying adopt not the typical resting position, but rather they now experience the ground much more and with this feel the oneness with the surface. A greater watchfulness can be noticed in this position than can exist in a normal supine position.

Experiencing the body's oneness with a surface encourages the contracting force in the second centre. At the same time the space around the head becomes freer and practitioners observe with greater watchfulness both their own painful tensions in the legs as well as the surrounding sphere above the surface. They look into the space as if with eyes located in the earth. From the vantage point of the earth, they perceive the air-space above them and leave the breath naturally free. This pose is equivalent to a particular kind of contemplation.

Now, however, practitioners move their arms above their head and begin to stretch lengthways. This stretch gives a feeling of the will subtly unfolding, and so it describes the deep striving that lives in the soul and can be understood as a striving towards the spirit. The body becomes narrower in this sensitive stretch, and practitioners increasingly forget the painful feeling in the legs. Thus there is a renouncement in this as well as in other positions, for practitioners leave the normal and comfortable supine position and approach a completely different planar formation. In the last stage they finally develop the almost liberating stretch lengthways, which ultimately opens up to them the feeling of the greatest possible release from the bodily structures. The lengthways stretch is reminiscent of the shaping processes of the warming beings operating in the sphere of Saturn.

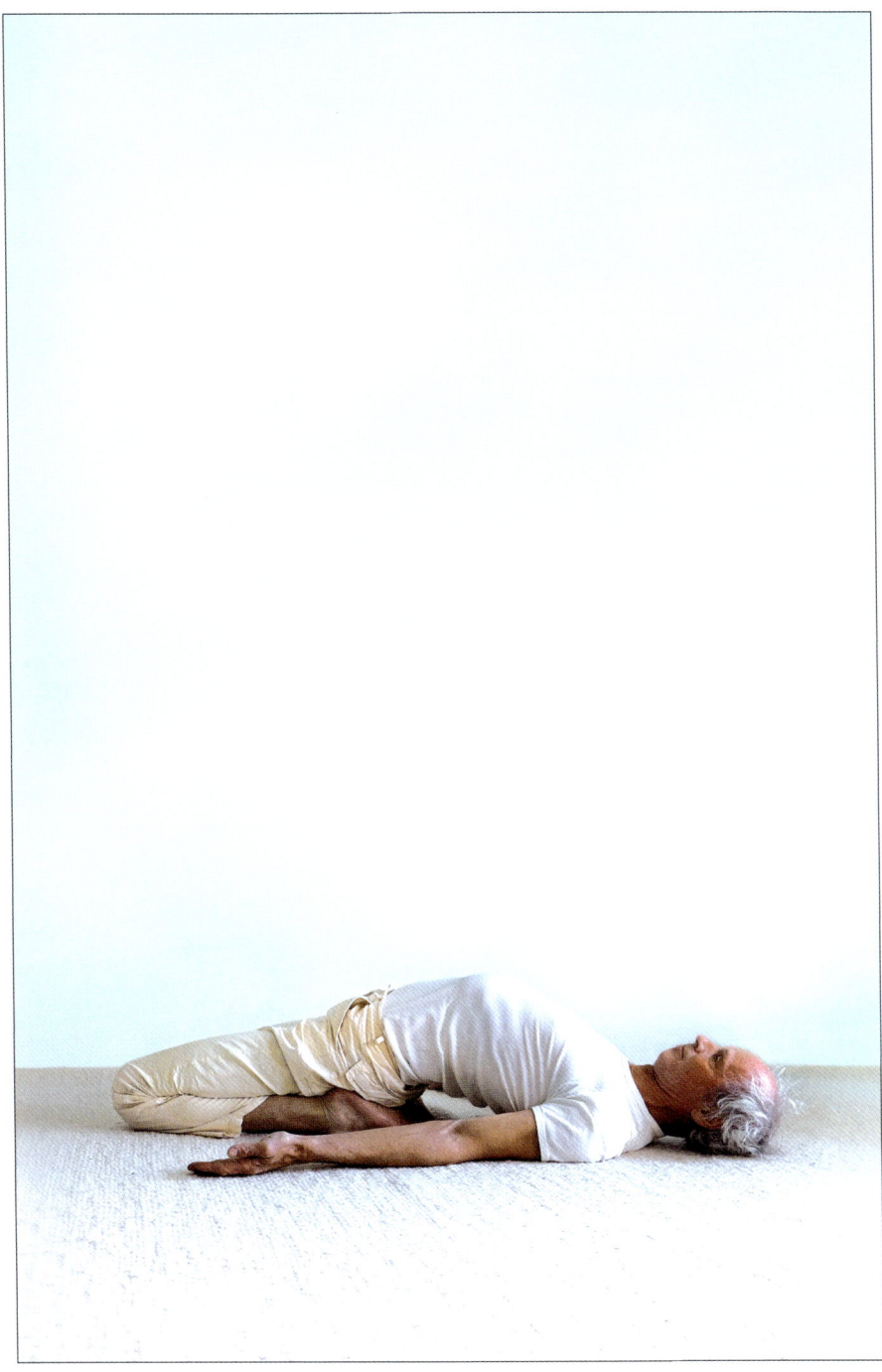

To practise

Take a kneeling position on your heels and then for a brief moment become sufficiently conscious of this position. Then supporting yourself on your elbows, move backwards and slowly approach the ground behind you. As far as the tensions in the legs allow, first the head and then the neck and shoulders can touch the ground. A slight, arched tension remains through the spine. In the sacrum there is a natural contraction.

First the arms lie next to the sides of the body and in this way encourage the experiencing of a surface. From below the eyes perceive the spacial sphere. Gradually the knees and feet become accustomed to the tension. Become conscious of your own body, which is now in a plane and almost merged with the ground, and become conscious of the given sphere of the etheric space, or in other words of the thought space, which exists in stillness above the surface of the ground.

Now lay your arms above your head, placing the palms together, and gently move into the stretch, beginning from your spine and moving upwards, so that through the will that hidden warmth element is silently stirred into effect. Whereas in the first position in the planar form you still felt more passively surrendered and one with the ground, now with the stretching of the arms above your head you experience yourself in a stimulating and independent unfolding of the will and in an independent striving which leads beyond the body. A certain transcendence particular to the seventh centre now occurs with *supta vajrāsana*.

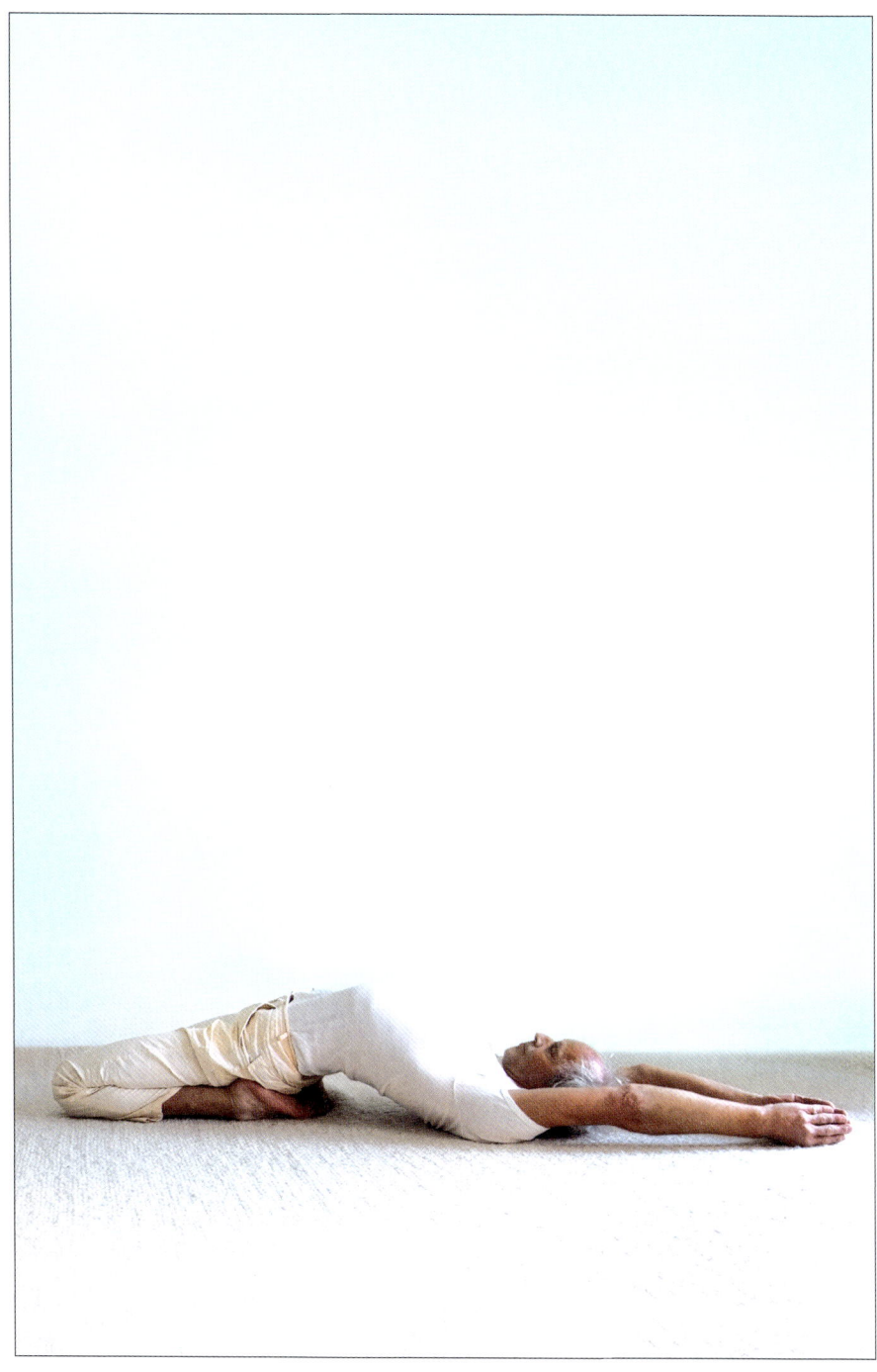

The scorpion
vṛścikāsana

The picture and the meaning of the exercise

The scorpion is a relatively difficult exercise, which begins with a daring, planned leap and finally reveals itself in a graceful gesture like a great, erected half moon. The head is lifted up relatively far from the ground and the legs float as if weightlessly in the half moon form in space. Practitioners actually experience themselves as if floating, released from the earth, abandoned to an unusual and new form. It is the principle of metamorphosis, which has a real existence in the soul and spiritual worlds, and transforms a lower form into one of a higher order. The half moon formed through the scorpion leap has the appearance of a so-called evolvent, a curve which begins from the head and constantly widens, and if continued would flow out into an infinite openness. This curve lends a graceful elegance, and once the pose has been mastered it bestows the feeling of an etheric dynamic and lightness. Whereas a straight line still represents more the physical, bodily nature, the graceful evolvent as a curve reveals an alive, sweeping etheric form. At the same time, in the truest sense, this form generated with the scorpion leap is barely touched by earthly forces. A kind of flame can be experienced in the innermost centre of this position as a sign of spiritual fire.

To practise

The scorpion is a very advanced pose which as its first step demands careful mental preparation for the new form to be adopted. In the kneeling position prepare for the daring leap into space. Once you have built up the mental image of the scorpion you can place your forearms on the ground and lunge up into the leap. The whole body is lifted far up into space. The head should remain raised right from the start. When you can manage the leap and hold the position to the right degree, you can extend the motionless period of the exercise up to one minute. It is good to attune yourself well to the new form, but also to practise falling.

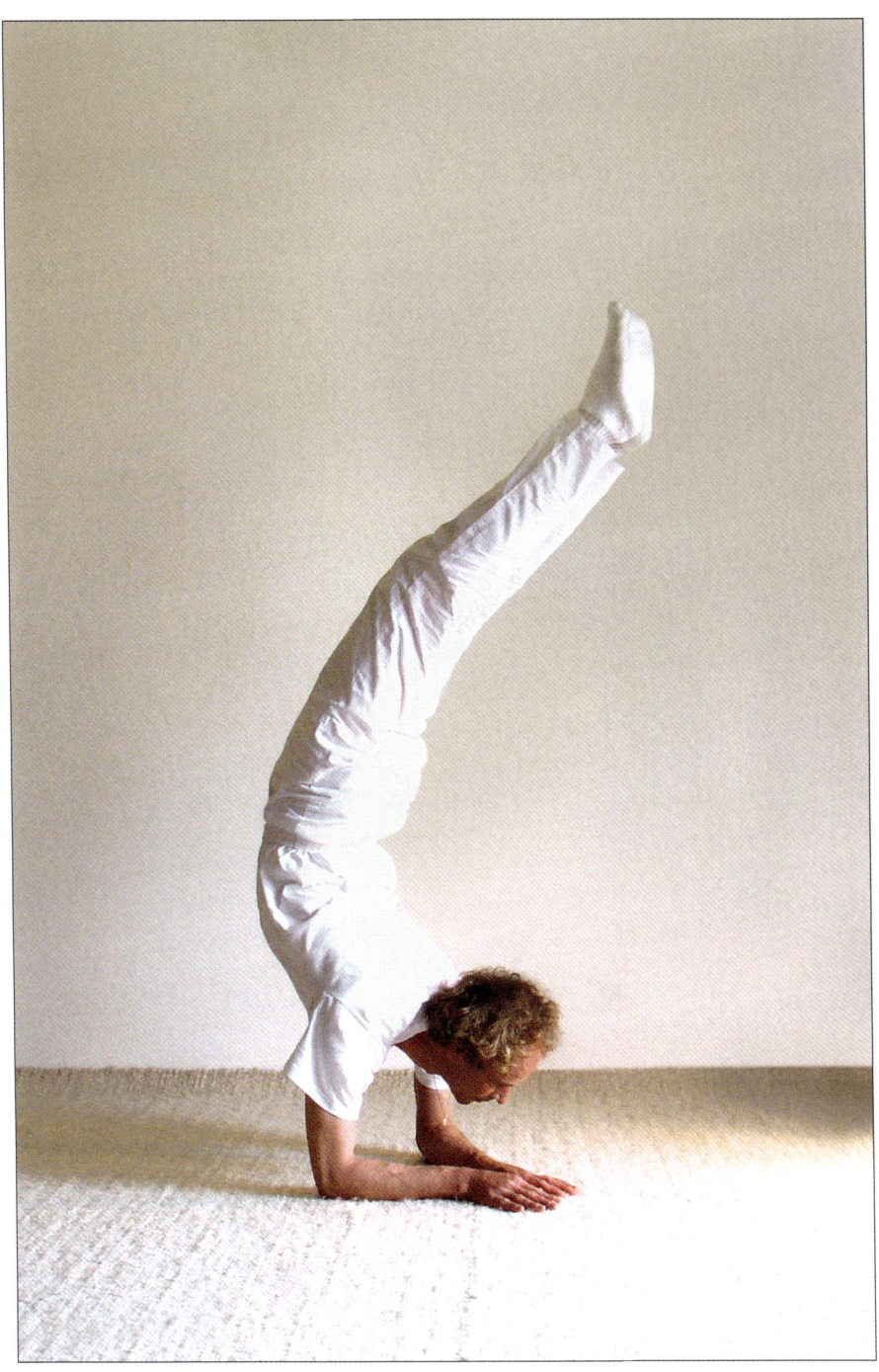

The horse
vātāyanāsana

The picture and the meaning of the exercise

Standing on both feet, naturally integrated in balance, stably grounded, with the torso and head upright, the human body moves forwards on the ground. In the pose *vātāyan-āsana*, which means "someone who runs like the wind", the body suddenly finds itself very released from the earth, in sensitive equilibrium, balancing on the mat with one knee and one foot, and out of this insecure, barely perceptible footing, it seeks to straighten up into the vertical dimension. With their limbs in these sensitive conditions of balance, practitioners can retain nothing fixed in reserve. They move into a kind of boldness of uncertain exposure, into a form of new equilibrium, which they find in a sphere that rests almost palpably distant from all earthly security.

The learning step that can be attained from the pictorial experience of the exercise is that now practitioners can realise what the soul and spiritual reality of life is actually like in its true existence. Reserves that come from earthly certainties can never support spiritual progress. It can even be observed that those people who are so very inclined to hold back earthly reserves for themselves and their secure life, finally after death, when they enter into a soul-spiritual realm, will experience a feeling of not belonging and not being able to collaborate in the building of creation. This feeling of making oneself free at the right time from earthly certainties, and advancing into new and daring spheres, unprotected and knowing solely of the spiritual realities, characterises in outline the expression of this pose.

If the horse is done with the maximum stretch of the arms upwards, it is reminiscent of the sphere of Saturn, whereas with folded hands in front of the chest it displays a clear centring at the heart. Experiencing the body pictorially gives a free sensory sphere.

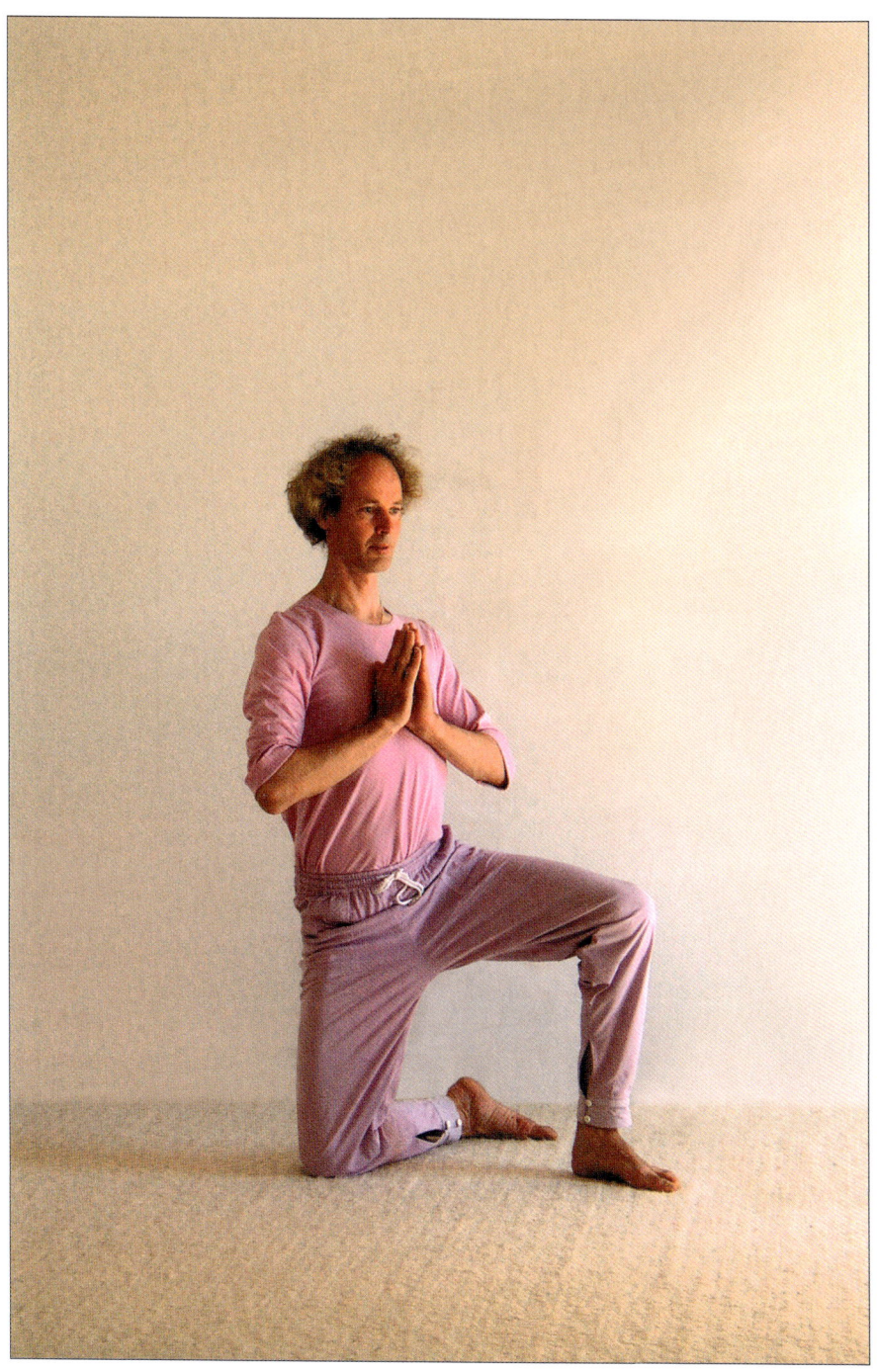

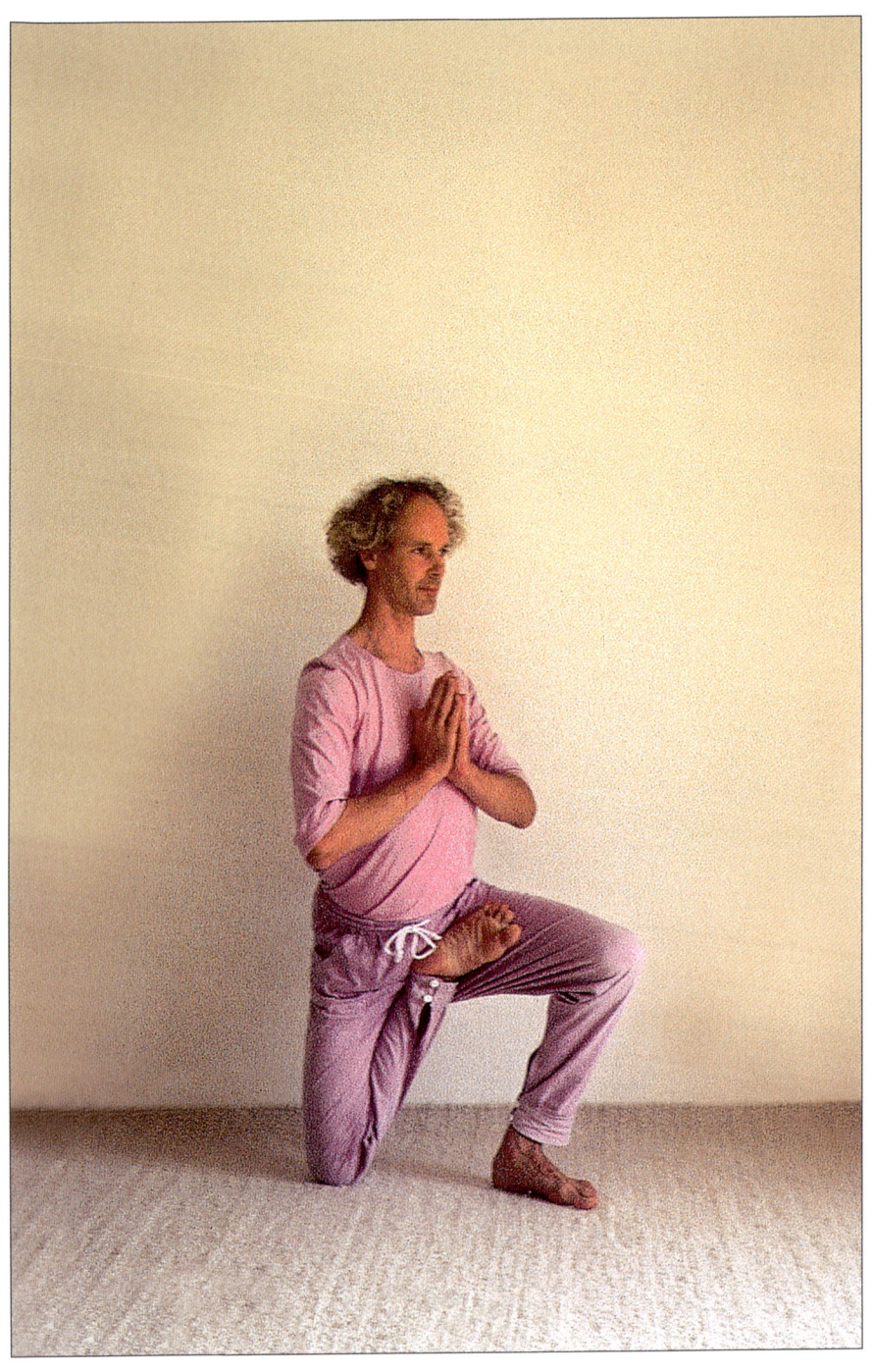

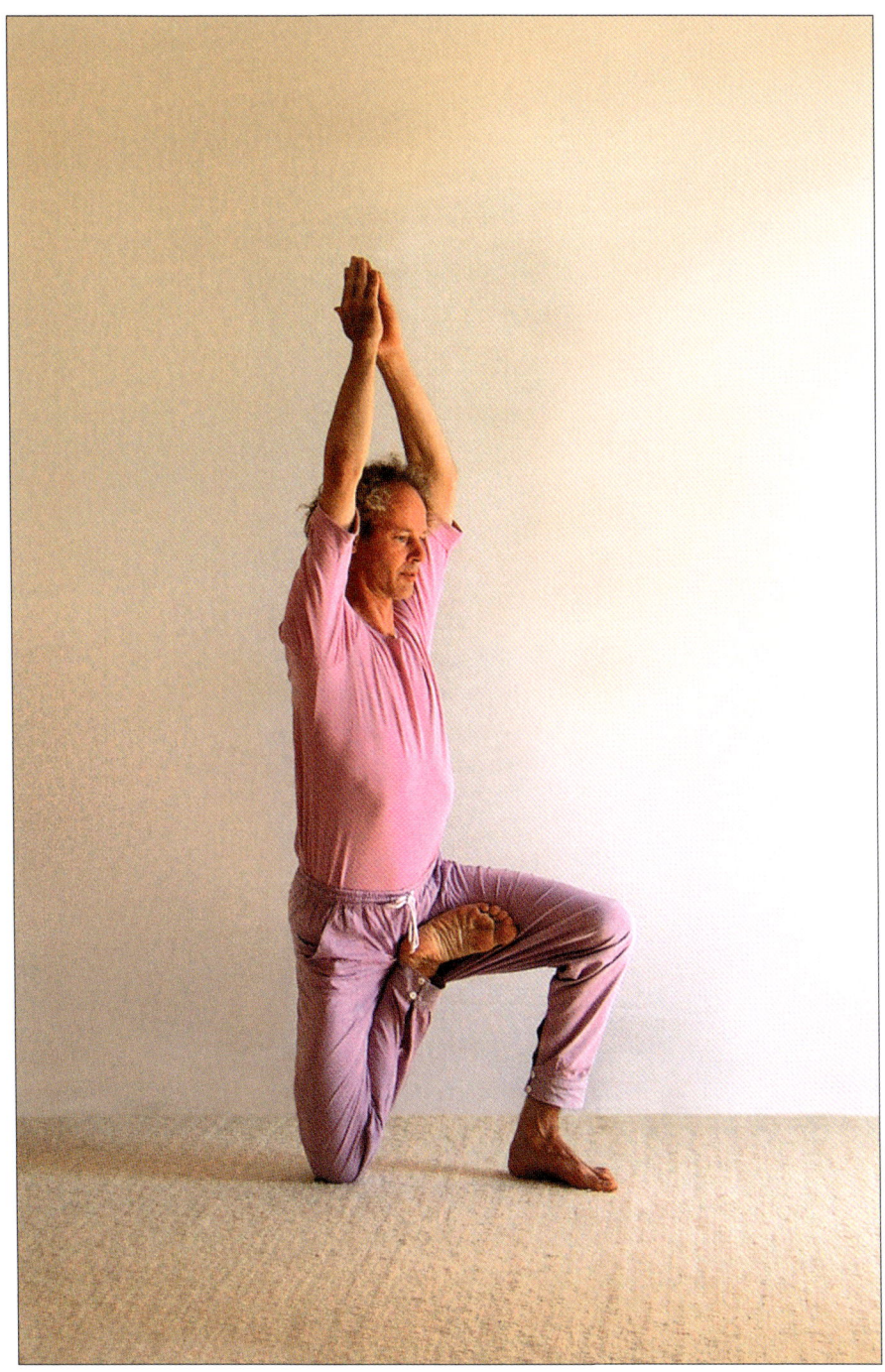

To practise

The normal standing position can be experienced as physical firmness. But now practitioners leave this stable and natural base and embark on a path of refinement by choosing a sensitive state of equilibrium. In doing this they feel as if they slip from one element to another, from an earthly element into an unprotected cosmic element and thus leave behind physical habits as well as reserves of security. They seem, in practising, to step out of the equilibrium of the physical body and to enter into a sensory sphere released from the earth.

The practice takes place from above to below, passing over from the standing position to standing sensitively on the knee. As with the tree pose, one leg is bent into the groin. Then reach down with your hands, seek the balance standing on the knee and on one foot and then straighten up the spine and head again vertically. Finally join your hands at the level of your heart to form *ātmāñjali-mudrā*. This position depicts the image of the heart centre.

The actual pose develops if you take your arms from *ātmāñjali-mudrā* straightened upwards over your head. In this position a higher challenge to the equilibrium now comes about, but precisely this position conveys that vertical line that corresponds to the effects of *sahasrāra-cakra* and symbolises that striving for the greatest possible freedom in the thought, through the fire within. The new and greater space is entered unprotected.

An easier variation, which does not demand such great hip flexibility, is possible if you do not bend the leg into the groin in half lotus, but extend it along the ground at an angle. This variation, however, only gives a hint of the reality without reserves. Practise each position on both sides (picture p. 305).

Rhythmically carry out the individual steps into the position and back out of the position again. At each individual stage the body is experienced pictorially and calmly. Through the pictorial experience a kind of sensitive freedom from the body occurs.

The crow
kākāsana

The picture and the meaning of the exercise

The crown centre, or *sahasrāra-cakra*, describes a greatest possible lightness while at the same time the attention is centred intensively on a particular region, like for example the spine, the head or another part of the body. In the experience of lightness, which becomes noticeable in contrast with the body, practitioners experience a first feeling of freedom from the body, which allows them greater alertness in the senses and in the general observation of the thought processes. The alertness of the senses increases through practising the crow poses. The seventh centre opens all sensory processes of the nervous system to a maximum extent and therefore bestows a consciousness that movement is not solely the expression of all motor impulses of the so-called efferent nerves, but that movement in its entirety represents a receiving gesture and in a particular way even makes a demand on the afferent nerves. Becoming conscious of this sensory receptivity in movement denotes one of the meanings of the crow poses.

In the two crow poses that follow, the attention is on the one hand on a careful technique and on the other hand on the position of the head. In the crow the whole head can be experienced as a dimension of its own, existing for itself, almost in opposition to the body. Described esoterically, the region of the head bears the cosmos of the most important sense organs.

To practise

The basic crow pose, in which practitioners come up onto their upper arms with their legs, and keep a well-dosed balance on their hands, is relatively simple if the technique is carefully applied, and can also be practised by the inexperienced without concerns. Squat on your toes and open your knees wide. Place your hands gently on the ground and put your elbows onto your shin bones as deeply and solidly beneath your knees as is technically possible for you. The subsequent movement into the balance begins by rising up onto your toes and skilfully transferring your whole body, particularly your head, forwards. Pay attention to the balance and to the solid stability of the hands. The head should not sink down too low. The neck and head are directed far out forwards into the horizontal. Hold this position, with flowing breath, for about half a minute and pay attention to the freedom of the senses and of the head.

A rather difficult variation of the crow is developed by straightening one leg and bending the other one over the thigh as in the lotus position. The foot that has been brought inwards is placed on the opposite upper arm and the body bends sideways, with the leg straightened, into the acrobatic horizontal position. Once again it is the head that becomes experienced as an extension free from the limbs and torso. Practise both sides for about fifteen seconds, applying the technique carefully (picture p. 312).

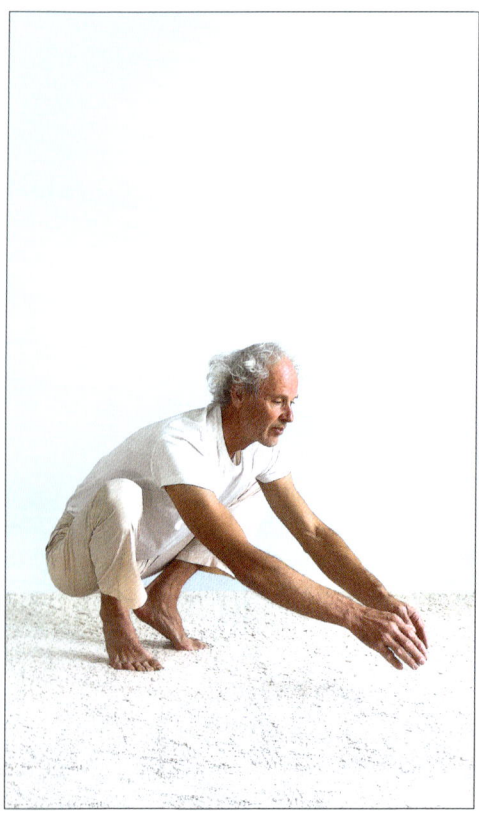

Right from the start of the exercise, the senses remain in an alert overview. The back is lifted and straightened with the help of the arms. As it straightens the head rises up naturally. The farther the initial stretch forwards happens, the easier it is to place the upper arms under the knees.

The movement up onto the extreme tips of the toes happens in the last dynamic phase, before the exercise moves over into the balance resting on the hands.

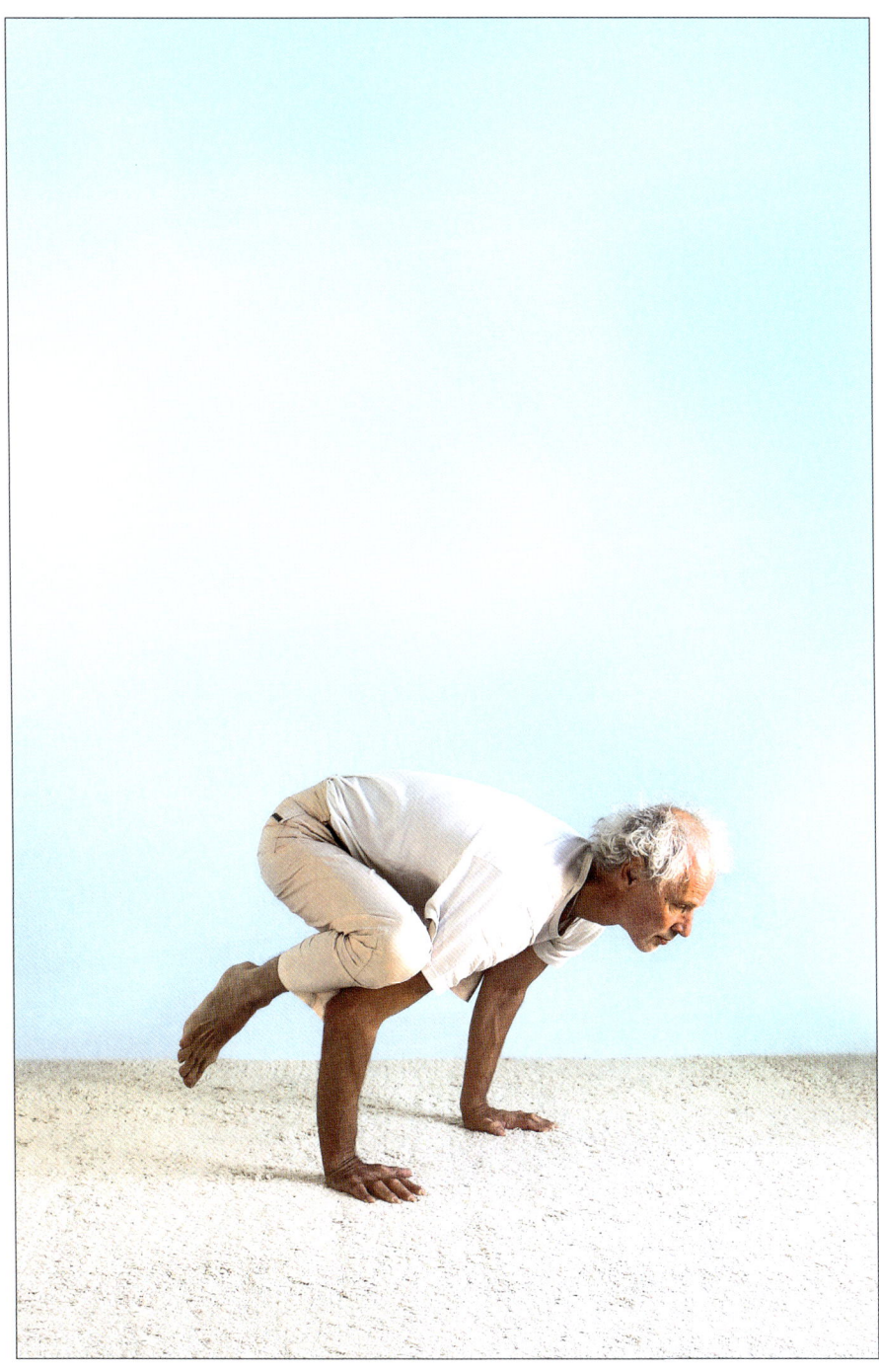

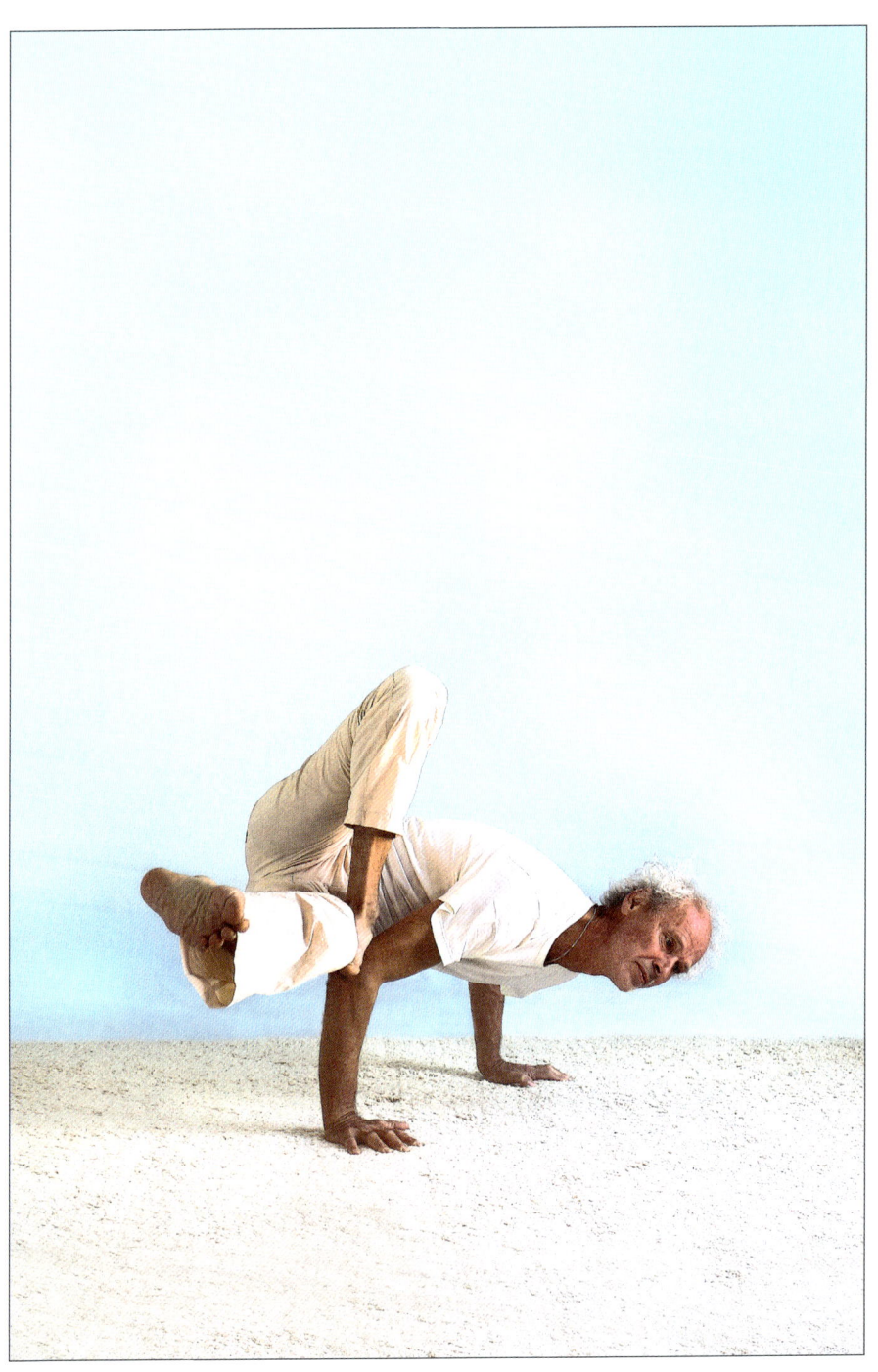

The scales
tulādaṇḍāsana

The picture and the meaning of the exercise

In all exercises that relate to the seventh centre, the meaning that the practitioner places into the *āsana* is key. The way the meaning is selected and put into practice determines the result in the exercise. *Yad bhāvan tad bhavati* takes on a real and practical form. The scales, *tulādaṇḍāsana*, is chosen here as an example for how the most differing meanings, relating to the various centres, can be thought and, through the practice, implemented. Here the scales is assigned to the crown centre, *sahasrāra-cakra*, but it could also be given an interpretation under other centres. It is a matter of personal freedom for practitioners which content they place into the exercise, how they think it and finally how they form it. Nonetheless to start with it is very good to orient oneself carefully to the guidelines and not to practise with too much intuitive spontaneity. A great deal of astral and consequently of nervous disorder would be likely to ensue if practitioners were to begin to build up a practice according to their personal feelings, without adequately developed knowledge, without guidelines or instructions. It would be roughly similar to allowing apprentice painters to mix the colours themselves immediately and paint houses in whatever way they feel. Thus, it is favourable if yoga practitioners orient themselves according to the instructions and make sure they implement these carefully.

Now in this exercise the significant content lies in individuals learning in their practice to picture different thoughts and to place these thoughts into the exercises in accordance with the individual lotus flowers. Thus the scales as an exercise becomes an example for the practice of each of the centres. The scales is in this sense an exercise that is suitable for independently studying and trying out the process of building thoughts and subsequently implementing them in practice. For this reason, the following description presents seven different steps with suggested content corresponding to the seven different centres.

To practice

Those who take the seventh centre, with a content, to their attention, can become conscious during practice of the orientation in space and of the arising feeling of space. Practitioners begin in a standing position and bring to consciousness the fact that they are entering with the body, in a more receded and detached way, into a very vast and free, new space. They place one foot forwards, step onto this foot clearly yet with a feeling of free and released lightness, and finally move with the whole body into a horizontal plane. They stretch the leg backwards (picture p. 316) and, preferably at the end, lead the arms in a relaxed way, with a free neck, into the horizontal line. With this extension, they become conscious of the dimension of the space that their body takes up in the horizontal span, and at the same time they develop a mental image that the body now becomes only a symbol for the inherent life of the soul with its subtle-feelings. This soul-life will one day occupy the entire universal space. It is not the body that can stretch out unendingly, but rather it is the soul that will one day move into this great macrocosmic span. The body actually becomes lighter and more receded. With this feeling of spacial experience, practitioners feel a hint of the greatest macrocosmic boundaries of space. It is good to hold the exercise for up to twenty seconds on each side.

If practitioners want to emphasise the sixth centre, they will start less from the feeling of macrocosmic space, but rather from the thought and the resulting experience of form. The content of consciousness that they now choose, and which can be characteristic of the sixth centre, lies on the one hand in the overseeing calmness and careful observation as well as attunement in the movement, and on the other hand in giving precise shape to a well-developed mental picture through the harmony of the form. The head remains lightly lifted, as it can be with the other centres too, so that a freer and more relaxed overview is possible (picture p. 319). While practising, practitioners also pay particular attention to a free neck and a fairly relaxed shoulder area. The exercise acquires a solid form developed in the body out of the clearly pictured and guided thought. It is a testimony to calmness and structure.

Viśuddha-cakra indicates beginning anew and releasing the old. If practitioners want to place a soul content into the scales appropriate to the process of this centre, they can devote themselves during the exercise to the mental image that with the strong, dynamic extension a new step is achieved. It is indeed a daring step, as balancing on one leg the body has to orient itself into a new, unusual and also strenuous movement. They leave behind the old, and adopt the new feeling in the extension of the movement. The standing leg is placed with particular consciousness, as this standing leg symbolises a kind of new step of incarnation.

When emphasising the fourth centre it is good if practitioners develop the variation in which they grow upwards in a precise way into the thoracic spine, as demonstrated in the picture (p. 318). This position is strenuous. Practitioners should maintain a sunny cheerfulness, even when the body trembles.

When centring at the *maṇipūra-cakra*, the third centre, practitioners decide upon the concentration point in the middle of the body and experience themselves in a strong, active extension from this point. They feel the limbs literally perfused by active dynamic strength and at the same time they notice a centre within themselves with an articulation outwards.

If practitioners want to emphasise the second centre they place the point of concentration more in the leg region and also in the inward pull of the leg. They work at rounding and forming in a specific dynamic way, through the gathering, contracting form of movement, which literally centres them in the sacrum and keeps them upwardly free.

When emphasising the first centre practitioners choose the greatest possible active dynamic strength while at the same time forgetting the body. The centre is at the lowest end of the spine and practitioners glide, in a very high yet unforced and thus decisive dynamic, into the horizontal.

Overall the scales depicts for the soul the picture of progress.

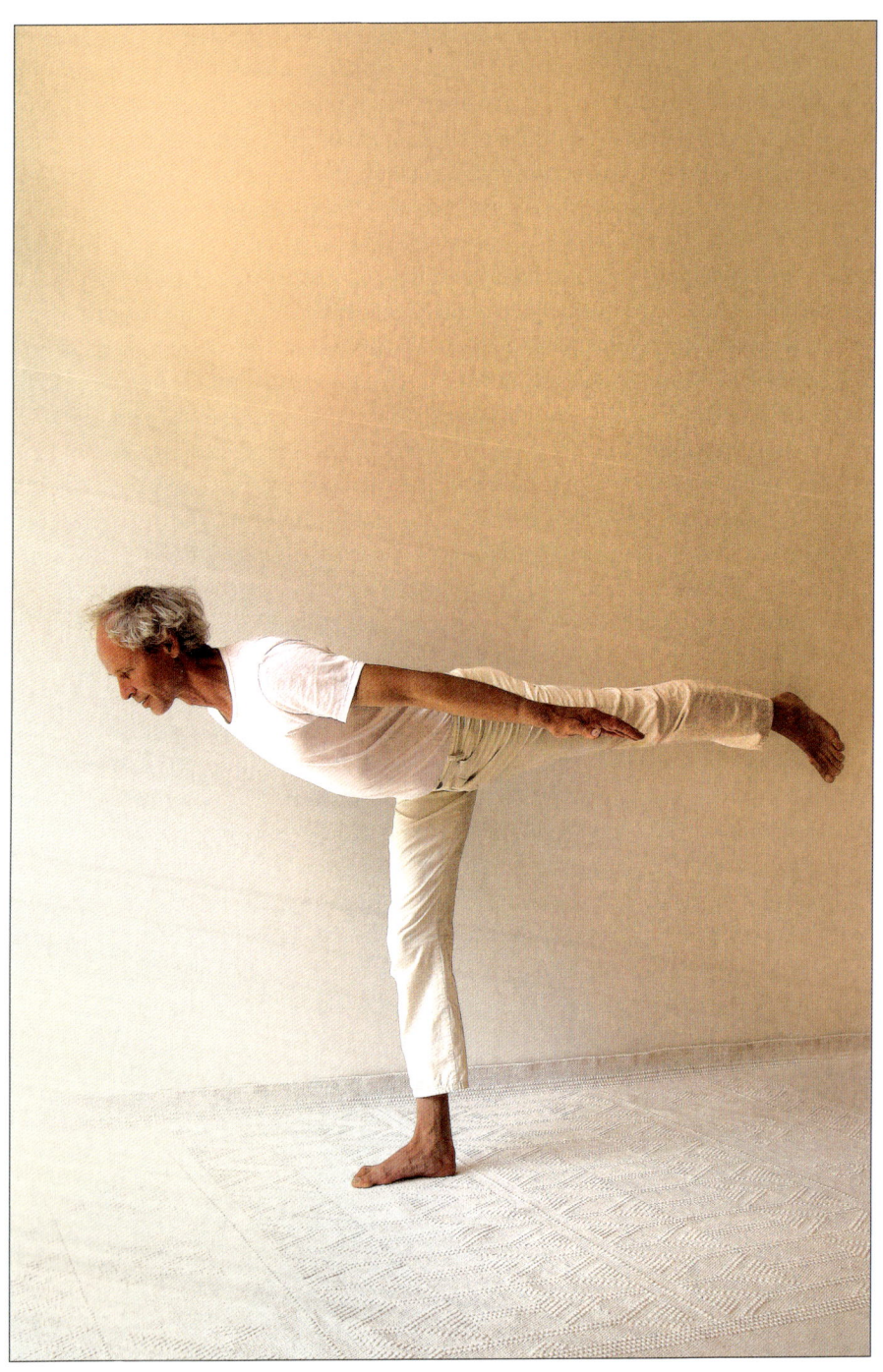

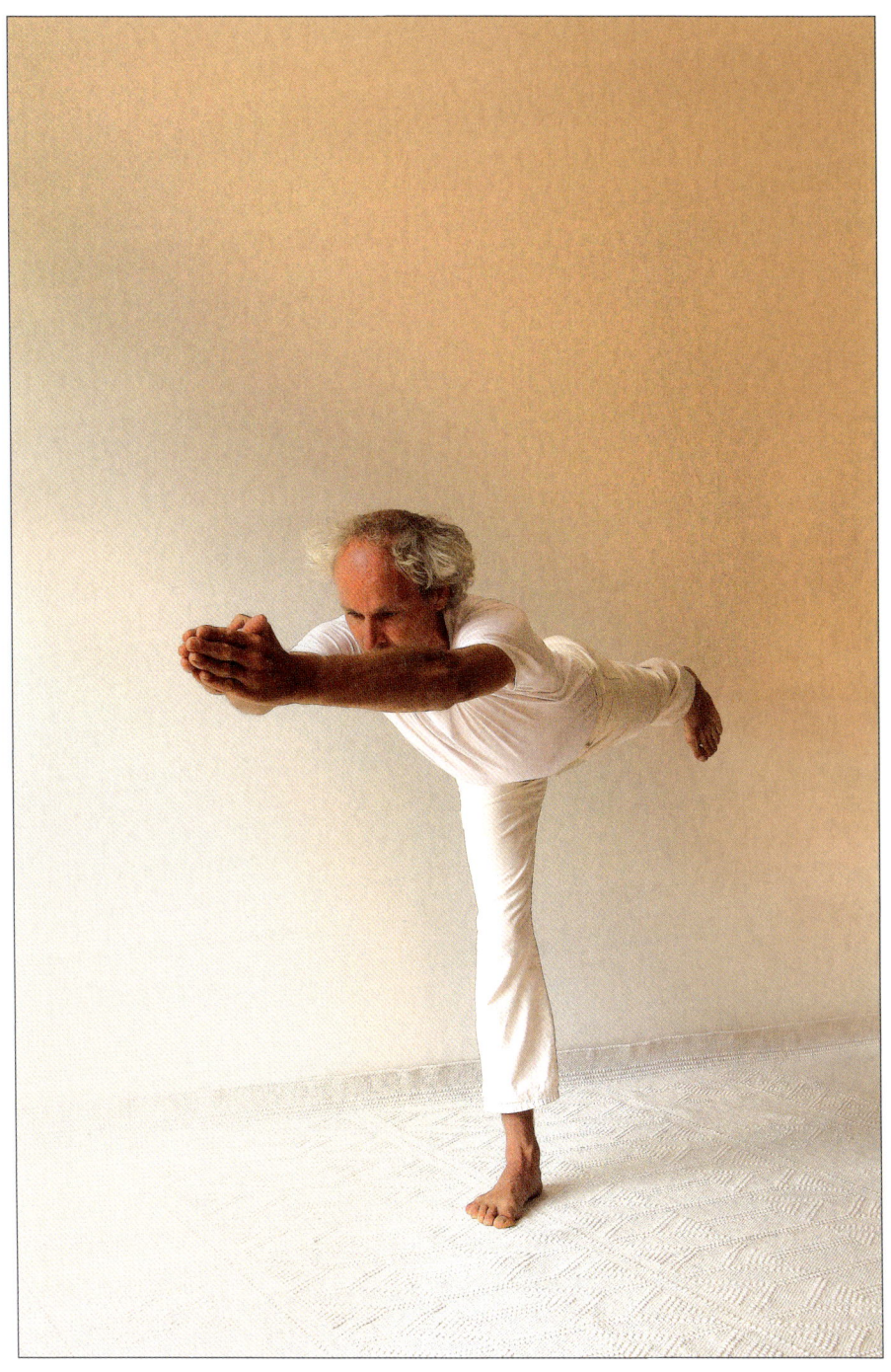

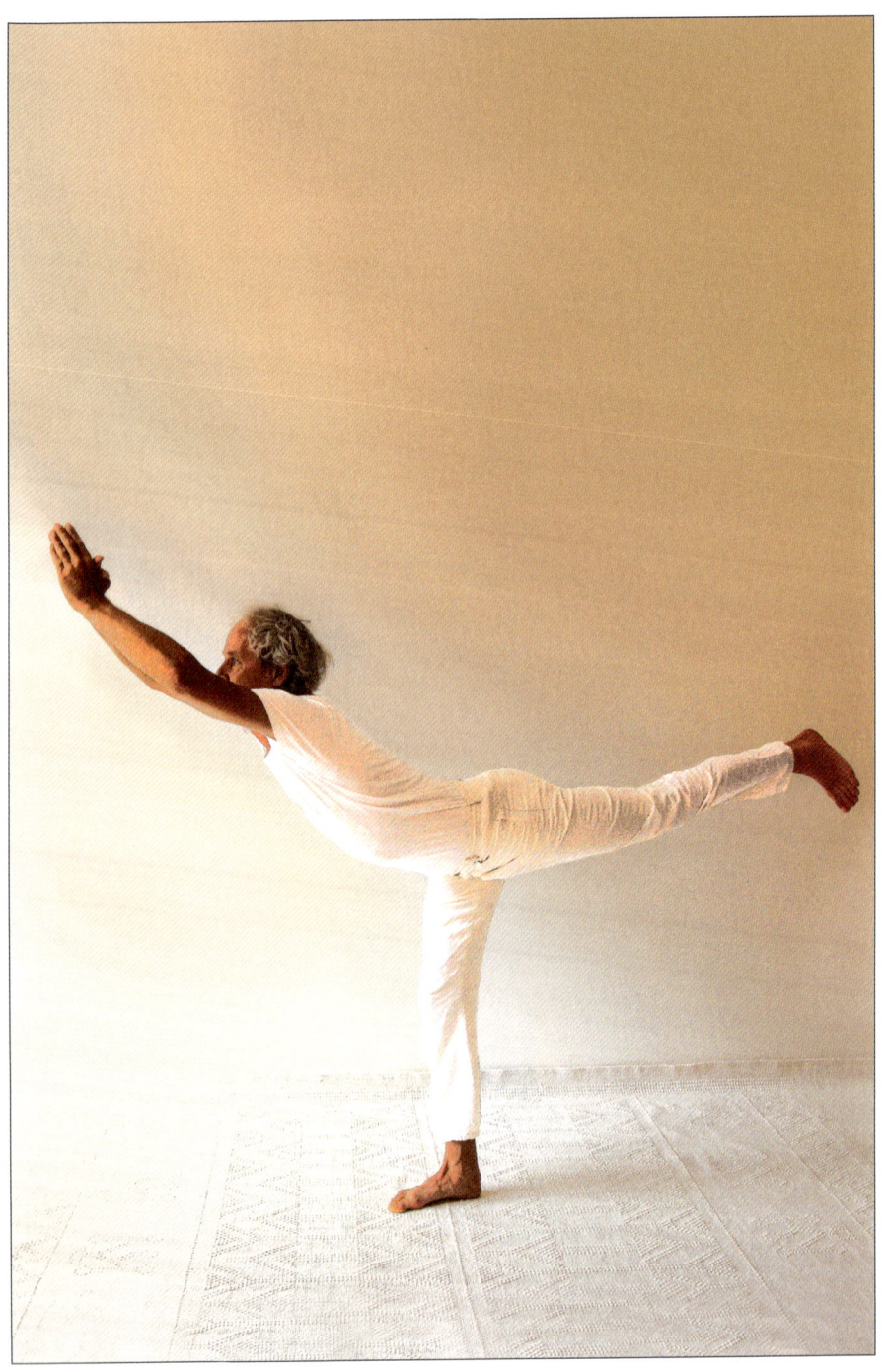

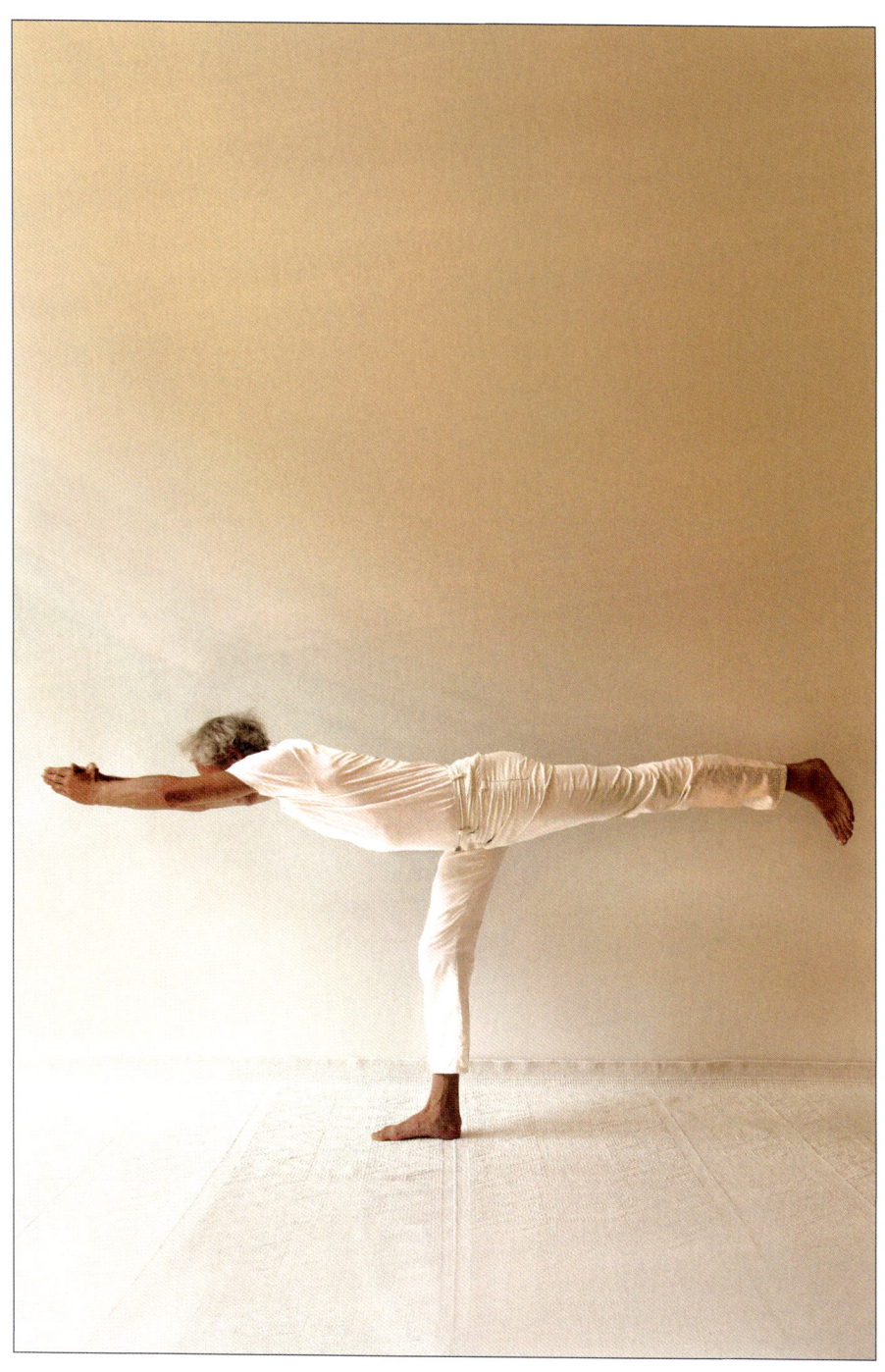

The dove
kapotāsana

The picture of the exercise

In this advanced exercise two big dimensions of movement combine. These consist of a horizontal direction, gliding outwards, inclined towards the earth, and a vertical dynamic, which glides towards the sky or the cosmos. Human life is directed on the one hand towards the so-called spiritual life, and towards striving for progress and development, and therefore carries in its heritage a vertical principle with a raised head. However, through the fact that the body is at the same time a part of the earth and has to connect itself with the earthly elements, the horizontal principle exists, expressing itself through closeness to the ground and even through an anchoring in the ground. With the legs and also with the metabolism, the human movement system connects intensively with the earthly elements.

The horizontal and the vertical depict two big directions of development, which each individual wants to achieve in life in a specific way. On the one hand the consciousness wants to experience knowledge about the celestial regions and the worlds beyond, and on the other hand it wants to penetrate into the various areas of interest that the world and its phenomena offer. Earthly and spiritual sciences motivate the human mind and carry it sometimes up more into the celestial regions and other times down into the earthly realms.

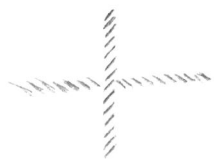

The two big opposites of the horizontal and vertical lines find their reconciliation in the life of the human soul and spirit. Neither escape into the higher worlds nor attachment to the earthly principles give the soul full satisfaction, but rather a striving, which encompasses the spiritual realities and from these is able to penetrate into the earthly conditions in a free way.

Harmony between these two directions of movement in a suitable form of synthesis can attain its beautiful and pictorial expression through a circle.

In the dove practitioners move with a leg-dynamic that glides out and also gathers, and they experience, even in the initial stages, a closeness to the ground on which they sit. This movement corresponds to the second centre and is significant for the universal mercurial forces of attraction, which actually give human beings the subtle-feeling of closeness and connectedness with the elements.

From this sitting position the entire back rises upwards dynamically, as if it is seeking the potential dimensions of a new, free and higher reality. This striving into the vertical demands of practitioners a certain effort, as they have to lift the spine out of the pelvis and then they even energise the thoracic spine with a dynamic to counter the unusual forces of gravity. The effort to straighten up in this way is one characteristic of *kapotāsana*.

The harmonious and perfect expression of the dove, however, finds its completion from the moment at which the foot is brought onto the back of the head, and the arms, as if turning inside out over the head, take hold of this foot. The whole body rests inside out in the backward bend and now forms not only the vertical line upwards, but a beautiful circular movement, which includes both the horizontal and the vertical striving of human beings. While the body rests close to the ground in balance, the chest opens wide and the whole body describes, in the completed circular movement, an openness to the cosmos and a connection to the earth.

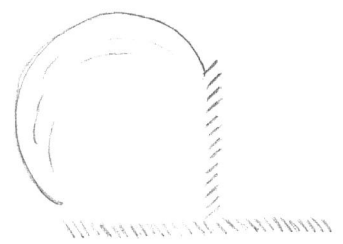

To practise

In this pose all seven centres are involved. Both strength as well as skill, extension, contraction, the ability to straighten up, balance, clear mental picturing, a forming of clear thoughts and also a certain letting go of tensions and bodily heaviness are necessary in this pose.

Start in a sitting position and bend one leg inwards, as in the pictures. It is a good idea to activate the backwardly stretched leg a few times dynamically by stretching and contracting the muscles, and, through several repetitions with alternating legs, gradually to lead the base towards the ground. The legs are literally drawn towards the pelvic floor and yet at the same time extended out again.

contraction

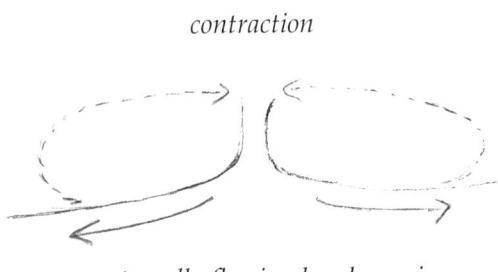

outwardly flowing leg-dynamic

To make it easier a cushion can be placed under the buttocks so as to raise the body slightly. The balance can be held more easily with the help of this levelling elevation.

Once the body is more or less in a straight line, practitioners begin to straighten up vertically. It is best to begin this first with one arm, then with both, in a rhythmic series, as shown in the following pictures. The thoracic spine is greatly stretched, lifted and in this way brought into an extension. However, the neck does not yet drop back.

At this stage it is helpful to lift up the lower leg and pull it forwards with the arms so that the legs find their way further into the stretch, and the sitting position slides towards the ground in the best way possible.

The movement over the head is extremely challenging. First one arm is led far into the stretch, the leg behind is lifted up, and then the toes are grasped above the forehead. Finally practitioners place the foot on the back of the head and take hold of it with the second hand. Resting in balance, paying attention to exact geometry and alignment, the whole body now draws together once again in the position. In the final stage there is hardly any tension in the arms; out of the leg-dynamic practitioners push the foot onto the head. The circle is now closed through its own dynamic and the arms merely hold the form. For about 15 seconds this position can be held in both the balance and the dynamic. The pose should always be practised on both sides.

As the movement over the head is very challenging, practitioners can turn the arm the other way up to take hold of the foot, and with one hand pull the leg towards the head. However, practitioners should take care not to position the upper body too extremely to one side, so that they do not deviate too far from the natural geometry of the position.

The four drawings on page 329 show the stages of the inverted handgrip. To start with practitioners can do the dove with just one arm, while keeping the other arm on the ground and holding the balance. The dove is a challenging balancing pose. It precisely stretches the thoracic spine.

This exercise is also recommended generally for people who cannot yet come into the far backward dynamic. It can be practised in individual stages to the point of a first straightening up into the vertical and a first stretching out into the horizontal.

The experience of the dove is sensitive and gives practitioners a first feeling for the two big dimensions of movement that are inherent as archetypes in their body.

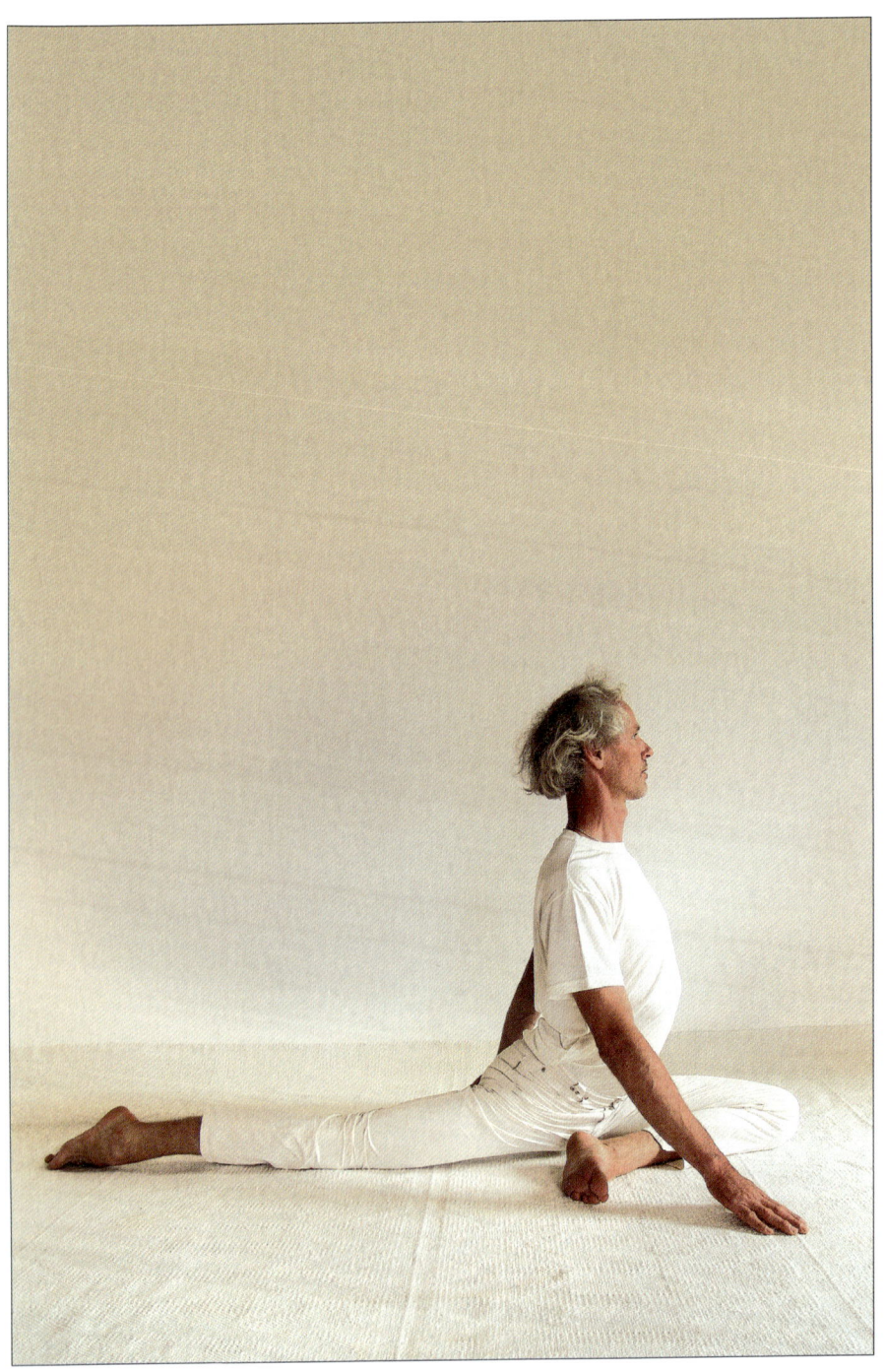

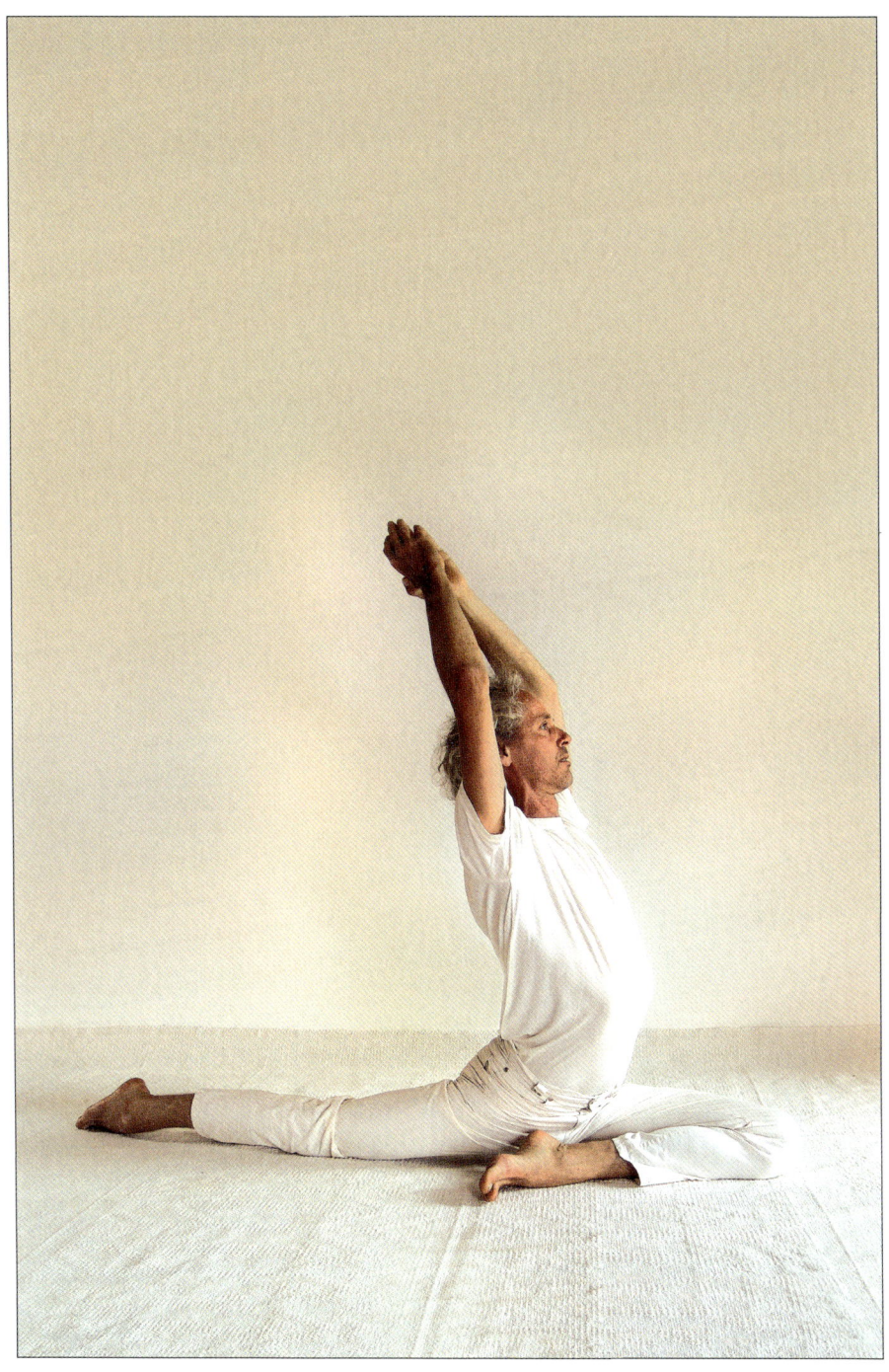

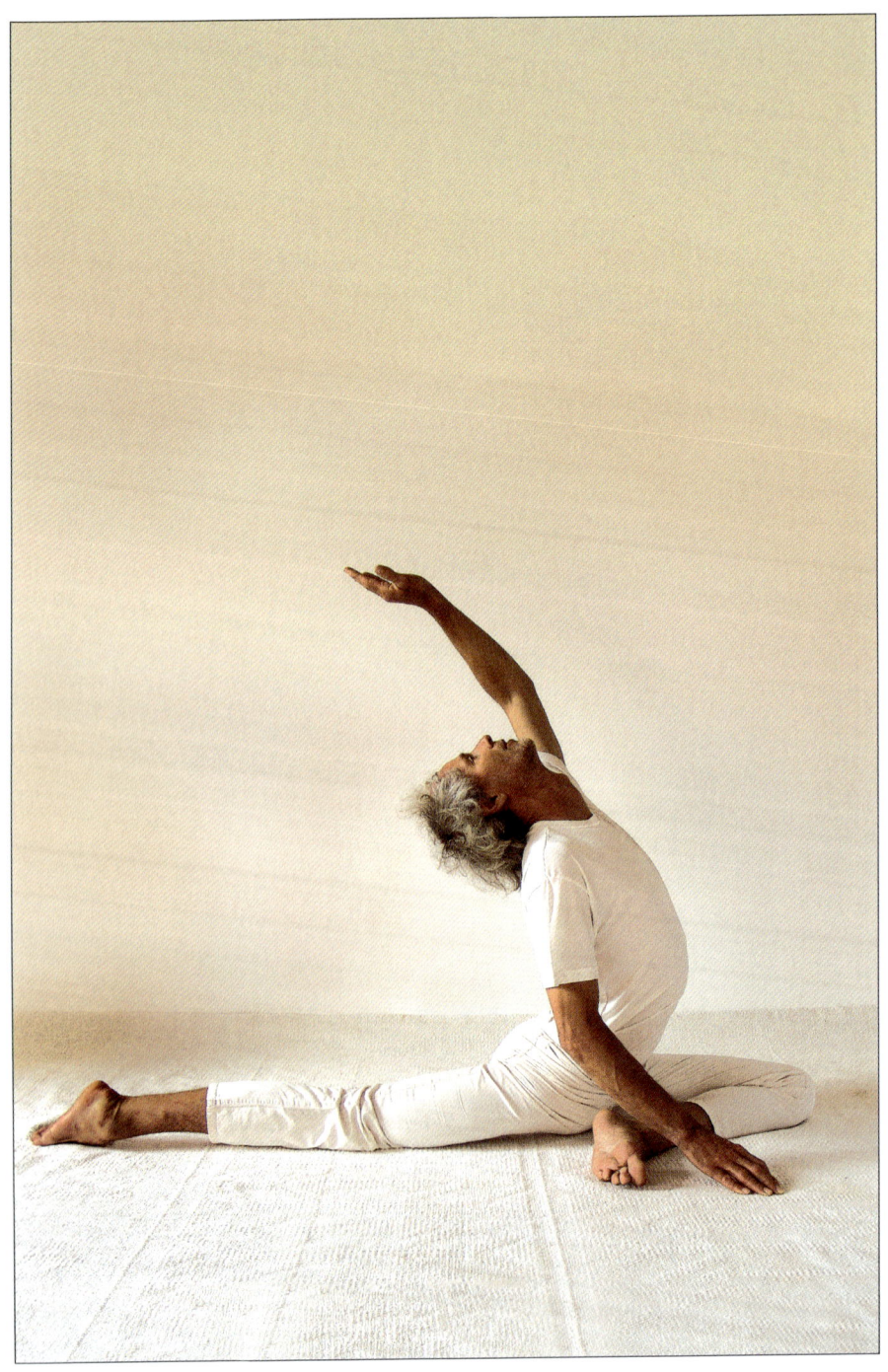

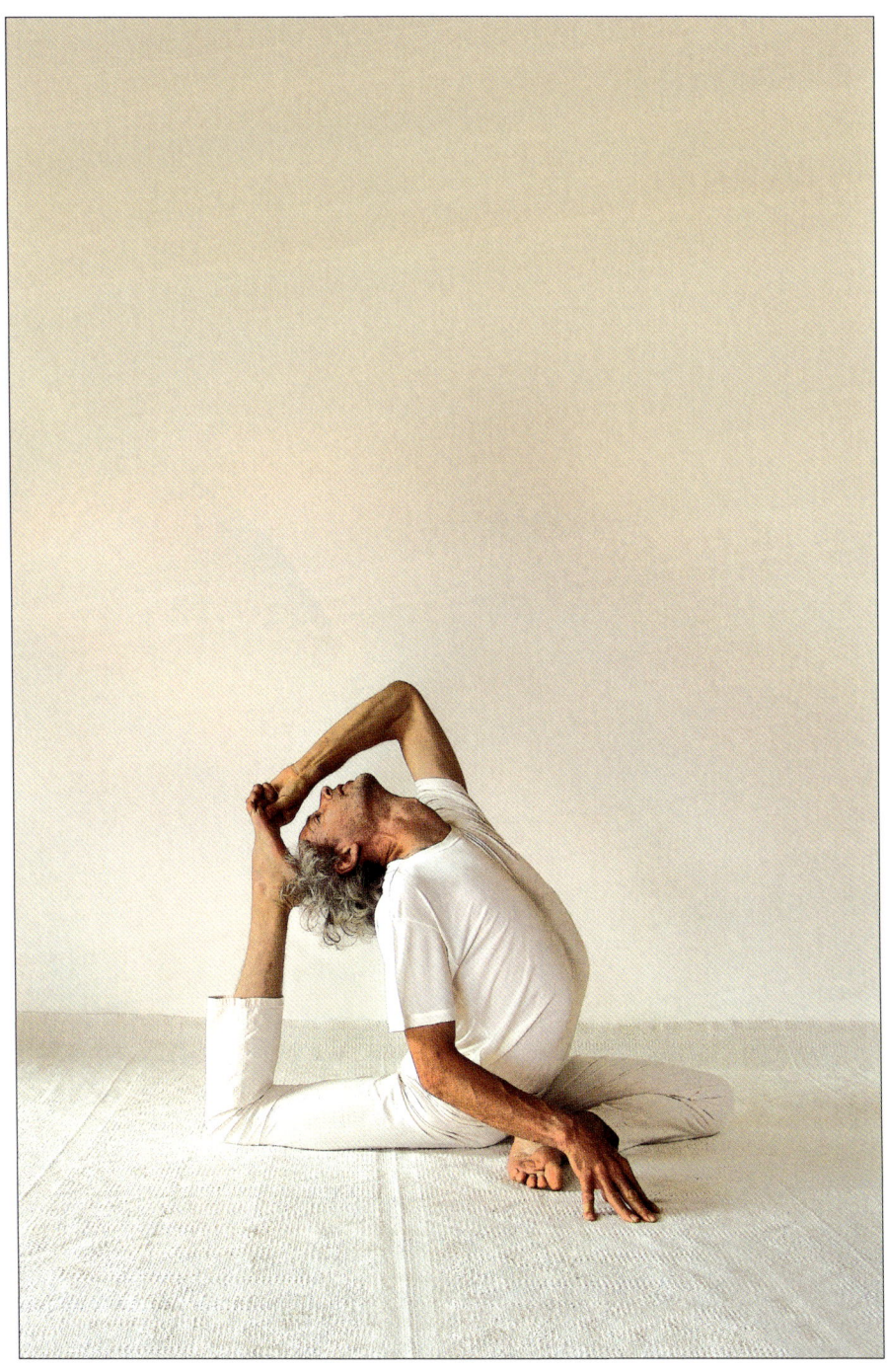

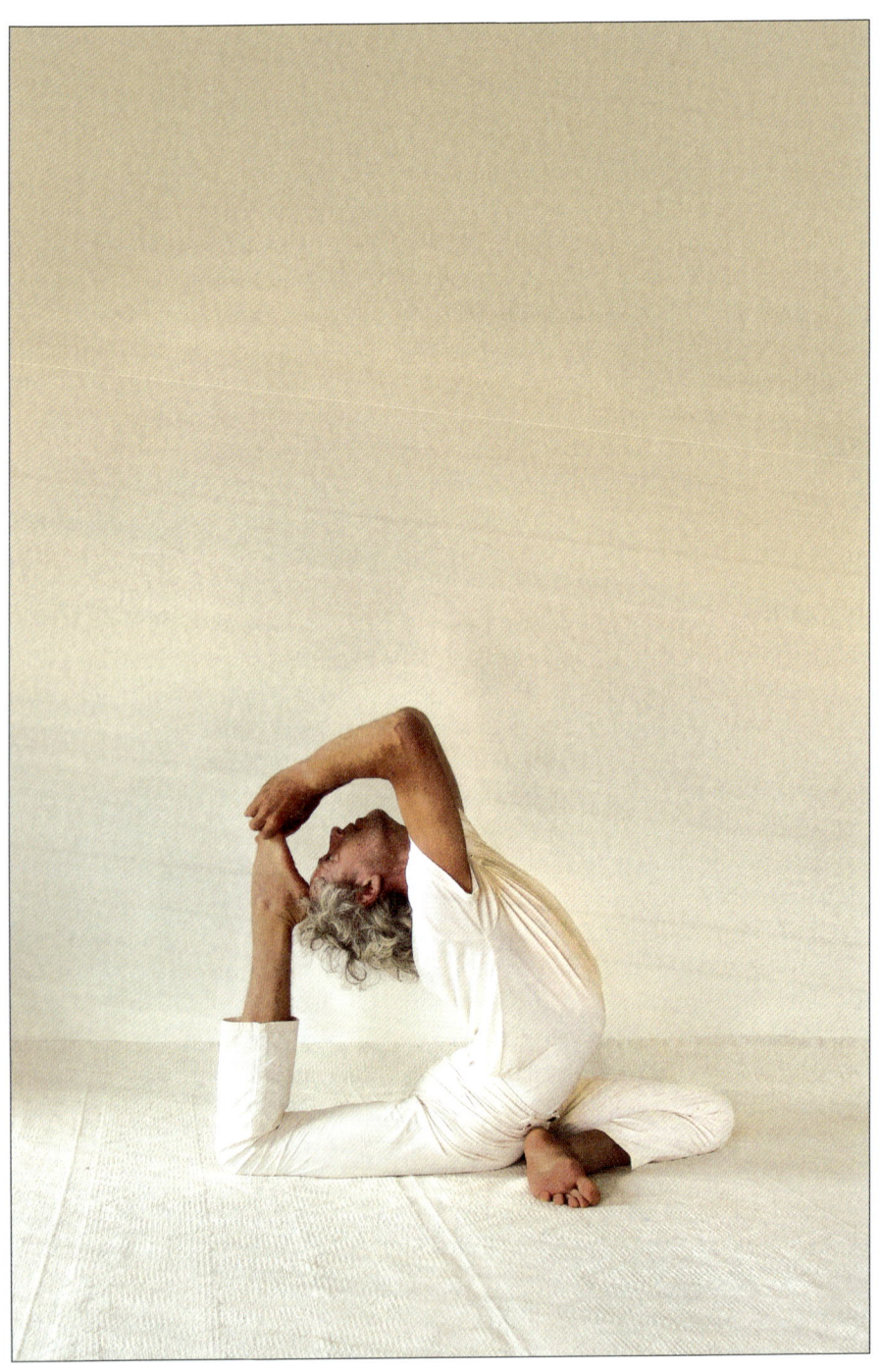

The backward-bending handgrip

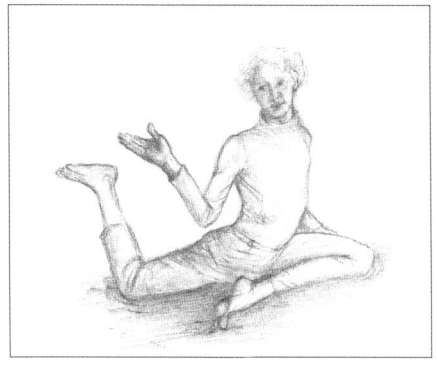
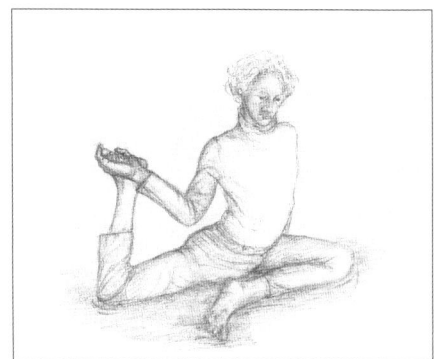

The hand is taken backwards in an unusual way with the hand facing upwards. Then practitioners take hold of the foot the other way round, with the fingers on the bridge of the foot and the thumb on the sole, pull the foot actively forward and invert their whole body in a great big movement. The spine plays an active part in this inversion.

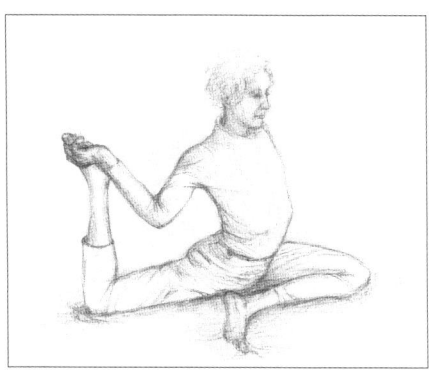
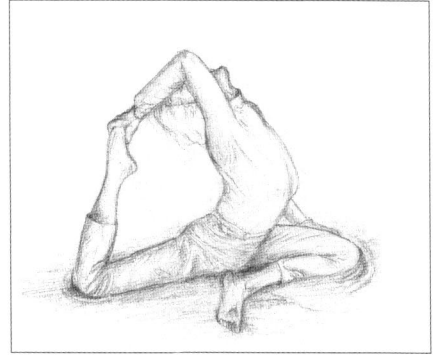

A methodical sequence with which to construct a practice session

The individual exercises described can now be put together to construct a systematic practice sequence that helps the consciousness work to discover some first qualities of the seven *cakrāḥ*. The first centre in this developmental process represents a new beginning, or the consciousness being born anew in the heart. Through the work with the soul dimension of yoga, completely new, foundational subtle-feelings and perceptions develop; life acquires a soul depth and a demonstrable, rejuvenating enlivenment. From this heart centre, which reveals the new birth of the individuality through developing a more elevated, soul-like existence, the impulses gradually flow to bring about the mastery of each of the subsequent lotus flowers. Proceeding from the heart, the third and fifth energy centres are integrated into the contextual meaning, then in a next intensification the second and the sixth centres, and finally, as the most difficult and greatest transformation, the first and seventh centres. However, it is now helpful to know that these centres are experienced more within an ordered context, and some first subtle-feelings related to these centres are lifted into conscious birth. A perfect development of the *cakrāḥ*, however, will not yet be possible through this way of practising. From the subtle streams of consciousness coming from the new birth in the heart, the first perceptible forms develop like connecting, circular radii, reaching into the deeper and higher lying *cakrāḥ*. From this natural, inner, soul-spiritual order, which brings forth its own being like a geometry, well-proportioned and linked together in precisely measured relationship, a practice sequence acquires its wisdom-filled meaning.

For example, you can practise a sequence as follows:

An exercise that leads the *anāhata-cakra* into experience,
for example: the tree – *tāḍāsana*

An exercise that enlivens the *maṇipūra-cakra*,
for example: the plough – *halāsana*

An exercise that sensitises the *viśuddha-cakra*,
for example: the half moon – *āñjaneyāsana*

An exercise that works to build consciousness for the second centre,
for example the wide stretch – *koṇāsana*

An exercise that addresses the *ājñā-cakra*
for example: the sitting twist – *ardha matsyendrāsana*

An exercise that incorporates the first centre
for example: the inclined plane – *pūrvottānāsana*

An exercise that grants a memory of the unity of the seventh centre,
for example: the lotus – *padmāsana*

By creating a whole cycle in this way with seven individual exercises, you notice deep down in the hidden soul, how via the activity of the consciousness, individual thoughts approach that spiritualisation so hard to describe, and want to manifest in the body. You then follow in your soul a path that wants to come from the spirit, from above to below, starting from a thought, from the first idea, to the deeper, subtle-feeling and finally to the manifestation in the will. The path through the individual lotus flowers is a path of etherising and spiritualising the body. The soul content that lies in the exercises, the deep meaning of the thoughts and subtle-feelings, wants to enrich existing life and manifest as a part of the personality.

For all exercises a strict systematic plan is not necessary. Very important is the development of an understanding for the individual lotus flowers, which are the subtle-matter gathering points for the soul's existence. Once you have acquainted yourself with the individual exercises, you can then also include several exercises for the centres. For example, you can practise the cycle given here, or introduce different exercises, such as, for example, in place of the tree the tiptoe pose, or at the point of the second centre you can also introduce several exercises. It is only important to understand how through actually thinking the individual thoughts and feeling the subtle-feelings, the work with the consciousness wants to come from above to below to manifestation.

The practice-sequence can be chosen freely by each person and different focal points for a single exercise can find their place within it. The schematic sequence serves more to stimulate a natural subtle-feeling, however the practice should not be pressed into a strict system. Practitioners get to know the movement of the individual lotus flowers, explore the subtle-feelings of the exercises and through repeated practice they acquire truer feelings for the identity of the soul, and these elevate and enrich life.

The sequence is built up in a rhythm conceived according to a clear order, and those who follow this rhythm notice how the order also becomes felt. Just as someone can immediately distinguish between an evenly shaped square and an uneven rectangle, so practitioners will also notice these first forms of order, which occur through the individual exercises and through the sequence. It is in fact literally a kind of geometric experience, which now comes into a harmony and attunement both with the body and also with the various thoughts that are decided upon for the exercises. A first and natural ordering of the astral body can enter in with these created forms of consciousness.

In the illustration, the planets are depicted in connection with the energy centres. If practitioners work at enriching and then transforming their entire soul-life, the energy centres can be said to unite with their existing connections. The lower centres shine onto the upper ones in rhythmic exchange, and the upper ones onto the lower ones. They give mirror images. The heart forms the centre, and the lively etheric streams flow down to the heart, via the upper centres, are penetrated from below and then suffuse all the lotus flowers again anew with subtle substances.

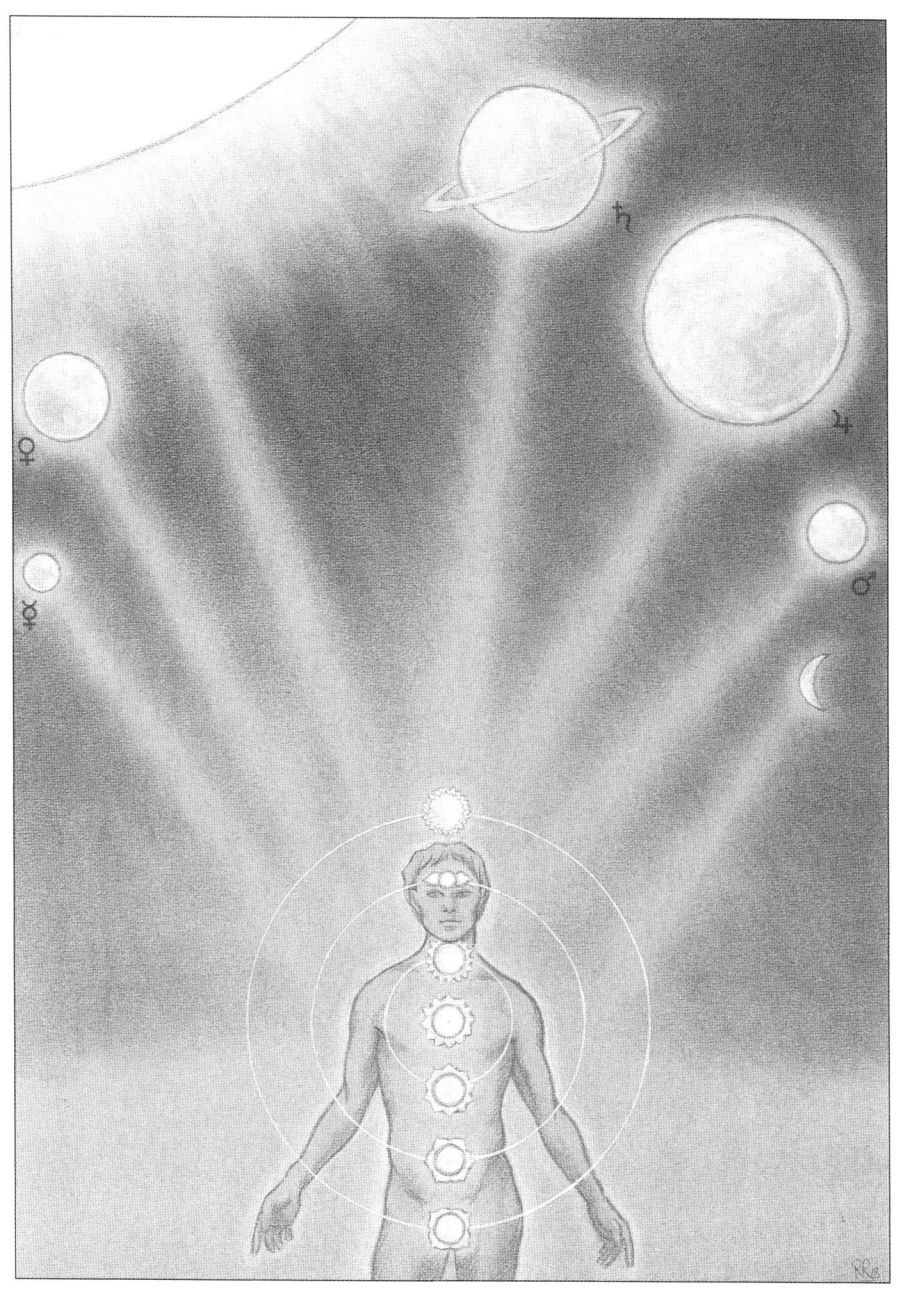

The sun prayer
sūrya namaskāra

This exercise cycle of twelve component movements helps to develop a regenerative dynamic strength in the spine and to warm up the body. The sun prayer is therefore a good gymnastic warming exercise that can be done at the beginning of a practice session.

You can most easily understand the soul-spiritual meaning of the sun prayer by equating the power of the sun, which traditionally is worshipped and revered, with the creative power of thought. What is the creative power of thought? It is not just an exclusive aptitude expressed by select artists in their field; even if it is usually underdeveloped, it is a part of the soul of every human being. The creative power of thought rests as a health-giving and spiritual potential in the innermost centre of every individuality.

If you think a high and noble thought today, with a sense of purpose and a need for realisation, then, in accordance with its nature of being, *bhāvan*, this thought will come to flow through the stages of development and attain realisation. Out of the Mother Earth, out of the creative, as yet undifferentiated origin, the thought comes to attain a fixed, experienceable and existent reality, which, naturally only after considerable time and after many interim experiences such as testings or true loyalty, becomes found with what in Christianity is termed the Godhead Father. The thought which has been realised in every part, right into the will, is not only symbolic, but in every way it is like the connection of the consciousness with something higher, or with universality, and this is described as Father.

In yoga mythology there is a feminine and also a masculine aspect, which are called *śakti* and *śiva* respectively. The force of *śakti*, which rests at the lower end of the spine and is feminine, is supposed to ascend to unite with the head, or with *śiva*, the masculine pole. It is the Mother Earth from which the thought grows and thrives and through its many experiential stages ascends to the level of Father or to highest, universal manifestation. It is in this sense, with the individual creative activity of forming thoughts, that the sun prayer is to be understood.

With this pictorial depiction, the twelve component movements can be combined with a mantra, each movement symbolically marking one month and together representing the time for the earth to orbit the sun.

Repeat one line of the mantra for each movement. Remain conscious of the image that every thought that has at some point been thought and purposefully wanted, month by month will come into realisation.

According to Copernicus the earth circles around the sun. But according to Ptolemy the sun orbits the earth. A thought, which in reality is of the sun, orbits life and at some point manifests itself in the individual heart. Month by month, the imagined, soul-felt and wanted thought descends into the personal nature. The consciousness may need an entire year before a demanding thought of spirituality is understood and realised in knowledge or in deed.

In this cyclical maturing of the life of thought and knowledge lies the meaning of the 12-part sun prayer.

The mantra goes:

Out of Mother Earth the self grows (1)
in sprouting energy, (2)
as a child (3)
becomes a pupil, (4)
whose learning (5)
leads to requesting, (6)
watching (7)
for the great testing, (8)
true loyalty(9)
in service, (10)
leads the youth (11)
to the Father. (12)

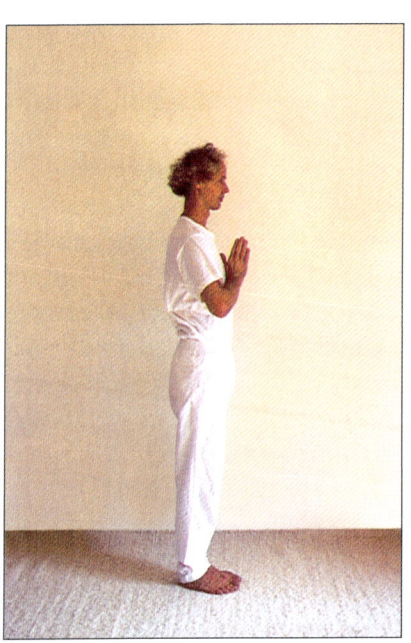

1 "Out of Mother Earth the self grows"

The hands are folded in front of the chest; the beginning takes place with the exhalation. If the initial gesture of the sun prayer is assigned a place in the yearly cycle, it corresponds to the deepest winter period, to December, Christmas time, which is the birth month of Christ and also the time in which the raw nights (iii) begin, the time in which the coming ideas for the year are sown.

2 "in sprouting energy"

The back arches, rising upwards, dynamically backwards; inhalation. The position corresponds to the month of January. The thought invisibly continues to germinate and mature inside.

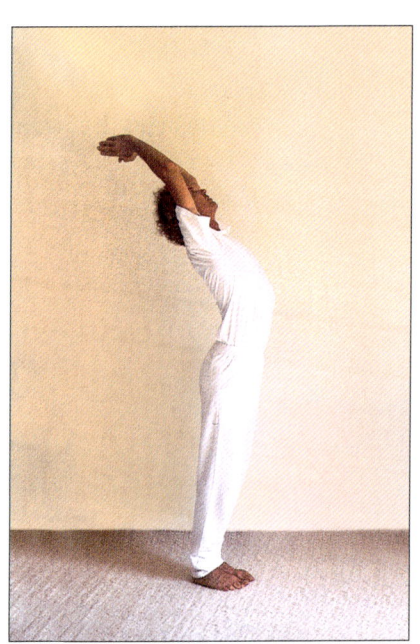

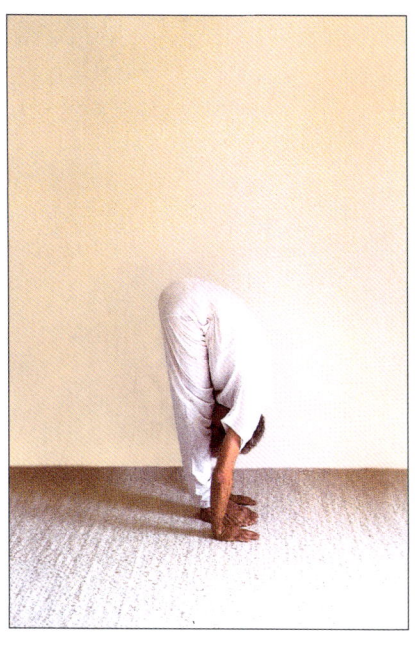

3 "as a child"

Intensive stretch forwards with simultaneous exhalation. The thought continues to mature in the month of February, but remains as yet unapparent like a germinating seed beneath the earth. The thought is like a child who has not yet attained the maturity and consciousness of life.

4 "becomes a pupil"

The position is developed further, in contrast to the classical form, and raised up to the half moon; inhalation. The month of March. The spring of thinking begins.

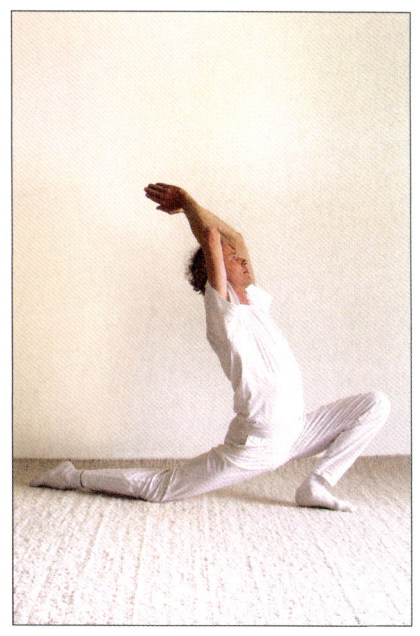

5 "whose learning"

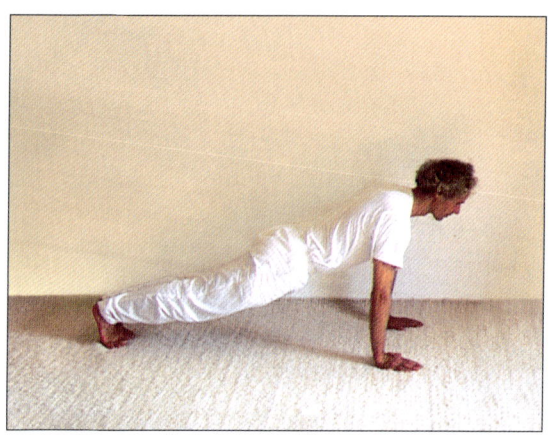

Hold the breath, keep the head in line in the inclined plane. The month of April. The thought awakens to a tangible form, emerges from its germinating, undifferentiated existence and becomes more concrete. It becomes experienced through learning.

6 "leads to requesting"

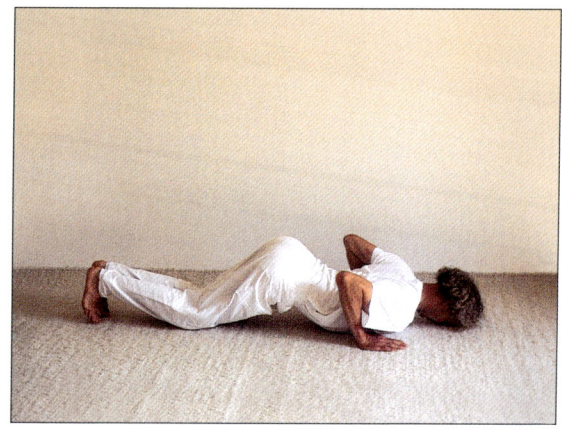

Exhale. Those who want to realise a thought, experience how without devotion and reverent requesting they can have no true success. The month of May.

7 "watching"

The spine curves dynamically into the cobra; inhalation. The month of June.

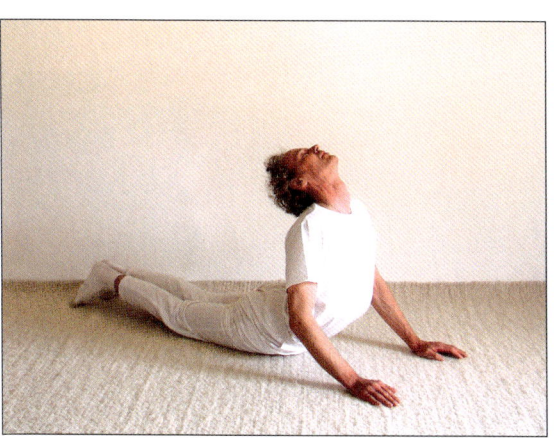

Vigilance on the path of realising a thought leads to differentiation and constitutes a stretch of the whole journey.

8 "for the great testing"

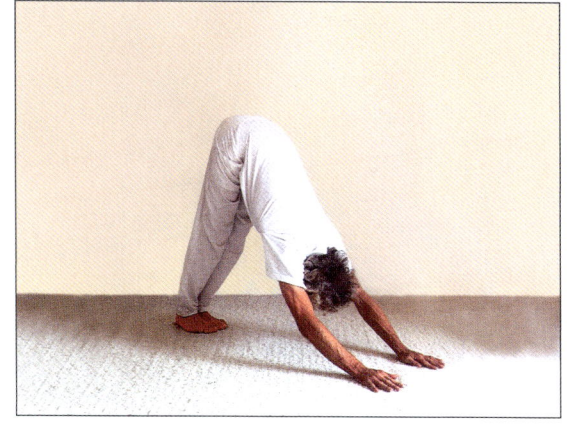

Along the way there are often decisive moments which have to be consciously recognised, interpreted and preserved. The month of July. The high point of the summer, of passion; exhalation.

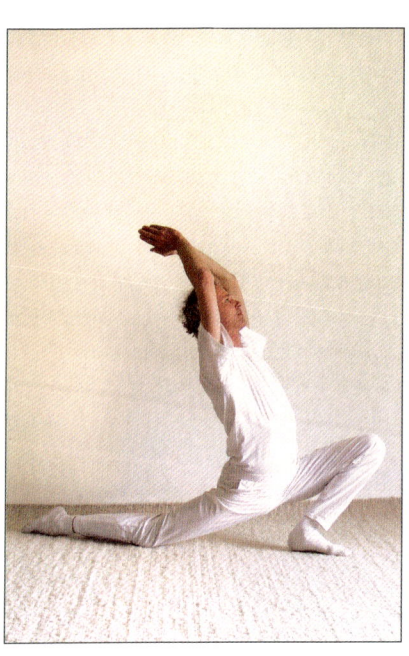

9 "true loyalty"

After the triangle comes inhalation and a repetition of the half moon base with the arms above the head. (In the classical practice the hands remain on the ground.) The month of August, the end of summer. Perseverance and loyalty to the aim are necessary along the way.

10 "in service"

Exhalation. Intensive stretch as in the third position. The month of September. Every thought is integrated into the social world plan and, beyond this, into the spiritually existing universal plan.

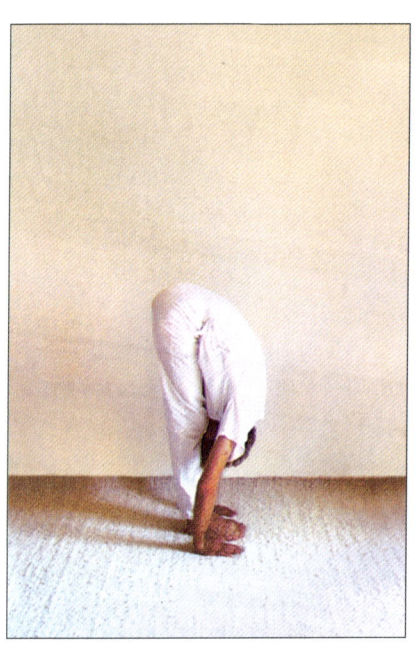

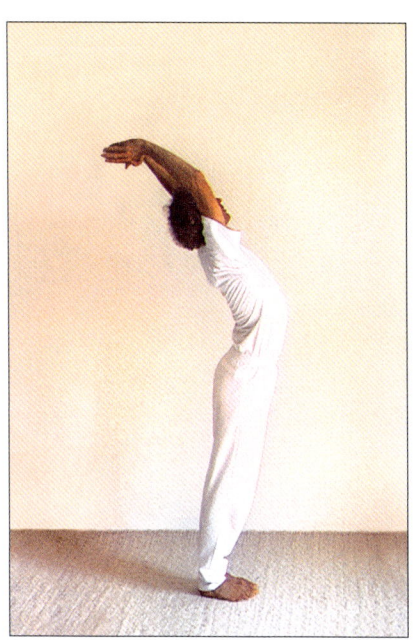

11 "leads the youth"

Inhalation and a big, dynamic stretch up into the half moon. The thought which, over the course of a year, continues to be thought, brought to life, researched, purposefully wanted and maintained in the idea of spirituality in a concentrated way, becomes evident as a youthful life-force. Mid-autumn, the month of October.

12 "to the Father"

Exhalation. The cycle ends in the normal standing position. Now the thought has matured within and practitioners feel their person to be one with the thought. The month of November, the deepest period of autumn.

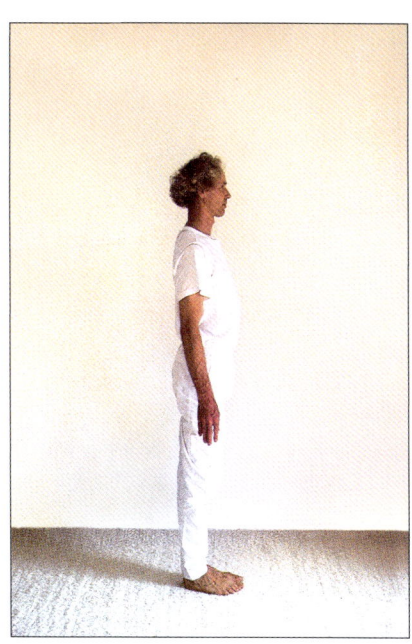

A meditation on the three circles

A direct, specific meditation should not take place on the individual energy centres, as in an isolated and monotone way they do not become addressed in their content-related and universal significance. The meditation described here opens up an initial understanding of how each centre corresponds to personal abilities, and how beyond this an everlasting influence out of cosmic, over-arching, spiritual spheres enlivens, nourishes and spiritualises these centres.

Participation I

For this meditation, first imagine a circle. The circle is a symbol for unity, eternity and an infinite flowing of spiritual, sun-radiant forces. Then once you have gained a sense for the meaning of the geometric symbol of a circle, develop a picture of the *āsana* we have called the "tip-toe pose", *pādāṅguṣṭhāsana*. This *āsana* now forms the tangible centre for the following mental images.

Now also conceive a big circle surrounding this pose of yours. The circle consists of the various people who make up your social and human environment: work colleagues, friends, acquaintances, family members, people with whom you are connected or have once been connected, perhaps even significant deceased people, as they also radiate with their soul into your close environment, as well as the current situations that you feel closely related to. All these people and the conditions linked to them you can connect into a circle that forms your individual social environment.

Think this circle like a living, fluid aura, which continuously radiates around you, and at every minute seeks a new mid-point precisely in the heart. Imagine the *āsana* surrounded by this circle. This centre at the heart, which forms itself out of the outer circle, is ultimately the heart centre or the centre of an initial feeling of self, *anāhata-cakra*.

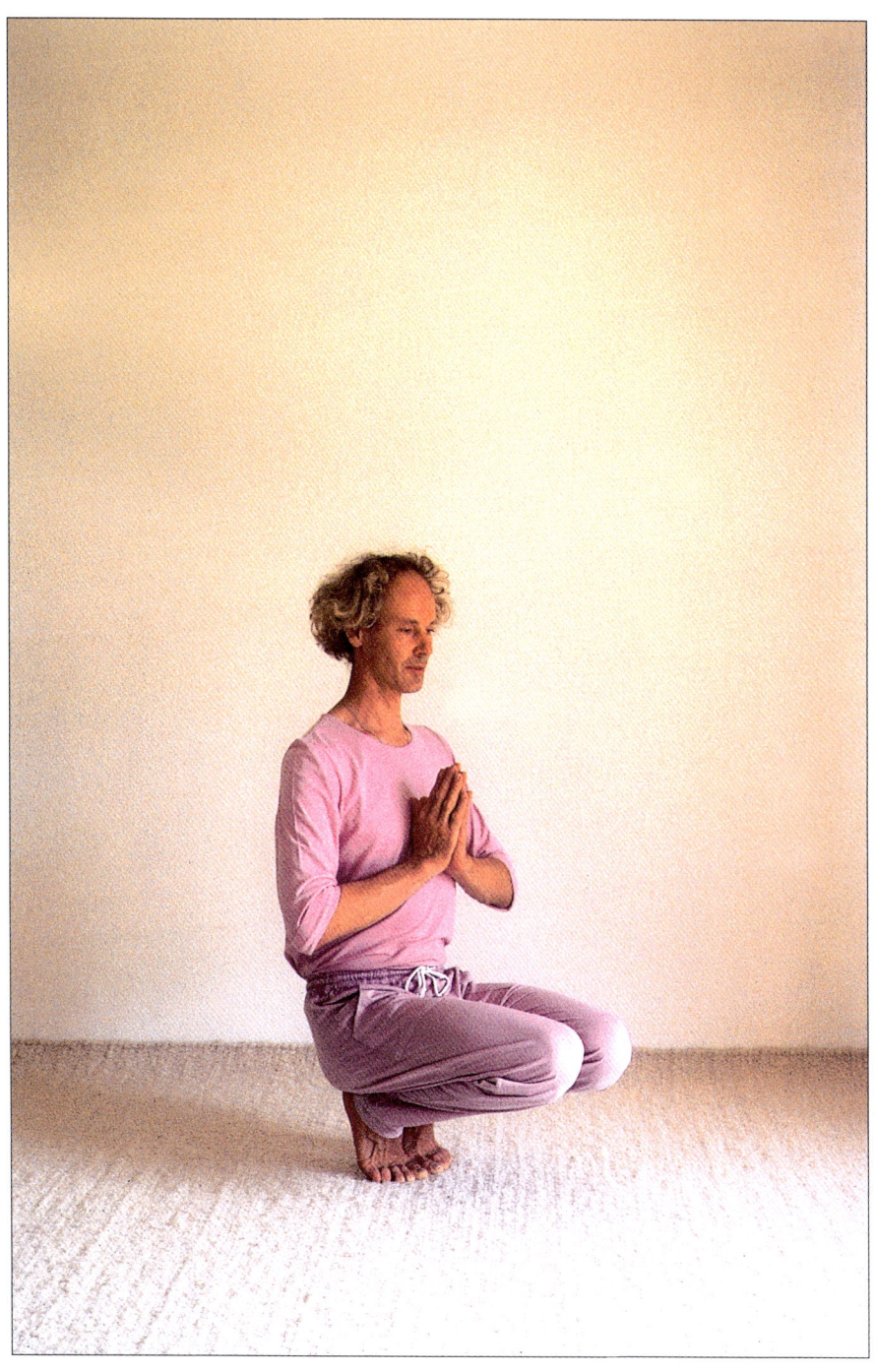

Participation II

When abstract ideas are considered and thought in precise pictures equating to the reality of universal forces, and then subtly felt with initial inner experiences, the understanding expands of the invisible and yet existing unity in which every human being, and the whole of humanity, weaves and lives with the higher realities of the cosmos. The idea itself is like a kind of law which is abstract yet, through the inner subtle-feeling, opens up a deep insight and consciousness in the personal realm of experience.

The heart centre develops in its harmony when, through independent activity, it becomes possible to order the personal, social environment and enrich it according to spiritual criteria.

The next centres to unfold in the development are the third and fifth centres, *maṇipūra-cakra* and *viśuddha-cakra*. These two centres belong together in a certain unity and can therefore be understood as a further abstract circle. As your mental image, take once again a typical *āsana*, which encompasses the consciousness of the third and fifth centres, for example the classical head to knee pose. Although this pose is characterised predominantly through the *maṇipūra-cakra*, nevertheless in its entirety and in its complete expression it represents the developed *manas*, the pure, pictorial, undeceived reality-thinking (Imagination), or in other words, the human thinking that is ensouled, oriented to the earth, to other people, to reverence and freedom. Take the mental image of a huge arc, which spans the whole earth, and imagine this arc then moving towards your body, gradually drawing inwards to the centre, and finally arching over the exercise *paścimottānāsana*. The third and fifth centres are connected with each other and the shaped arc itself connects not only these centres, but the whole person with the sphere around the earth.

When these two centres have unfolded harmoniously, you take up, within the surrounding sphere, the soul of the whole earth, and with subtle-feelings you can have an ordering influence on your own astral body and on that of others.

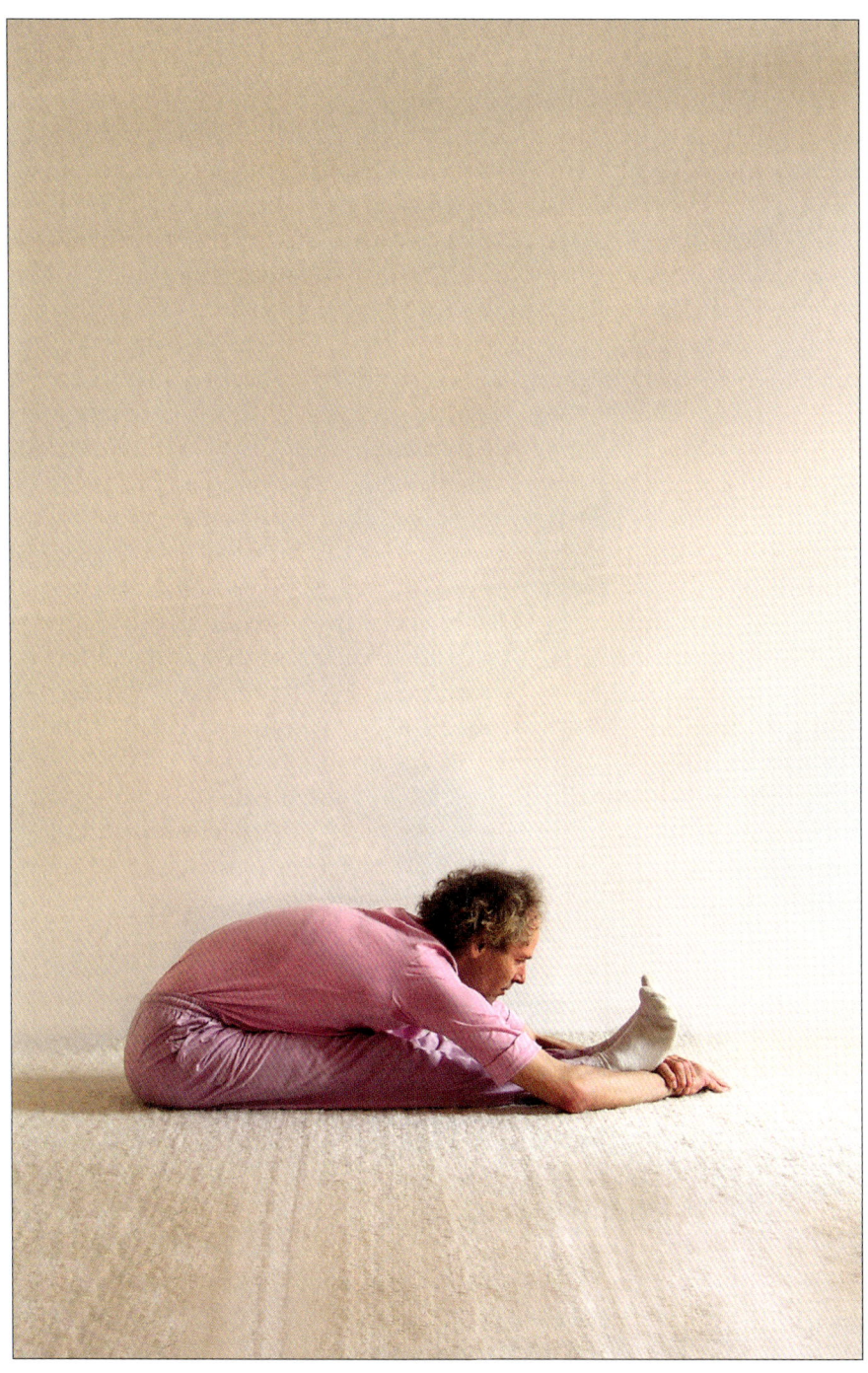

Participation III

Then continue the exercise by imagining a new circle, which is as big as the movement of the sun around the earth. Start quite consciously from the Ptolemaic world view, which maintains that the sun circuits around the earth and considers the earth to be at the centre. Imagine this great circuit of the sun pervaded with luminous beings and once again choose an *āsana* that corresponds to the action of forces that is alive in this area. The best example of such an *āsana* is the cobra. As a meditation model, even the complete cobra is suitable, as this *āsana* represents cosmic, sun-radiant love. It is an expression for the newly enlivened creative forces in the sixth centre, *ājñā-cakra*, and in the second centre, *svādhiṣṭhāna-cakra*, which when developed constitute fire and love for the real feeling-capacity of meditation. Living forces of concentration flow in these centres and effect in human beings the power for creative, receptive inspiration and for the healing radiation of the feeling for other beings.

In your imagination let the circle move ever closer to the *āsana*, until it finally condenses out of the wide, over-arching spacial sphere of the sun and finds its rest centred in the second and sixth centres. Out of the sun and its vast sphere, there radiate, through the thoughts, crystal-forming beings. The sun's course with its radiation carries the thought beings and these create a transparency at the human body, so that in every minute, through the light itself, this human body is founded in a new and alive way. The thoughts work in the light and form the basis for the physical. The circle itself, however, remains preserved in its unified completeness, it is far and near, open and closed, macrocosmic and microcosmic, warm and alive.

If both *cakrāḥ* are completely, integrally and consciously developed, the degree of realisation in the so-called *buddhi* is well-advanced. Human beings feel themselves united with the essence of the sun's course through the capacity of their own developed thinking, and have a healing action right into the etheric body, their own and that of others.

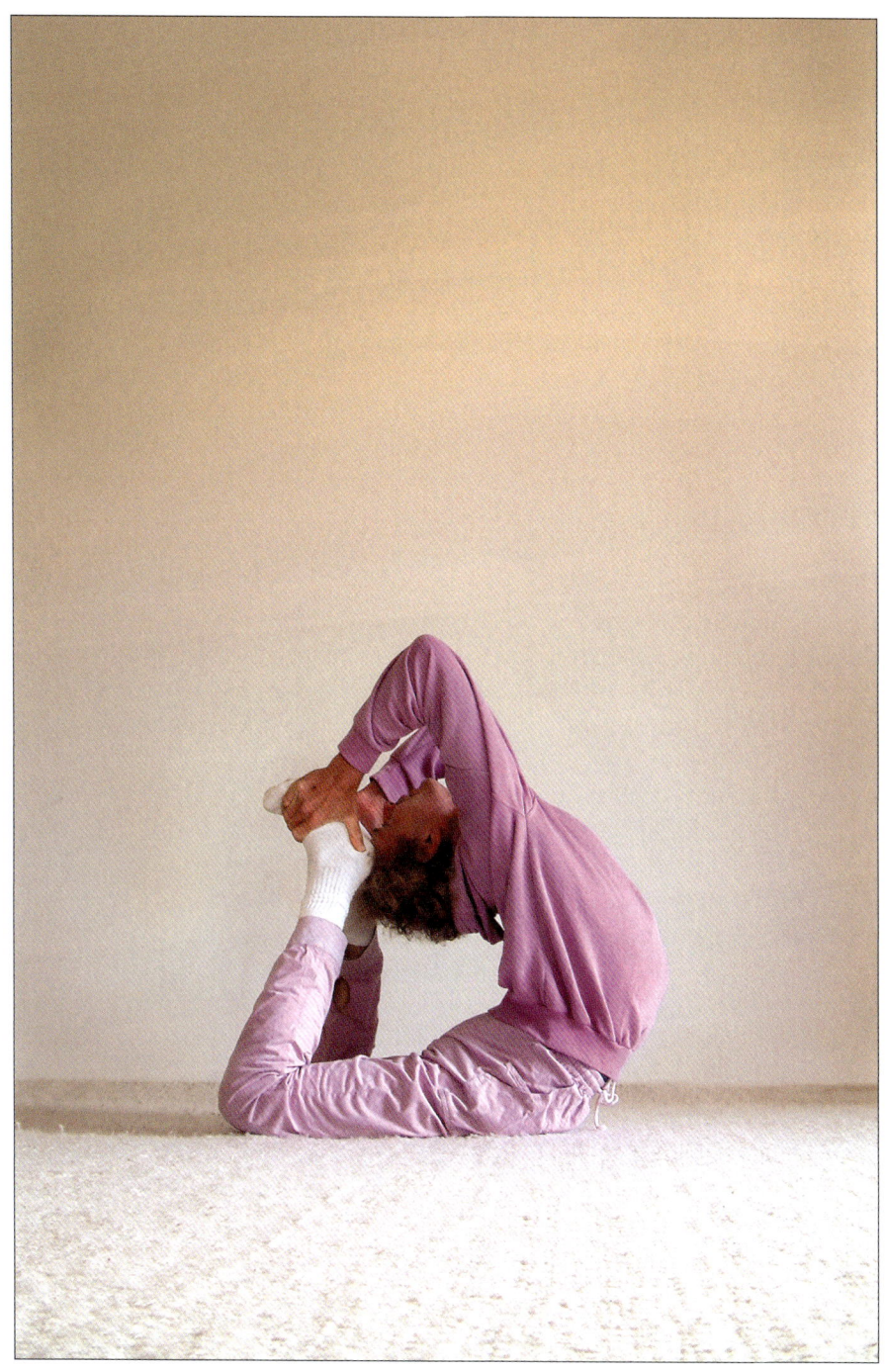

347

Participation IV

The last and most demanding step in the realisation of life is the spiritualisation, which reaches right into the cells of the physical body. Imagine an even bigger circle, which reaches beyond the path of the sun right to distant Saturn. Saturn is the planet that stands for universal *karma* and universal justice. The time Saturn takes to orbit is very long.

Choose a suitable *āsana*; for example the leg pose with complete uprightness. The leg pose in its perfected aesthetic expression stands symbolically for the developed seventh and the developed first centres. However, do not make the mistake of thinking that if, through flexibility, you can perform the leg pose with technical perfection, you will also have developed the seventh and first centres. For the development of these centres, as for the other centres, it is necessary to study the universal principles in a spiritual way, to purify life from flaws and to develop new abilities for creative, health-giving growth on the basis of the whole of spiritual life. All development happens out of the spirit and that is why the meditation is directed to the vast circle of an inconceivable sphere. Out of this higher circle, finally the imprint forms of the personal life in the will, and gives shape to the first and seventh centres.

By meditatively cultivating these mental images, the petty-minded, worry-laden fears about the physical, mortal body are lost and you will notice that your attention and view are to be directed far into space, so that out of the greater oneness the associated subtle-feeling can be experienced within. In the will you are in fact connected with this great sphere of a universal setting. The actual body forms merely a mid-point in itself, which is created out of this setting as vast as the cosmos. After death the soul will enter into this vast cosmic sphere and according to the zeal and courage, the wisdom and empathy that it has realised, it will participate in the free reality associated with the greatest possible sphere of space. You can experience the body in the vertical line of the will also at the same time like an open vessel.

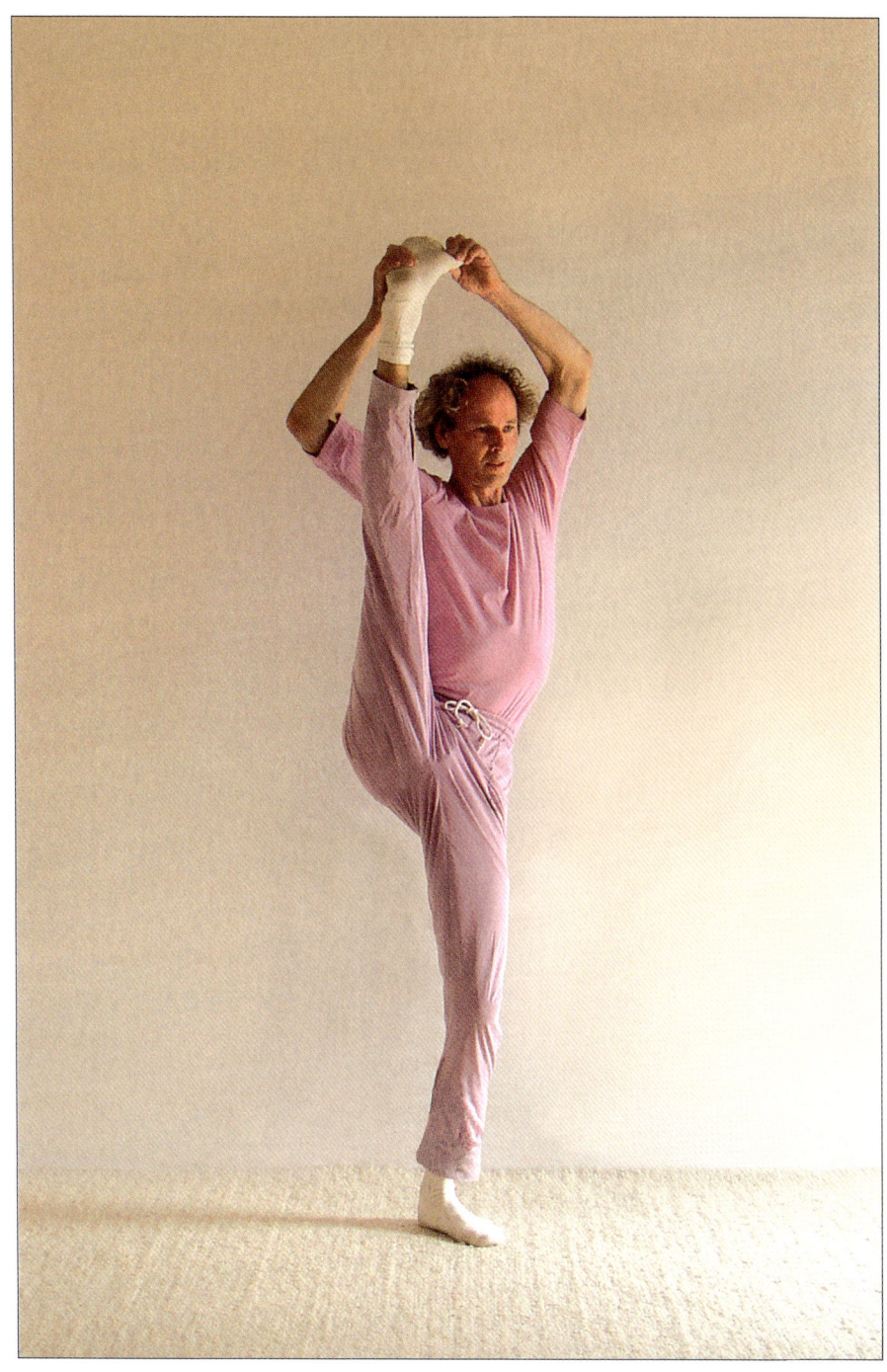

Author's notes

1 A conscious and targeted intervention into the will is of course necessary at various educational stages of life. In *prāṇāyāma*, however, there is an intervention into the manifested fabric of the will, or to be more specific, into the autonomic nervous system. By altering the rhythm of the breath in a particular and targeted way, practitioners also change the inner circumstances of their will. As a result they do not intervene into the will in external life with appropriate educational steps, but they begin to alter the manifested, individual conditions in the body and therefore in so doing they are manipulating the underlying set-up of the will. This set-up, however, is not accessible to normal consciousness and so from this understanding *prāṇāyāma* should not be practised. (p. 28)

2 The full implications of the *prāṇāyāma* methods are no longer understood adequately today. A great number of yoga schools practise the *prāṇāyāma* methods with relatively few concerns. However, to practise *prāṇāyāma*, students ought already to be free from all worldly dependencies and for this they ought to possess a very strong, overseeing I-power, so that they can integrate all the forces they build with *prāṇāyāma* into life meaningfully. To a certain extent, students ought also to have some capacity to see spiritually, so that they perceive the various astral forces which are connected to the flow of breath. Then with this method they would be able to establish order in their inner bodies, from an I-self. (p. 28)

3 In the autonomously established breath process there also lies the person's *karma*. It could be said that in these breath processes the legacy of an earlier life is accumulated. You will find more precise explanations of this in the book "Harmony in Breathing", and also in the lecture series by Rudolf Steiner "Broken Vessels", GA 318, lecture 6 onwards. (p. 29)

4 The breath process can and should naturally experience a certain strengthening through the practice of an *āsana*. The typical *prāṇāyāma*-practice of yoga would, however, lead to the releasing of a stand-alone, isolated consciousness, and practitioners cannot usually recognise that this has risen up from the past. (p. 30)

5 The circumstances of one's own subjective will are subject to the so-called *karma*, to previous life, while the work of consciousness that is possible through forming mental pictures and thoughts can be free from these subjective circumstances. Working with the will via the consciousness requires a certain freedom from the body and therefore also free breath. (p. 31)

6 *Cakrāsana* means "wheel" and should not be brought into connection with the seven *cakrāḥ*. Detailed instruction and description of the two poses in the pictures is not given here. The images are merely intended to illustrate the dynamic that arises from the third centre as will-activity in its articulated form. A more detailed description of *cakrāsana* can be found in my book "The Spiritualising of the Body". (p. 50)

7   This fire is different from the fire in *ājñā-cakra* or *sahasrāra-cakra*. In the heart it is predominantly the so-called warmth ether that is active, described in Sanskrit by the term *agni*. (p. 54)

8   In his various medical discourses, Rudolf Steiner defined both a physical heart and also an etheric heart. Each organ has its own ether force and is therefore pulsated with life. However, particularly in relation to the heart it is significant to speak of a developing etheric heart, as this will develop in the future almost like an independent organ in its own right. The realised heart centre will become a kind of etheric heart through which human beings, thinking and feeling, can ensoul their entire life. The heart itself will then become a very physically functioning organ through an increasing amount of striated muscle, and the so-called etheric heart nearby will adopt an independent spiritual function. Spiritual development with high ideals promotes the development of this etheric heart. (p. 112)

9   The kind of experience described here should not so much indicate the physical body. When practitioners affect the outside world by emanating metrical and expanding forms into it, this is such a subtle and metaphysical effect that it can never be perceived with the eyes, but develops entirely in the sense in which the thought is experienced as a form. (p. 125)

10 The literal translation of *tāḍāsana* is "mountain", however the *āsana* corresponds more to the symbol of the tree, hence this translation used. (p. 126)

11 Chapter III of the Bhagavad Gītā describes in a relatively clear, ascetic sense the human being's release from desires, and in various verses it expounds a discipline of will, which aims to express the so-called action in inaction, or in other words action which is entirely free. To a certain extent, dealing with the first centre, with its very strong, free, wilful orientation, is related to these statements. (p. 280)

12 This fire element, which lives in the direct thought, is represented in the plane of Saturn through the ability to be inspired. As the word "inspiring" expresses, it is a strong motive force of the spirit itself. (p. 294)

Translator's notes from the text

(i)   Rudolf Steiner – Lecture given on November 30, 1919: The Mission of the Archangel Michael, The Ancient Yoga Culture and the New Yoga Will.
      The Michael Culture of the Future. GA 0194.
      Available at https://wn.rsarchive.org/Lectures/19191130p01.html

(ii) Bede Griffiths – Universal Wisdom ISBN 0-00-627815-9
      Bede Griffiths – The Cosmic Revelation ISBN 0-00-599957

(iii) This period refers to the 12 nights between Christmas and Epiphany. It is also called the rough nights or holy nights in English.

General notes on the translation

In this translation we have attempted to remain as close as possible to the original German in the way the sentences and paragraphs are built up. This is because it has become evident to us that Heinz Grill uses language in an artistic way, and the rhythm of the words is as important as their actual meaning. The language is used as a vehicle to convey thoughts and also feelings for qualities inherent in the spiritual worlds, and in this sense it falls somewhere between prose and poetry. Some sentences or words might therefore appear atypical, and this is also the case in the German.

There are some words that play an important role throughout the book in that they aim to open up new subtle-feelings and experiences to the reader, that were unknown before. We have mainly been consistent in our translation of these words so that readers can develop a feeling for their meaning. Some of these are listed here:

Anschauung

Heinz Grill teaches the process of looking very clearly and objectively at an object or phenomenon, in order to see what is really there. The result of this looking process is an objective seeing in which personal subjective interpretation has no part. In the translation we have mainly used the term "seeing".

Empfindung

Dictionaries generally give the words feeling, perception, sensation or sentiment. Heinz Grill uses this term in quite a specific way to indicate a subtle-feeling for the quality of something. Whereas an emotion rises up from within a person, an *Empfindung* comes towards a person from the thing being observed and is experienced outside the body. It experienced with the soul as a kind of subtle awareness and could be described as a soul feeling. We have adopted the following terms in the translation:

Empfindung   -   subtle-feeling or feeling
Empfinden   -   to feel or sense
Empfindsam   -   sensitive

Erbauen

The dictionary translation is edify which is usually used in the English language to mean to instruct or improve someone morally, intellectually or spiritually. Our understanding is that Heinz Grill means a whole strengthening, development and growth of one's being right down to the physical level. We have decided to retain the term "edify" but readers should be aware that it has this expanded meaning.

Erkenntnis

In everyday language this is generally used to mean recognition, realisation, understanding or insight. Here we have chosen the words "insight", "knowledge" or "insightful knowledge". They refer here not to the intellectual accumulation of facts, but rather to a deep, authentic recognition of profound truths.

Gliedern
The verb *gliedern* means to articulate something, in the sense of dividing or separating out its distinct parts. Heinz Grill uses the term both for the soul, in which the thinking, the feeling and the will are separated from each other, and for the body, where different parts of the body play different roles within a yoga exercise. In the translation we have used the word "articulate".

Spannkraft
This is made up of two words:
Spannen can mean to stretch out (as in the case of an elastic band), or to tense (as in tightening muscles). Interestingly many of the yoga movements involve both a tightening at the centre and a simultaneous stretching out into the periphery. *Kraft* means strength, power, force or vigour.
Thus Spannkraft means the strength to stretch out, tense or tighten, and Heinz Grill uses the term to depict a particularly dynamic form of movement. We have generally chosen the following English terms:
Spannkraft   -   dynamic strength
Spannung   -   tension

Sympathie und Antipathie
These two words can be understood to mean liking and disliking. They form two basic polar qualities of the soul, as described in the chapter entitled "The different regions of the soul-life". For this reason, we have translated them as "sympathy and antipathy".

Vitale
We have translated the German word *vitale* directly with the English word "vital" but readers should note that this does not have the usual English meaning of "essential", but rather the more physical meaning of lively, full of energy, spirited, belonging to life.

A note about Sanskrit pronunciation

The Sanskrit script is used for Sanskrit words throughout the book, and all Sanskrit words are printed in italics. For some letters the Sanskrit pronunciation is different to that of English – e.g. the word *cakra* is pronounced "shakra".

Recommended literature

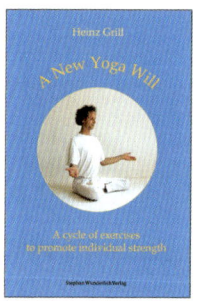

Heinz Grill
A New Yoga Will
A cycle of exercises to promote individual strength
Available from
www.yogainsomerset.co.uk

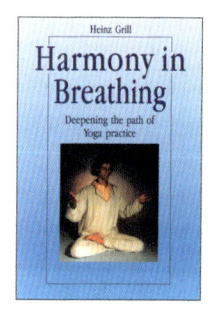

Heinz Grill
Harmony in Breathing
Deepening the path of yoga practice
ISBN 3-98042-304-2

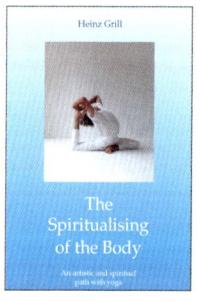

Heinz Grill
The Spiritualising of the Body
An artistic and spiritual path with yoga
ISBN 3-935925-58-1

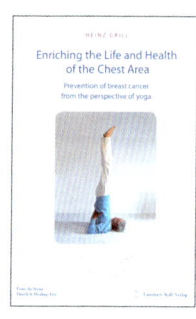

Heinz Grill
Enriching the Life and Health of the Chest Area
ISBN 978-3-935925-34-1

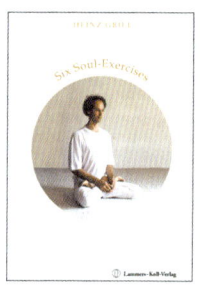

Heinz Grill
Six Soul exercises
ISBN 978-3-935925-51-8

Heinz Grill
Nutrition and the Inner Sense of Giving
The spiritual meaning of food
ISBN 978-3-935925-53-2

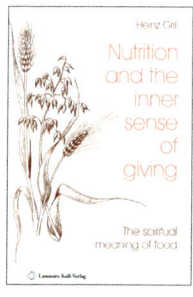

About Heinz Grill

Heinz Grill is a spiritual teacher and researcher, lecturer, mountaineer, healing practitioner, and author of around 150 books on topics including yoga, the development of the consciousness, medicine and health, nutrition, architecture and mountaineering. Born in Bavaria in 1960, he established his first yoga school and began training yoga teachers in 1989. He moved to Italy in 1999 where he has set up the so-called "Sun Oasis", a centre where spiritual thoughts are fostered and can radiate out to society. Over the years, more that 100 000 people have participated in his teaching.

Whilst his fields of activity are many and varied, the essence of all Heinz Grill's work is to bring alive those deep spiritual truths of existence which have lasting validity. His teaching and his books enable others to develop their own inner feeling for these truths, and to give them expression in their chosen field of work or life. His aim is to enrich the visible forms of society with inner, invisible spiritual content. Thus the practice of yoga too is seen not merely as a means towards personal well-being, but as a vehicle for giving profound spiritual principles an outer, physical expression.

Heinz Grill's ideas have a huge power to inspire people. This is because his words, whether written or spoken, always carry within them not just factual information, but an invisible aliveness which gives them a genuine authenticity. He is authentic not only in the sense that he knows what he is teaching, but in the sense that what he is teaching carries in it a truth that is universally valid. Thus those reading or hearing his words have the sense "I always knew that, but I could not have put it into words myself". His words carry within them a substance which directly awakens the soul, triggering in his audience an inner development to new realisation and maturity.